ENDOCARDITIS

Edited by **Francisco Ramón Breijo-Márquez**

Endocarditis
Edited by Francisco Ramón Breijo-Márquez

Published by InTech
Janeza Trdine 9, 51000 Rijeka, Croatia

Publishing Process Manager Martina Durovic

Technical Editor Teodora Smiljanic

Cover Designer InTech Design Team

Additional hard copies can be obtained from orders@intechopen.com

Endocarditis, Edited by Francisco Ramón Breijo-Márquez
p. cm.
ISBN 978-953-307-901-1

For EU product safety concerns:
IN TECH d.o.o., Prolaz Marije Krucifikse Kozulić 3, 51000 Rijeka, Croatia,
info@intechopen.com or visit our website at intechopen.com.

Meet the editor

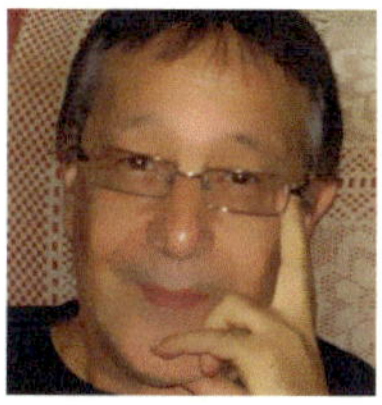

Dr Francisco Ramón Breijo-Márquez is an expert in Internal Medicine and Cardiology. Currently, he holds the position of Titular Professor of Clinical and Experimental Cardiology, Boston, Massachusetts (USA). He is a Board Member of several scientific committees and a member of Editorial Board of several international journals specialized in Cardiology, such as International Journal of Cardiology, Journal of Electrocardiology, Advances in Cardiology, Cardiology in the Young, Heart and Rhythm, Insights Clinical Medicine: Cardiology and Portalesmedicos. Dr. Breijo-Márquez has published many clinical works on Cardiology and has served as a doctor advisor and reviewer in many cardiology related journals.

Contents

Preface

The book coversthe most prevalent causes and current treatments of endocarditis, as well as the cases when the organs remote from the heart are affected by this disease.

As we know, endocarditis is an inflammation of the lining of the heart chambers and valves (endocardium) caused either by infectious or non-infectious diseases. Endocarditis can also involve the heart muscle, valves or lining of the heart. Most people who develop endocarditis have had a heart valve abnormality. Risk factors for developing endocarditis can be various and include injection drug use, placement of permanent access roads in the veins, after valve surgery, recent dental surgery, and weakened valves. Bacterial infection is the most common source of endocarditis. It can also be caused by fungi, although in some cases no cause can be identified.

From my standpoint, all these topics have been covered comprehensively in this book. I fervently hope that reading it would be as enjoyable and informative for the readers as it has been for me.

Prof. Dr Francisco Ramón Breijo-Márquez
Titular Professor of Clinical and Experimental Cardiology
Commemorative Hospital
Boston, Massachusetts,
U.S.A.

1

An Overview on Endocarditis

Breijo-Marquez and M. Pardo Rios
Commemorative Hospital, Boston, Massachusetts;
Catholic University, Murcia;
[1]USA
[2]Spain

1. Introduction

The endocardium is the innermost layer of tissue that lines the chambers of the heart. Its cells are embryologically and biologically similar to the endothelial cells that line blood vessels.

The endocardium underlies the much more voluminous myocardium, the muscular tissue responsible for the contraction of the heart. The outer layer of the heart is termed epicardium. Whole heart is surrounded by a small amount of fluid enclosed by a fibrous pouch called the pericardium.

Recently, it has become evident that the endocardium, which is primarily made up of endothelial cells, can have control over myocardial function. This modulating role is separate from the homeometric and heterometric regulatory mechanisms that control some myocardial contractility. Furthermore, the endothelium of the myocardial (heart muscle) and capillaries, which is also closely appositioned to the cardiomyocytes (heart muscle cells) are involved in this modulatory role. Thus, the cardiac endothelium (both the endocardial endothelium and the endothelium of the myocardial capillaries) controls the development of the heart in the embryo as well as in the adult, for example during cardiac hypertrophy. Additionally, the contractility and electrophysiological environment of the cardiomyocytes are regulated by the cardiac endothelium. This function recently known, it is extremely important to us when there are some injuries cardiac affecting to the myocardial infarction.

The endocardial endothelium may also act as a kind of blood-heart barrier (analogous to the blood-brain barrier), thus controlling the ionic composition of the extra-cellular fluid in which the cardiomyocytes bathe.

All inflammation of the endocardium is called, therefore, endocarditis.

Depending on how extensive of the inflammation, endocarditis can be: localized (most often) or generalized.

As in every inflammation, the cause of endocarditis can be infectious (virus, bacteria, parasites and so...) - bacteria is the most common - or non-infectious.

During depolarization, the impulse is carried from endocardium to epicardium, and during repolarization, the impulse moves from epicardium to endocardium. In infective endocarditis, the endocardium (especially the endocardium lining the heart valves) is affected by originating agent, (The majority, an infectious agent).

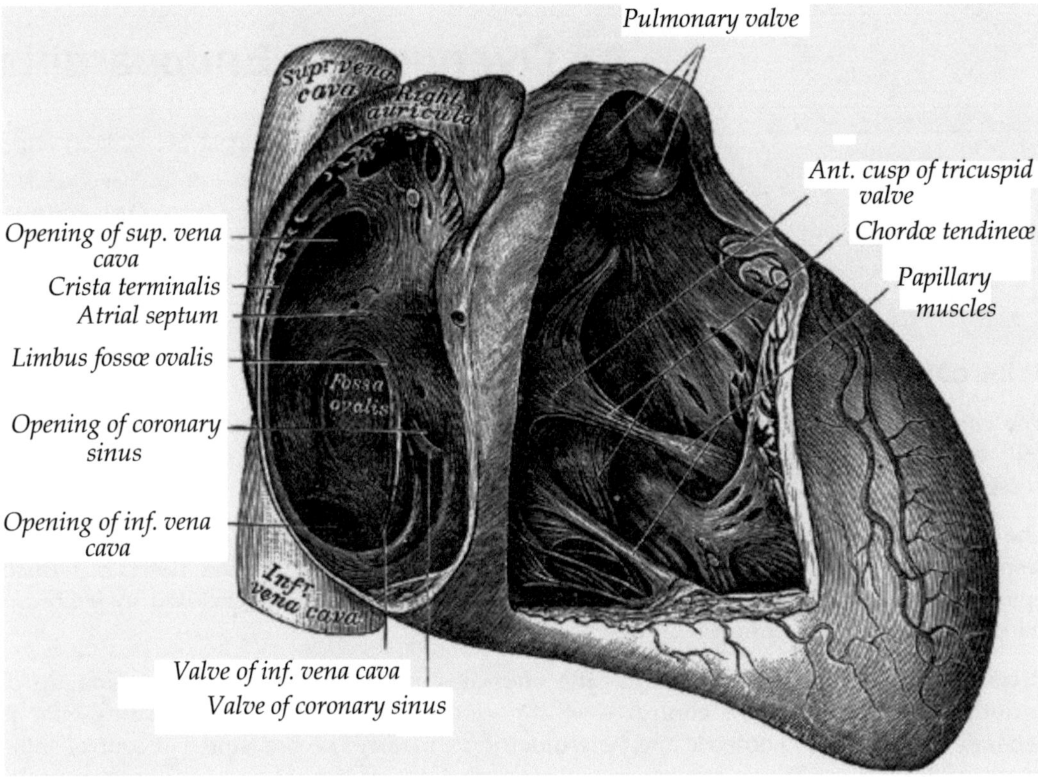

Fig. 1. Interior of right side of heart. (modified from Gray's)

Infective endocarditis is the most common form of endocarditis and its valves, the most affected structures, over all the mitral valve: The agents are usually bacterial, but other organisms can also be responsible.

The valves of the heart do not receive any dedicated blood supply. As a result, defensive immune mechanisms (such as white blood cells) cannot directly reach the valves via the bloodstream. If an organism (such as bacteria) attaches to valve surface and forms vegetation, the host immune response is blunted. The lack of blood supply to the valves also has implications on treatment, since drugs also have difficulty reaching the infected valve.

Normally, blood flows smoothly through these valves. If they have been damaged - from rheumatic fever, for example - the risk of bacterial attachment is increased.

Historically, infective endocarditis has been clinically divided into *acute* and subacute presentations (because untreated patients tended to livelonger with the subacute as opposed to the acute form). This classifies both the rate of progression and severity of disease.

Subacute bacterial endocarditis (SBE) is often due to streptococci of low virulence and mild to moderate disease, which progresses slowly over weeks and months and has low propensity to haematogenous seed extracardiac sites.

Acute bacterial endocarditis (ABE) is a fulminant infection over days to weeks, and is more likely due to Staphylococcus aureus which has much greater virulence, or disease-producing capacity and frequently causes metastatic infection. (Currently, the terms short incubation -meaning less than about six weeks-, and long incubation -greater than about six weeks- are preferred).

Infective endocarditis may also be classified as culture-positive or culture-negative. Culture-negative endocarditis can be due to micro-organisms that require a longer period of time to be identified in the laboratory, such organisms are said to be fastidious because they have demanding growth requirements, or due to absence of an organism as in marantic endocarditis. Some pathogens responsible for culture-negative endocarditis include Aspergillus species, Brucella species, Coxiella burnetii, Chlamydia species, and HACEK bacteria. Another possible reason for culture negativity, even with the more typical pathogens, is prior antibiotic treatment.

Endocarditis can also be classified by the side of the heart affected:

Patients who inject narcotics or other drugs intravenously may introduce infection, which will travel to the right side of the heart classically affecting the tricuspid valve, and most often caused by S. aureus.

In other patients without a history of intravenous exposure, endocarditis is more frequently left-sided. Another form of endocarditis is nosocomial endocarditis which is when the patient is diagnosed with endocarditis and has had hospital care one month prior to the incident and is usually secondary to IV catheters, Total parenteral nutrition lines, pacemakers, and so.

Besides, Endocarditis can have a classification according its affected valve types: The distinction between native-valve endocarditis and prosthetic-valve endocarditis is clinically important. Prosthetic valve endocarditis can be early (< 60 days of valvular surgery) or late (> 60 days of valvular surgery).

Early prosthetic-valve endocarditis is usually due to intraoperative contamination or a postoperative bacterial contamination, which is usually nosocomial in nature. Late prosthetic valve endocarditis is usually due to community acquired microorganisms.

In a healthy individual, a bacteraemia (where bacteria get into the blood stream through a minor cut or wound) would normally be cleared quickly with no adverse consequences. If a heart valve is damaged and covered with a piece of a blood clot, the valve provides a place for the bacteria to attach themselves and an infection can be established.

In the past, bacteremia caused by dental procedures (in most cases due to viridans streptococci, which reside in oral cavity), such as a cleaning or extraction of a tooth was thought to be more clinically significant than it actually was. However, it is important that a dentist or a dental hygienist be told of any heart problems before commencing treatment. Antibiotics are administered to patients with certain heart conditions as a precaution, although this practice has changed in the US, with new American Heart Association guidelines released in 2007, and in the UK as of March 2008 due to new NICE guidelines. Everyday tooth brushing and flossing will similarly cause bacteremia. Although there is little evidence to support antibiotic prophylaxis for dental treatment, the current American Heart Association guidelines are highly accepted by clinicians and patients.

Another group of causes results from a high number of bacteria getting into the bloodstream. Colorectal cancer (mostly Streptococcus bovis), serious urinary tract infections (mostly enterococci), and drug injection (*S. aureus*) can all introduce large numbers of bacteria. With a large number of bacteria, even a normal heart valve may be infected.

A more virulent organism (such as *S.* aureus, but see below for others) is usually responsible for infecting a normal valve.

Intravenous drug users tend to get their right-sided heart valves infected because the veins that are injected enter the right side of the heart, so they will have injured valves on that side that the bacteria can bind to. In rheumatic heart disease infection occurs on the aortic and the mitral valves, on the left side of the heart.

Other factors that increase the risk of developing infective endocarditis are low levels of white blood cells, immunodeficiency or immunosuppression, malignancy, diabetes, and alcohol abuse.

As we have already said, altered blood flow around the valves is a risk factor for obtaining endocarditis. The valves may be damaged congenitally, from surgery, from auto-immune mechanisms, or simply as a consequence of old age. The damaged part of a heart valve becomes covered with a blood clot, a condition known as non-bacterial thrombotic endocarditis (NBTE). Altered blood flow, and thus infective endocarditis, is more likely in high pressure areas.

Consequently, ventricular septal defects create more susceptibility than atrial septal defects. Damaged vascular endothelium will also promote platelet and fibrin deposition, upon which bacteria can take hold. Valvular lesions are a major cause of such damage, as are jet lesions resulting from ventricular septal defects or patent ductus arteriosus.

All patients should fulfill the Duke criteria in order to establish the diagnosis of endocarditis. As the Duke criteria rely heavily on the results of echocardiography, research has addressed when to order an echocardiogram by using signs and symptoms to predict occult endocarditis among patients with intravenous drug abuse and among non drug-abusing patients. Unfortunately, this research is over 20 years old and it is possible that changes in the epidemiology of endocarditis and bacteria such as staphylococci can make the following estimates incorrect.

2. Duke criteria

Established in 1994 by the Duke Endocarditis Society and revised in 2000, the Duke criteria are a collection of major and minor criteria used to establish a diagnosis of endocarditis. A diagnosis can be reached in any of three ways: two major criteria, one major and three minor criteria, or five minor criteria.

Major criteria include:

Positive blood culture with typical IE microorganism, defined as one of the following:

Typical microorganism consistent with IE from 2 separate blood cultures, as noted below:
Viridans-group streptococci, or
S. bovis including nutritional variant strains, or
HACEK group, or
S. aureus, or
Community-acquired enterococci, in the absence of a primary focus
Microorganisms consistent with IE from persistently positive blood cultures defined as:
Two positive cultures of blood samples drawn >12 hours apart, or
All of 3 or a majority of 4 separate cultures of blood (with first and last sample drawn 1 hour apart)
Coxiella burnetii detected by at least one positive blood culture or antiphase I IgG antibody titer >1:800
Evidence of endocardial involvement with positive echocardiogram defined as
Oscillating intracardiac mass on valve or supporting structures, in the path of regurgitant jets, or on implanted material in the absence of an alternative anatomic explanation, or
Abscess, or
New partial dehiscence of prosthetic valve or new valvular regurgitation (worsening or changing of pre-existing murmur not sufficient)

Minor criteria include:

Predisposing factor: known cardiac lesion, recreational drug injection
Fever >38°C
Evidence of embolism: arterial emboli, pulmonary infarcts, Janeway lesions, conjunctival hemorrhage
Immunological problems: glomerulonephritis, Osler's nodes
Positive blood culture (that doesn't meet a major criterion) or serologic evidence of infection with organism consistent with IE but not satisfying major criterion

High dose antibiotics are administered by the intravenous route to maximize diffusion of antibiotic molecules into vegetation(s) from the blood filling the chambers of the heart. This is necessary because neither the heart valves nor the vegetations adherent to them are supplied by blood vessels. Antibiotics are continued for a long time, typically two to six weeks. Specific drug regimens differ depending on the classification of the endocarditis as acute or subacute (acute necessitating treating for S. aureus with oxacillin or vancomycin in addition to gram-negative coverage). Fungal endocarditis requires specific anti-fungal treatment, such as amphotericin B. In acute endocarditis, due to the fulminant inflammation empirical antibiotic therapy is started immediately after the blood has been drawn for culture. This usually includes oxacillin and gentamicin IV infusions until the culture sensitivity report with the minimum inhibitory concentration comes, when the therapy can be modified to tailor to the microorganism.

There should be noted that the routine use of gentamicin to treat Staphylocococcal endocarditis has been questioned, given the lack of evidence to support its use and the high rate of complications.

In subacute endocarditis, antibiotic treatment is based on the micro organism involved, requiring the culture sensitivity report.

So immediate therapy is mainly focused on symptomatic treatment.

The most common organism responsible for infective endocarditis is viridans-group streptococci, which are highly sensitive to penicillin. High dose IV crystalline penicillin every 4hrs for 2 weeks is recommended and still remains the drug of choice.

Again it is important to note that antibiotic therapy hinges upon the culture sensitivity report.

The short course treatment in patients where the blood culture reveals the causative organism, culture sensitivity reports should be followed to treat the patient,

In addition to usage of two bactericidal antibiotics for a minimum of two weeks as a combination therapy.

Surgical debridement of infected material and replacement of the valve with a mechanical or bioprosthetic artificial heart valve is necessary in patients who fail to clear micro-organisms from their blood in response to antibiotic therapy, or in patients who develop cardiac failure resulting from destruction of a valve by infection. other indications to consider surgery include:

- unstable prosthetic valve or obstruction
- recurrent septic emboli, mycotic aneurysm
- large vegetations
- abscess formation
- early closure of mitral valve
- gram negative species

Infective endocarditis is associated with 25% mortality.

3. Non-infective endocarditis

Nonbacterial thrombic endocarditis (NBTE) or marantic endocarditis is most commonly found on previously undamaged valves.

As opposed to infective endocarditis, the vegetations in NBTE are small, sterile, and tend to aggregate along the edges of the valve or the cusps.

Also unlike infective endocarditis, NBTE does not cause an inflammation response from the body (confusing, as the suffix "-itis" refers to inflammation).

NBTE usually occurs during a hypercoagulable state such as system wide bacterial infection, or pregnancy, though it is also sometimes seen in patients with venous catheters. NBTE may also occur in patients with cancers, particularly mucinous adenocarcinoma (where Trousseau syndrome can be encountered). Typically NBTE does not cause many problems on its own, but parts of the vegetations may break off and embolize to the heart or brain, or they may serve as a focus where bacteria can lodge, thus causing infective endocarditis.

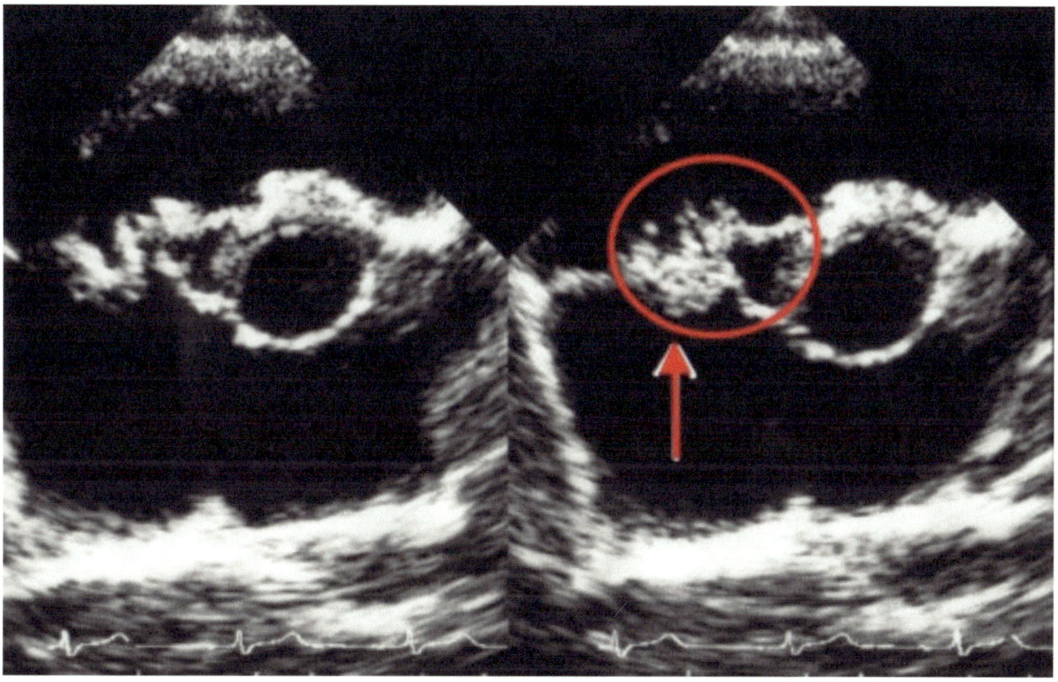

Fig. 2.Vegetation on the tricuspid valve by echocardiography. (Arrow denotes the vegetation)

Another form of sterile endocarditis, is termed LibmanSacks endocarditis; this form occurs more often in patients with lupus erythematosus and is thought to be due to the deposition of immune complexes. Like NBTE, LibmanSacks endocarditis involves small vegetations, while infective endocarditis is composed of large vegetations. These immune complexes precipitate an inflammation reaction, which helps to differentiate it from NBTE. Also unlike NBTE, LibmanSacks endocarditis does not seem to have a preferred location of deposition and may form on the under surfaces of the valves or even on the endocardium.] Prognosis:

Features suggestive of a worse prognosis are Acute endocarditis (Staphylococcus aureus), heart failure, IV drug abuse (often left and right sided disease), prosthetic valve infection, infection of the aortic rather than mitral valve, associated rhythm disturbance.

Subacute bacterial endocarditis (Streptococcus viridans) has a better prognosis.

4. References

[1] Mitchell RS, Kumar V, Robbins SL, Abbas AK, Fausto N (2007). *Robbins Basic Pathology* (8th ed.). Saunders/Elsevier. pp. 406–8.

[2] Morris AM (January 2006). "How best to deal with endocarditis". *Curr Infect Dis Rep* 8 (1): 14–22.

[3] Kasper DL, Brunwald E, Fauci AS, Hauser S, Longo DL, Jameson JL (May 2005). Harrison's Principles of Internal Medicine. McGraw-Hill. Pp

[4] Amal Mattu; Deepi Goyal; Barrett, Jeffrey W.; Joshua Broder; DeAngelis, Michael; Peter Deblieux; Gus M. Garmel; Richard Harrigan; David Karras; Anita L'Italien; David

Manthey (2007). Emergency medicine: avoiding the pitfalls and improving the outcomes. Malden, Mass: Blackwell Pub./BMJ Books. pp. 63.

[5] Taubert KA, Gewitz M, et al. (October 2007). "Prevention of infective endocarditis: guidelines from the American Heart Association". *Circulation* 116(15): 1736–54.

[6] Findler M, Livne S, et al. (December 2008). "Dentists' knowledge and implementation of the 2007 American Heart Association guidelines for prevention of infective endocarditis". *Oral Surg Oral Med Oral Pathol Oral Radiol Endod* 106(6): e16-9.

[7] Elad S, Binenfeld-Alon E, Zadik Y, Aharoni M, Findler M. (March 2011). of acceptance of the 2007 American Heart Association Guidelines for the prevention of infective endocarditis: A pilot study "Survey of acceptance of the 2007 American Heart Association guidelines for the prevention of infective endocarditis: a pilot study". *Quintessence Int* 42 (3): 243–51.

[8] Gold, JS; Bayar, S, Salem, RR (2004 Jul). "Association of Streptococcus bovis bacteremia with colonic neoplasia and extracolonic malignancy". Archives of surgery (Chicago, Ill. : 1960) 139 (7): 760-5.

[9] Durack D, Lukes A, Bright D (1994). "New criteria for diagnosis of infective endocarditis: utilization of specific echocardiographic findings. Duke Endocarditis Service". *Am J Med* 96 (3): 200–9.

[10] Weisse A, Heller D, Schimenti R, Montgomery R, Kapila R (1993). "The febrile parenteral drug user: a prospective study in 121 patients". *Am J Med* 94 (3): 274–80.

[11] Samet J, Shevitz A, Fowle J, Singer D (1990). "Hospitalization decision in febrile intravenous drug users". *Am J Med* 89 (1): 53–7.

[12] Marantz P, Linzer M, Feiner C, Feinstein S, Kozin A, Friedland G (1987). "Inability to predict diagnosis in febrile intravenous drug abusers". *Ann Intern Med* 106 (6): 823–8.

[13] Leibovici L, Cohen O, Wysenbeek A (1990). "Occult bacterial infection in adults with unexplained fever. Validation of a diagnostic index". *Arch Intern Med* 150 (6): 1270–2.

[14] Mellors J, Horwitz R, Harvey M, Horwitz S (1987). "A simple index to identify occult bacterial infection in adults with acute unexplained fever". *Arch Intern Med* 147 (4): 666–71.

[15] Kaech C, Elzi L, Sendi P, et al. (2006). "Course and outcome of Staphylococcus aureus bacteraemia: a retrospective analysis of 308 episodes in a Swiss tertiary-care centre". *Clin Microbiol Infect* 12 (4): 345–52.

2

Infective Endocarditis in the Elderly

Lucy Miller and Jim George
Department of Medicine for the Elderly,
Cumberland Infirmary, Carlisle,
U.K.

1. Introduction

In the 21st century, despite advanced diagnostic imaging, improved antibiotic treatment, and widely available surgery, the incidence of infective endocarditis (IE) has not reduced in recent years, and continues to have high morbidity and mortality (Prendergast, 2005). Over the years there have been changes in the natural history, predisposing factors, sequelae and causative organisms. In particular, rheumatic heart disease is an uncommon predisposing factor, and now degenerative valve disease is much more common in the elderly population. As with many conditions, elderly patients with IE can present in very non-specific ways, making diagnosis more difficult, leading to delays in treatment. IE in elderly patients is associated with a poor prognosis. Fewer patients receive valve surgery, due to higher operative risk, but this does still remain a treatment option for suitable patients. Our knowledge and understanding of endocarditis in the elderly, compared to younger patients, is predominantly influenced by important case series reports in the literature (Table 1) and these will be referred to in the text. European Guidelines are available for guidance in management of IE in all age groups (European Society of Cardiology, 2009).

2. Epidemiology

Elderly patients are predisposed to infectious diseases for multiple reasons; impairment of innate and adaptive immunity, increased comorbidities, increased functional limitations, increased instrumentation and implantation of prosthetic devices, and increased numbers of patients living in care homes (High et al, 2005). These factors result in an increase in adverse outcomes in the elderly. It therefore stands to reason that the incidence of IE has been shown to increase with age, and the incidence amongst elderly patients is also increasing (Dhawan, 2002). So with the ageing population, IE in the elderly is at an all time high. In the European Heart Survey, 26% of cases of IE were in elderly patients (>70 years old) (Iung et al, 2003), and in a French survey 33% of IE patients were over 67 years of age (Delahaye et al, 1999). In further French studies, the incidence of IE peaked between the ages of 70 and 80 years (Hoen et al, 2002). The risk of IE in the elderly has been found to be 4.6 times higher than in the general population. Reasons for this may include a high prevalence of undiagnosed degenerative valve disease, and again higher rates of invasive procedures and implanted devices compared to younger patients.

Author	Patients	Clinical features	Prosthetic devices (e.g. pacemakers or valves)	Causes	Surgery	Mortality
Selton-Suty et al (1997)	Total 114 Over 70 25 Under 70 89	Younger patients more embolic complications 28% v 8% (p< 0.05)	52% elderly v 25% young (p< 0.05)	Portal of entry more often digestive in older patients 50% v 17% (p=0.01)	Older patients less often operated on 24% v 43% (p=0.07)	Mortality higher in older patients 28% v 13% (p=0.08)
Di Salvo et al (2003)	Total 315 Over 70 87 50-70 111 Under 50 117	Clinical features similar between 3 groups except anaemia less common in patients under 50 years	Pacemaker endocarditis commoner in over 70's, but prosthetic valve endocarditis similar in both groups	Older patients more often digestive or urinary portal of entry	50% under 50 years, 52% 50-70, 41% over 70 (p=0.35)	10% under 50 years, 7% 50-70, 17% over 70 (p=0.02)
Durante-Mangoni et al (2008)	Total 2759 Over 65 1056 Under 65 1703	Mitral valve involvement more common in older people. Fewer vegetations and more abscesses in older patients. Vascular and immune mediated phenomena, including embolisation, less common in older people (p<0.001). Chronic illnesses, including diabetes and cancer, commoner in older people. Rate of complications lower in older people.	More commonly prosthetic devices or pacemakers in older people (p<0.001)	MRSA, Strep bovis and enterococci more common in older patients	38.5% older v 53.5% younger (p<0.001)	24.9% older v 12.8% younger. Age an independent predictor of mortality.
Remadi et al (2009)	Total 348 Over 75 75 Under 75 273	Older patients more severely ill and more comorbidities. No difference in embolism risk.	Pacemakers and prosthetic valve endocarditis significantly more common in older patients (p<0.001)	Similar between older and younger patients	29% older v 56% younger (p=0.001)	No significant difference between young and old
Ramirez-Duque et al (2011)	Total 961 Over 65 356 Under 65 605	Comorbidity, renal failure and septic shock more common in older patients	25% older patients v 23% young patients (NS)	Nosocomial acquisition commoner in older patients (p<0.01)	36% older v 51% younger (p<0.01)	42% older v 26% younger (p0.01)

Table 1. Case series of infective endocarditis in older people compared to the young

It has been previously reported that IE in the elderly is associated with a poor prognosis and high complication rate. The onset is usually insidious, sometimes the presenting symptoms are less severe, and diagnosis is sometimes therefore delayed, as well as more aggressive pathogens causing the infection. Age has been shown to be an independent prognostic factor for in-hospital mortality (Durante-Mangoni et al, 2008).

3. Causes

Historically, previous rheumatic heart disease was a very common predisposing factor for IE (Prendergast, 2005). However, this is now rarely a factor. Older people are particularly prone to develop mitral annular calcium (MAC). This is a chronic degenerative process that occurs in older persons, particularly women, and often results in mitral regurgitation (Roberts and Perloff, 1972). Older people with MAC have a high incidence of atrial fibrillation and are especially at risk of developing endocarditis (Mambo et al, 1978). The avascular nature of the mitral annulus prevents antibiotics reaching the bacteria, predisposing to peri annular abscesses and a poor prognosis. Aronow et al (1990) demonstrated at follow up of 39 months a 3% incidence of bacterial endocarditis in 526 older persons with MAC and only a 1% incidence in 450 older persons without MAC. In IE in the elderly, gastrointestinal sources of bacteria are more common. Group D streptococcus (Streptococcus bovis) is frequently implicated (Vahanian, 2003). This is associated with colonic pathology, in particular neoplasia, as well as the involvement of multiple valves and embolic complications. Enterococcus is also more common in the elderly. However, it has also been reported that vegetations in the elderly are generally smaller, with a lower embolic risk (Selton-Suty et al, 1997). Pathogens are more commonly of urinary origin as well. It is thought that this is due to the higher proportion of urethral and prostatic procedures performed in the elderly (Di Salvo et al, 2003). Pacemaker endocarditis is commoner amongst the elderly, as would be expected as the number of patients with pacemakers increases with age (Remadi et al, 2009). Pacemaker endocarditis has been associated with even more difficult and delayed diagnosis, resulting in a poor prognosis.

4. Diagnosis

The clinical diagnosis of IE is based on Duke criteria, which includes positive blood cultures, suggestive features on echocardiography, predisposing heart disease, fever, and vascular and immunological phenomena (Prendergast, 2005). The St Thomas modifications include serology, elevated inflammatory markers, and other clinical signs including splenomegaly, haematuria, splinter haemorrhages and rashes (Prendergast, 2005). However, the onset of IE can be acute or insidious, and the presence of classical signs as described by Duke criteria are often absent, particularly in the elderly (Vahanian, 2003). Therefore, in the presence of signs of sepsis with no obvious source, IE should always be considered in the elderly. Table 2 lists the many common presentations in older people. Overall, the elderly report fewer symptoms (Selton-Suty, 1997). Fever is less common than with younger patients, but anaemia is more common, probably due to the presence of Streptococcus bovis and colonic pathology, resulting in bleeding and anaemia. Delirium is also a more prominent feature. Murmurs are often thought to be insignificant in the elderly, so do not necessarily raise suspicion of IE. New or changing murmurs are heard less frequently in the elderly. Positive blood cultures remain the main diagnostic tool (Prendergast, 2005). At least three sets of cultures should be taken prior to the administration of any antibiotics, and ideally both aerobic and anaerobic cultures should be incubated. Negative cultures most frequently occur after prior antibiotic administration, but increasingly due to fastidious organisms. In particular, negative cultures occur in IE related to prosthetic valves and pacemakers, which are more common in the elderly. Transthoracic and transoesophageal echocardiography (TTE and TOE respectively) are now commonly used in the diagnosis and management of IE (Prendergast, 2005). It has been reported that the detection of vegetations in the elderly is lower with TTE, so TOE should be used as it is more sensitive and specific. In general, TTE is performed first, then TOE performed when TTE is negative, but there is a high clinical suspicion of IE. TOE has revolutionised the diagnosis of IE in the elderly by increasing the diagnostic yield by 45% (Dhawan, 2002).

Sepsis of unknown origin (especially if associated with known infective endocarditis causative organism). New regurgitant murmur. Embolic events of unknown origin. Fever if associated with:

- Intracardiac prosthetic material, including pacemakers
- Previous valvular heart disease
- Congestive cardiac failure
- Recent medical interventions with bacteraemia New cardiac conduction disturbance
- Positive blood cultures with IE causative organism
- Peripheral abscesses of unknown cause
- Non specific neurological symptoms or signs
- Previous history of IE

Table 2. Clinical presentations of infective endocarditis in the elderly

5. Management

Successful treatment of IE in the elderly requires close cooperation between the geriatrician, cardiologist, microbiologist, and cardiac surgeon. Regular review of the patient is required to assess for progression or development of complications (Prendergast, 2005). International guidelines have been published to provide recommendations on the treatment of IE (European Society of Cardiology, 2009). Rapid administration of antibiotics is critical in the initial management of IE (Dhawan, 2002). Antibiotics in high serum concentrations are essential to ensure penetration into the vegetations, and prolonged treatment (4-6 weeks) is required to kill dormant bacteria (Prendergast, 2005). Intravenous antibiotics as an in-patient is the preferred method, but with increasing provision for the administration of intravenous antibiotics in the community, this is becoming an increasingly popular option after the initial two week treatment period when the complication rate is highest. However, this may not be a suitable option in elderly patients who may require in-patient care for the full duration of treatment. Usual initial treatment is broad spectrum, with a combination of a penicillin and an aminoglycoside. In the presence of a prosthetic valve vancomycin or gentamicin is usually used, with or without rifampicin (Dhawan, 2002). There is no evidence for the use of oral antibiotics after the completion of the intravenous course (Prendergast, 2005). When IE is suspected, and after blood cultures have been taken, broad spectrum intravenous antibiotics should be administered until the results of the cultures and sensitivities is known, then a more specific antibiotic can be commenced (Prendergast, 2005). Prosthetic valve and pacemaker endocarditis, which is more common in the elderly requires 4-6 weeks of intravenous antibiotics, as well as removal of the prosthesis if possible (Prendergast, 2005). Repeat valve surgery is recommended in early prosthetic valve endocarditis. Surgery can be life saving in cases of IE and has been shown to be of benefit in suitable elderly patients. Often elderly patients are more unwell with multiple comorbidities and therefore may be deemed unsuitable for surgery (Prendergast, 2005). In one study (Di Salvo et al, 2003) surgery was performed only slightly less frequently than in younger patients and the operated group had a lower mortality. Of course this may reflect the fact that the patients suitable for surgery are generally fitter. Elderly patients may also refuse surgery. In a recent study of 961 patients with endocarditis in Spain (Ramírez-Duque, 2011) significantly fewer elderly patients underwent cardiac surgery (Table 1). The three main indications for surgery are heart failure, uncontrolled infection, and prevention of embolic events (European Society of Cardiology, 2009). In the Spanish study (Ramírez-Duque, 2011), compared with medical treatment, surgery showed lower mortality in the younger patients (less than 65 years), but a high mortality was observed with both medical and surgical treatment in the elderly (over 65 years). Overall in Europe, surgery is undertaken in around 50% of patients with IE with long-term survival rates of around 70% (Prendergast and Tornos, 2010). Surgery is better undertaken early before cardiac tissue damage has occurred and there is a general deterioration in the patients condition. Delay in surgery may contribute to poor outcomes in older patients.

6. Culture negative endocarditis in the elderly

Culture negative endocarditis is particularly common in older patients. The definition of culture negative endocarditis is endocarditis which fulfils established diagnostic criteria for endocarditis, but at least three independent blood cultures are negative after seven days of incubation and subculturing (Raoult et al, 2005). A two year multicentre prospective study in Italy found that 25% of patients with a definite diagnosis of endocarditis by Duke criteria were culture-negative (Cecchi et al, 2004). Cultures are negative in endocarditis for three major reasons: i) previous administration of antibiotics; ii) inadequate microbiological techniques, or iii) infection with highly fastidious bacteria or non-bacterial pathogens (e.g. fungi). Risk factors for culture negative endocarditis include underlying valvular heart disease, presence of a pacemaker and exposure to fastidious organisms. HACEK organisms (Haemophilus aphrophilus; Actinobacillus actinomycetemcomitans; Cardiobacterium hominis; Eikenella corrodens and Kingella Kingae) were originally thought to be the most common cause. However, better laboratory techniques have now led to the more successful isolation of these organisms. In a prospective study of 348 patients with culture negative endocarditis 275 (79%) aetiological agents were identified using serological tests, and polymerase chain reaction (PCR) techniques (Houpikian and Raoult, 2005). The commonest agents found were coxiella burnetti (Q fever) and bartonella species. Serology and PCR on blood samples or removed valves can therefore help considerably in identifying fastidious organisms. Fungi are particularly common pathogens in early prosthetic valve endocarditis (Thuny et al, 2010). Clinically if it is not possible to identify the aetiological agent then treatment may have to be directed either at the most likely source if the patient has already been on antibiotics, or as broad spectrum as possible while closely monitoring clinical response. The long-term prognosis of negative blood culture IE in the elderly is similar to patients with positive blood cultures (Peréz de Isla et al, 2007). A specific form of culture negative endocarditis can occur in older people and cause diagnostic uncertainty. Non-bacterial thrombotic endocarditis (NBTE), or marantic endocarditis, is a rare condition associated with cancer and other illnesses where there is an increased thrombotic tendency, for example septicaemia (Clough et al, 2010). Clinical features of NBTE are very small, multiple valvular vegetations which may be only visible on TOE and multiple small, medium and large disseminated emboli in patients with an underlying cause for NBTE , and multiple negative blood cultures and serology. NBTE, unlike IE, may benefit from anticoagulation, but the outlook is poor, usually because of the underlying cause.

7. Complications and outcomes of infective endocarditis in the elderly

Complications of infective endocarditis can be categorised as:

i. cardiac;
ii. septic;
iii. embolic;
iv. neurological;
v. musculoskeletal;
vi. renal;
vii. associated with medical treatment.

Cardiac complications are the most common complication in older patients. The most common of these is heart failure which is also the most common cause of death in IE. The usual cause of heart failure is infection-induced valvular damage for which cardiac surgery may be lifesaving. Embolisation seems less common in older people (Selton-Suty, 1997), but can occur resulting in stroke, splenic or renal infarction or myocardial infarction. The risk of embolisation is reduced by prompt antibiotic therapy. Apart from embolic stroke, other neurological complications include brain abscesses, seizures, meningitis and encephalitis. Renal failure may result from renal infarction, but also from glomerulonephritis and rarely renal abscesses. Musculoskeletal complications include vertebral osteomyelitis or discitis and septic arthritis. Finally, older patients with IE can develop complications associated with prolonged antibiotic treatment – for example ototoxicity and nephrotoxicity. It is widely accepted that age is an independent predictor of mortality in IE (Durante-Mangoni et al, 2008). Other factors associated with poor outcome are listed in Table 3 and include diabetes, significant comorbidities, heart failure and echocardiographic findings of poor left ventricular function, severe valve regurgitation and large vegetations. However, prognostic predictions should be made with caution in individual patients and many of these factors may be correctable with surgery.

8. Prevention of endocarditis in the elderly

It has previously been recommended that antibiotic prophylaxis should be given to the majority of patients with congenital and valvular heart disease before any dental or surgical procedure. However, this recommendation has now been narrowed to only high risk patients, including patients with prosthetic heart valves or with a previous history of IE and only for high risk procedures. High risk procedures include dental procedures that involve manipulation of gingival tissue, or the peri-apical region of the teeth, or perforation of the oral mucosa and also procedures in patients with ongoing gastrointestinal or genito-urinary infections. Interestingly, the NICE guidelines for England and Wales do not advocate antibiotics, even for high risk patients undergoing dental procedures (Chambers et al, 2011). This is because of lack of convincing trial evidence for antibiotic prophylaxis, even in this high risk group, and the risk of anaphylaxis with antibiotics and the potential development of antibiotic resistance. However, this is contrary to the European guidelines (European Society of Cardiology, 2009) and the usual practice of most clinicians who are influenced by the high mortality rate of high risk patients if they develop endocarditis, even though it may be a rare complication.

Older age Prosthetic valve endocarditis Diabetes Comorbidity (frailty, renal or pulmonary disease) Complications - heart failure - renal failure - stroke - septic shock Infecting organisms - staphylococcus aureus - fungi - gram negative bacilli Echocardiographic findings - large vegetations - pulmonary hypertension - periannular complications - poor left ventricular ejection fraction - severe left sided valve regurgitation or severe prosthetic dysfunction

Table 3. Predictors of poor outcome in older patients with infective endocarditis

9. Conclusion

IE is a very important and atypical illness in older people. Firstly, its incidence seems to be increasing because of the increase in degenerative valvular disease and the increasing use of cardiac prosthetic devices. Secondly, it can present in a variety of different ways depending on the underlying cardiac disease and the microorganisms involved and the underlying patient comorbidities and resistance to infection. It therefore requires a collaborative approach involving physicians, geriatricians, cardiologists, cardiac surgeons and microbiologists. Thirdly, the evidence for its clinical manifestations, treatment and prognosis comes from clinical case series rather than from clinical trials or meta-analyses. Five important case series predominantly from Europe have been published and are summarised in Table 1, comparing older patients with younger patients with IE. Consistently older patients tend to have a higher mortality, are less likely to have surgery and more likely to have prosthetic devices and be infected with bacteria from the gut or urinary tract. Older people are more likely to present insidiously with smaller vegetations and less embolic manifestations. It can be argued that IE is a completely different disease in the older person and deserves a different, more aggressive approach in both treatment and prevention because of its high morbidity and mortality.

10. References

Aronow, W.S., Koenigsberg, M., Kronzon, I. et al (1990). "Association of mitral annular calcification with new thromboembolic stroke and cardiac events at 39-month follow up in elderly patients." *Am J Cardiol;* 65: 1511-1512. Cecchi, E., Forno, D., Imazio, M., Migliardi,

A., Gnavi, R., Dal Conte, I. & Trinchero, R. (2004). "New trends in the epidemiological and clinical features of infective endocarditis: results of a multicenter prospective study." *Ital Heart ;J* Apr;5(4): 249-56.

Chambers, J.B., Shanson, D., Hall, R., Pepper, J., Graham V. & McGurk, M. (2011). "Antibiotic prophylaxis of endocarditis: the rest of the world and NICE." *J R Soc Med;* 104: 138-140.

Clough, H., George, J. & Duncan, A. (2010). "Psychosis due to non-bacterial thrombotic endocarditis." *Age and Ageing;* 39: 276-277.

Delahye, F., Rial, M.O., de Gevigney, G., Ecochard, R. & Delaye, J. (1999). "A critical appraisal of the quality of the management of infective endocarditis." *J Am Coll Cardiol;* 33: 788-793.

Di Salvo, G., Thuny, F., Rosenberg, V., Pergola, V., Belliard, O., Derumeaux, G., Cohen, A., Larussi, D., Giorgi, R., Casalta, J.P., Caso, P. & Habib, G. (2003). "Endocarditis in the elderly: clinical echocardiographic, and prognostic features." *European Heart Journal;* 24: 1576-1583.

Dhawan, V.K. (2002). "Infective Endocarditis in Elderly Patients." *Clinical Infectious Diseases;* 34 (15 March): 806-812.

Durante-Mangoni, E., Bradley, S., Selton-Suty, C., Gripodi, M.F., Barsic, B., Bouza, E., Cabell, C.H., de Oliveira Ramos, A.I., Fowler, V., Hoen, B., Konecny, P., Morena, A., Murdoch, D., Pappas, P., Sexton, D.J., Spelman, D., Tattevin, P., Miró, J.M., van der Meer, J.T.M. & Utili, R. (2008). "Current Features of Infective Endocarditis in Elderly Patients." *Arch Intern Med;* 168(19): 2095-2103.

European Society of Cardiology' (2009). "Guidelines on the prevention, diagnosis, and treatment of infective endocarditis (new version 2009)." *European Heart Journal;* 30: 2369-2413.

High, K.P., Bradley, S., Loeb, M., Palmer, R., Quagiarello, V. & Yoshikawa, T. (2005). "A New Paradigm for Clinical Investigation of Infectious Syndromes in Older Adults: Assessment of Functional Status as a Risk Factor and Outcome Measure." *Clinical Infectious Diseases;* 40: 114-122.

Hoen, B., Alla, F., Selton-Suty, C., Beguinot, I., Bouvet, A., Briancon, S., Casalta, J.P., Danchin, N., Delahaye, F., Etienne, J., LeMoing, V., Leport, C., Mainard, J.C., Rulmy, R. & Vandenesch, F. (2002). "Changing profile of infective endocarditis: results of a 1-year survey in France." *JAMA;* 288: 75-81.

Houpikian, P. & Raoult, D. (2005). "Blood culture-negative endocarditis in a reference center: etiologic diagnosis of 348 cases." *Medicine (Baltimore),* May; 84(3): 162-173.

Iung, B., Baron, G., Butchart, E.G., Delahaye, F., Gohlke-Barwolf, C., Levang, O.W., Tornos, P., Vanoverschelde, J.L., Vermeer, F., Boersma, E., Ravaud, P. & Vahanian, A. (2003). "A prospective survey of patients with valvular heart disease in Europe: the Euro Heart Survey on Valvular Heart Disease. *Eur Heart J;* 24: 1231- 1243.

Mambo, W.C., Silver, M.D., Brunsdon, D.F.V. (1978). "Bacterial endocarditis of the mitral valve associated with annular calcification." *Can Med Assoc J;* 119: 323-326.

Peréz de Isla, L., Zamorano, J., Lennie, V., Vázquez, J., Ribera, J.M. & Macaya, C. (2007). "Negative Blood Culture Infective Endocarditis in the Elderly: Long-Term Follow Up." *Gerontology;* 53: 245-249.

Prendergast, B.D. (2006). "The changing face of infective endocarditis.". *Heart;* 92: 879-885.

Prendergast, B.D. & Tornos, P. (2010). "Surgery for Infective Endocarditis: Who and When?" *Circulation;* 121: 1141-1152.

Ramírez-Duque, E., Carcía-Cabrera, R., Ivanova-Georgieva, R., Noureddine, M., Lomas, J.M., Hidalgo-Tenorio, A., Plata, J., Gálvez-Acebal, J., Ruíz-Morales, J., de la Torre-Lima, J., Reguera, J.M., Martínez-Marcos, F.J. & de Alarcón, A. (2011). "Surgical treatment for infective endocarditis in elderly patients." *Journal of Infection;* 63: 131-138.

Raoult, D., Casalta, J.P., Richet, H., Khan, M., Bernit, E., Rovery, C., Branger, S., Gouriet, F., Imbert, G., Bothello, E., Cocllart, F. & Habib, G. (2005). "Contribution of systematic serological testing in diagnosis of infective endocarditis." *J Clin Microbiol.,* Oct:43(10): 5238-5242.

Remadi, J.P., Nadji, G., Goissen, T., Zomvuama, N.A., Sorel, C. & Tribouilloy, C. (2009). "Infective endocarditis in elderly patients: clinical characteristics and outcome." *Eur J Cardiothorac Surg;* 35: 123-129.

Roberts, W.C., Perloff, J.K. (1972). "Mitral valvular disease. A clinicopathologic survey of the conditions causing the mitral valve to function normally." *Ann Intern Med;* 77: 939-975.

Selton-Suty, C., Hoen, B., Grentzinger, A., Houplon, P., Maignan, M., Juilliére, Y., Danchin, N., Canton, P. & Cherrier, F. (1997). "Clinical and bacteriological characteristics of infective endocarditis in the elderly." *Heart;* 77: 260-263.

Thuny, F., Fournier, P.E., Casalta, J.P., Gouriet, F., Lepidi, H., Riberi, A., Collart, F., Habib, G. & Raoult, D. (2010). "Investigation of blood culture-negative early

prosthetic valve endocarditis reveals high prevalence of fungi." *Heart,* May;96(10): 743-747.
Vahanian, A. (2003). "The growing burden of infective endocarditis in the elderly." *European Heart Journal;* 24: 1539-1540.

3

Pathogenesis of Endocarditis – Bacteraemia of Oral Origin

Inmaculada Tomás-Carmona[1] and M. Álvarez-Fernández[2]
[1]*Santiago de Compostela University*
[2]*Xeral-Cíes Hospital (Vigo)*
Spain

1. Introduction

Bacteraemia is defined as the presence of bacteria in the blood. A feature that is unique to the oral bacterial biofilm, particularly the subgingival plaque biofilm, is its close proximity to a highly vascularised milieu. Any disruption of the natural integrity between the biofilm and the subgingival epithelium, which is at most about 10 cell layers thick, could lead to a bacteraemic state (Parahitiyawa et al., 2009). For several decades, the haematogenous spread of bacteria from the oral cavity has been considered a decisive factor in the pathogenesis of 10% to 15% of cases of infective endocarditis (IE); certain dental procedures may therefore carry a significant risk (Carmona et al., 2002). However, this statement has come under question, its detractors argue that not all patients with heart valves infected by bacteria that typically colonize ecological niches of the oral cavity have undergone dental procedures. Furthermore, there is as yet little evidence of genetic similarity between bacteria isolated from the heart valves, the bloodstream, and the oral cavity of patients with IE (Pallasch, 2003; Seymour et al., 2000).

Apart from its possible role in the onset of episodes of IE, bacteraemia of oral origin has attracted particular interest in the past two decades due to its possible involvement in the progression of atherosclerosis and its consequent implication in the development of ischaemic disease; however, the mechanism of action has not yet been fully elucidated (Beck et al., 1996; DeStefano et al., 1993; Olsen, 2008). A number of recently published clinical studies have demonstrated an association between periodontal disease and cardiovascular disease (Dietrich et al., 2008; Monteiro et al., 2009; Stein et al., 2009), and oral bacteria have been detected in atherosclerotic plaques, heart valves and aortic aneurysms (Gaetti-Jardim et al., 2009; Nakano et al., 2009; Pucar et al., 2007).

This chapter first provides a historical perspective of IE of oral origin. The models of the onset of IE of oral origin and the diagnostic methods for the detection and identification of oral bacteraemia are then discussed. This is followed by a critical review of bacteraemia secondary to dental procedures, focusing on prevalence, duration, magnitude and bacterial diversity, also analyzing factors that could favour the onset of bacteraemia. For this purpose, dental procedures have been divided into surgical and non-surgical, as invasive procedures are more likely to carry a higher risk. As the periodontal space is considered to be the principal portal of entry of bacteria into the bloodstream (Fig. 1), an independent analysis is performed of the dental procedures involving this anatomical region (periodontal procedures). Several authors have demonstrated that certain activities of daily living, such as chewing or toothbrushing, can also cause bacteraemia of oral origin; the importance of this observation is that these activities can significantly increase the number of episodes of bacteraemia compared to those produced exclusively by dental treatments. It has thus appeared appropriate to include a section on bacteraemia after everyday oral activities, including the concept known as "cumulative exposure", which encompasses this interesting aspect of bacteraemia of oral origin. The chapter concludes with a discussion of how current scientific evidence in the field of oral bacteraemia has influenced clinical practice guidelines on prophylaxis for IE of oral origin.

2. Historical perspective on infective endocarditis of oral origin

A focal infection is "a localised or generalised infection caused by the dissemination of microorganisms or toxic products from a focus of infection" (Easlick, 1951). The idea that many systemic infections could originate from infections of the oral cavity and that conservative dental treatment could favour this process took on special importance at the beginning of the 20th century. In 1900, William Hunter wrote: "Gold fillings, crowns and bridges built on and about diseased tooth roots form a veritable mausoleum over a mass of sepsis to which there is no parallel in the whole realm of medicine or surgery…" (Hunter, 1900).

Frank Billings was a key person in elaborating the concept and later dissemination of the theory of focal infection (Billings, 1916). He suggested that there was a possible relationship between the focus of infection, positive blood cultures and cardiac disease (Billings, 1909). Furthermore, this theory explained the origin of many acute systemic diseases and of a number of chronic diseases such as arthritis and nephritis (Billings, 1912). The microbiologist Edward Rosenow was Billings' most outstanding pupil, and his experiments on animal models permitted new theories to be elaborated which supported the importance of focal infection, including "bacterial transmutation" and "elective localisation" (Rosenow, 1914).

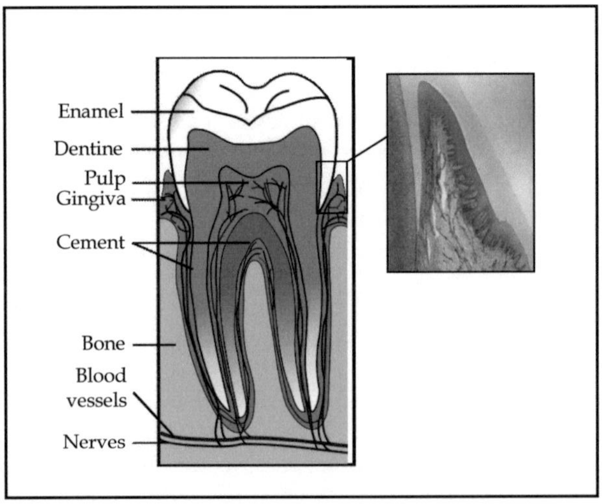

Fig. 1. Dental anatomy and histology of the critical area through which oral bacteria enter the bloodstream

After a period of popularity of the theory of focal infection, leading to the application of so-called "therapeutic edentulism" to many patients, the first detractors to this theory appeared in the 1930s (Holman, 1928). Reimann & Havens strenuously criticised Rosenow's experiments on the basis that, in many cases, the infectious agents had not been identified and that the patient's systemic disease did not reliably improve after dental extraction or tonsillectomy (Reimann & Havens, 1940).

However, in the forties and fifties there was a resurgence of the theory of focal infection, based mainly on the appearance in the medical literature of many cases of IE of oral origin (Bernstein, 1932; Brown, 1932; Geiger, 1942) and on epidemiological studies which revealed that the practice of dental extractions represented an important cause of IE (Kelson & White, 1945; Northrop & Crowley, 1943).

Okell & Elliott were the first authors to report bacteraemia after performing dental extractions; in a study of 138 patients undergoing such procedures, they detected bacteraemia due to *Streptococcus* species in 64% of cases (Okell & Elliott, 1935). A year later, Burket & Burn inoculated pigmented *Serratia marcescens* into the gingival sulcus of 90 patients before performing a dental extraction, isolating this bacterium in 20% of post-manipulation blood cultures. These results confirmed that microorganisms from the oral cavity could enter the bloodstream when performing a dental extraction (Burket & Burn, 1937). Between the mid 1930s and early 1950s numerous studies were published on the prevalence of post-extraction bacteraemia, reporting frequencies between 2% and 83% (Bender & Pressman, 1945; Hopkins, 1939; Palmer & Kempf, 1939; Rhoads et al., 1950; Robinson et al., 1950).

With respect to other oral activities, Richards performed a curious experiment in 1932 based on demonstrating whether "massage of a focus of infection" (located in joints, tonsils, gums, prostate or boils) caused the passage of bacteria into the bloodstream. In the case of the gums, the author selected 17 patients with gingivitis or the presence of periapical infection (confirmed by x-ray study) and massaged the gums or "moved" the teeth for 10 minutes; post-massage bacteraemia was detected in 3 cases (18%) (Richards, 1932) In 1941, Murray & Moosnick published an interesting study consisting of the extraction of blood cultures from patients with oral infections (active caries and/or periodontal disease) after chewing paraffin for 30 minutes. The blood cultures were positive for *Streptococcus* species in 185 (55%) of the 336 participants in this experiment (Murray & Moosnick, 1941).

In the early 1930s attention started to be paid to the need for IE prophylaxis in patients with valvular heart disease undergoing certain dental manipulations. Abrahamson & Brown, two of the pioneers of this idea, recommended the prophylactic use of autogenous vaccines (Abrahamson, 1931; Brown, 1932). In 1938, Feldman & Trace suggested cleaning and scraping the teeth prior to the manipulation in order to reduce contamination of the operating field, performing only 1 or 2 dental extractions per session, following the procedure with curettage and antiseptic irrigation of the periodontal pockets (Feldman & Trace, 1938). A year later, Elliott proposed perialveolar cauterization of the gingiva after dental extraction as a prophylactic measure, as this technique not only sterilized the sulcus but also sealed the gingival capillaries, thus preventing the passage of microorganisms into the bloodstream (Elliott, 1939). The practice of dental extractions under local infiltration anaesthesia with epinephrine was also recommended, as some authors had shown that this type of anaesthesia and this mode of administration acted as a barrier, preventing vascular invasion by the bacterial inoculum (Burket & Burn, 1937; Feldman & Trace, 1938). Fish &

Maclean recommended that the teeth of patients with IE be filled with cotton-wool soaked in a paste of zinc oxide and oil of cloves and that this was renewed every few days; those authors also recommended the administration of a dose of "prontosil" (azosulfamide) prior to dental extraction, in addition to cauterization of the gingiva (Fish & Maclean, 1936).

The first guidelines for antibiotic prophylaxis for IE associated with dental manipulations in patients with valvular heart disease were soon developed, and were based on the use of different sulfonamides (Hupp, 1993; Thomas et al., 1941). In 1948, Hirsh et al. were the first authors to investigate the effect of penicillin on the prevalence of post-extraction bacteraemia. The study group was composed of 65 control patients and 65 study patients, the latter group receiving 600,000 IU of penicillin intramuscularly 3 to 4 hours before the dental extraction; blood samples were taken immediately after the completion of surgery and at 10 and 30 minutes. Although the overall percentage of bacteraemia did not decline significantly (46% in controls *versus* 37% in those who received penicillin), the prevalence of streptococcal species in the positive blood cultures was significantly lower in patients who received prophylaxis compared with controls (15% *versus* 34%), confirming that penicillin was effective in reducing the prevalence of streptococcal bacteraemia, although not bacteraemia caused by other microorganisms (Hirsh et al., 1948).

In 1955, the American Heart Association (AHA), which at that time was formed by only seven physicians, developed its first protocol for IE prophylaxis before dental procedures. That protocol was recommended in patients with congenital or rheumatic heart disease who were undergoing dental extractions or other manipulations affecting the gingival tissues. Those experts considered that the fundamental principle of prophylaxis was to make high concentrations of antibiotic available in the bloodstream at the time of the manipulation and to maintain those levels for several days in order to eliminate the bacteria that had adhered to the heart valves during the bacteraemic episode. Their method of choice was based on the intramuscular injection of aqueous penicillin, 600,000 IU, and procaine penicillin, 600,000 IU, dissolved in oil with 2% aluminum monostearate and administered 30 minutes before the dental procedure. Alternatively (although less desirable), they proposed the oral administration of 250,000 IU to 500,000 IU of penicillin 30 minutes before each meal and before bedtime, starting 24 hours before the dental treatment and continuing for five days, with the administration of an extra dose of 250,000 IU of penicillin immediately before the procedure. For patients with a history of allergy to penicillin, the AHA recommended the use of other antibiotics such as oxytetracycline, chlortetracycline or erythromycin for five days starting the day before dental treatment (American Heart Association [AHA], 1955).

Later, several international committees, made up mainly of cardiologists, specialists in infectious diseases and pharmacologists, drew up alternative prophylactic regimens for IE in the context of dental procedures, describing the profile of the "susceptible patient" and the "at-risk" dental procedures. Those protocols have generated controversy and a degree of confusion.

3. Models of the development of infective endocarditis of oral origin

The classical model of the development of IE of oral origin is that the lesions occur in areas of damaged valvular endothelium, with accumulation of fibrin and platelet deposits constituting a so-called nonbacterial thrombotic endocarditis. This vegetation is sterile until invaded by oral microorganisms as a consequence of bacteraemia, with the subsequent onset of IE (Drangsholt, 1998) (Fig. 2).

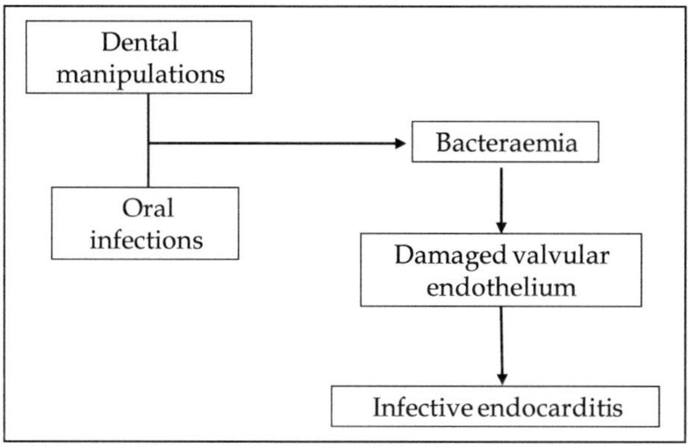

Fig. 2. Classical model of the development of infective endocarditis of oral origin

Several authors have demonstrated that bacteraemia of oral origin can play a significant role in the onset of atherosclerosis (Beck et al., 1996; DeStefano et al., 1993) and, based on these considerations, Drangsholt suggested that bacteraemia of oral origin, instead of directly inducing the onset of IE, could favour the initial thickening of the cardiac valves due to atherosclerosis, making them more susceptible to bacterial adherence and subsequent colonisation. He therefore proposed a new model for the pathogenesis of IE of oral origin, in which initially several episodes of bacteraemia would affect the endothelial surface of the cardiac valves over a long period of time, until finally a bacteraemic episode with a duration of days or weeks led to bacterial adherence and colonisation of the affected valve, culminating in an established cardiac infection (Drangsholt, 1998) (Fig. 3).

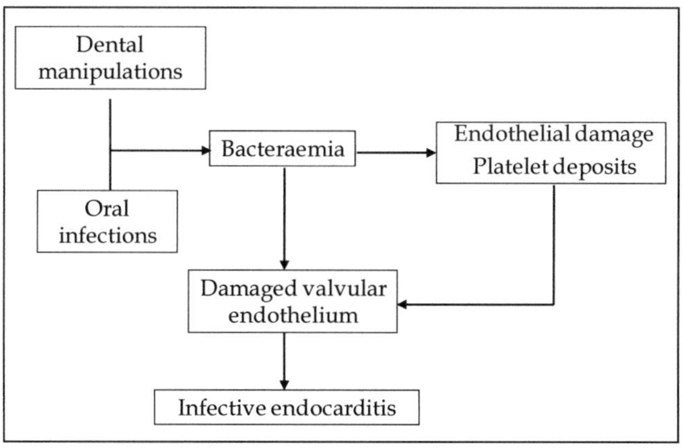

Fig. 3. A more recent model for the development of infective endocarditis of oral origin

Rather than an acute infectious disorder, this model describes IE of oral origin as a chronic disease with a long latency period and a number of well-defined stages. However, there is little evidence to support this model and few studies have been performed in experimental animals on the long-term effect of low-intensity bacteraemia of oral origin on the endothelial surface of the heart valves (Cohen et al., 2004).

4. Diagnostic methods for the detection and identification of bacteraemia of oral origin

There are several procedures for the microbiological analysis of blood cultures taken after dental procedures (Loza Fernández de Bobadilla et al., 2003; Romero et al., 1993). Early studies used quantitative methods that enabled the number of bacteria per millilitre of blood cultured to be determined; this technique was based on extending the blood sample on nutrient agar and then incubating (Elliott & Dunbar, 1968). However, it is recognized that this method is complex and requires expert staff, that it must be done at the time bacteraemia is suspected and the blood drawn and that it is not effective for the isolation of anaerobic bacteria (Romero et al., 1993).

In more recent papers on bacteraemia of oral origin, other authors used a lysis-centrifugation technique (Heimdahl et al., 1990), which is based on the collection and centrifugation of blood in a "Vacutainer system" tube with saponins that break down blood cells, followed by cultivation of the resulting pellet directly on the culture plates (Loza Fernández de Bobadilla et al., 2003; Romero et al., 1993). A variant of this technique is called lysis-filtration, in which, after the initial lysis stage, the blood is filtered and it is the filters that are cultivated directly on the culture plates (Hall et al., 1993). These two techniques enable semi-quantitative estimation to be performed by counting the colonies isolated, although it has been suggested that manipulation of the sample could increase the possibility of contamination (Loza Fernández de Bobadilla et al., 2003; Romero et al., 1993).

Qualitative methods have been used in many studies. In this method, blood is cultured in bottles with liquid or biphasic media (Roberts et al., 1997; Roberts et al., 1998b; Tomás et al., 2007). The culture medium must be examined each day to detect signs of bacterial growth. Although the conventional method involves daily visual inspection of the bottles, automated reading systems now exist based on the detection of the CO_2 produced by bacterial growth using radiometric or fluorimetric techniques, infrared spectroscopy, changes in pH, etc. (Loza Fernández de Bobadilla et al., 2003; Romero et al., 1993).

In 2002, Lucas et al. compared two techniques, lysis-filtration and the BACTEC system, for the analysis of post-dental extraction blood cultures in children. The results revealed that the BACTEC system is a quicker and more efficient method for the detection of both aerobic and anaerobic bacteria, particularly *Staphylococcus* spp. and some species of *Streptococcus,* and that it is able to detect extremely low levels of bacteraemia (Lucas et al., 2002a). Although the lysis-filtration technique allows the intensity of bacteraemia to be estimated, it requires immediate processing, whereas processing with the BACTEC system may be delayed up to 48 hours without affecting the bacterial detection rate (Chapin & Lauderdale, 1996). Nevertheless, after reviewing the literature on bacteraemia of oral origin, significant differences were detected between studies in relation not only to the microbiological technique applied, but also to the transport and culture media, atmosphere and incubation times used, as well as the characteristics of the phenotypic identification of the isolates (Diz et al., 2011; Tomás et al., 2011). All these factors could affect bacterial isolation and identification, particularly of fastidious oral bacteria. Some authors have therefore stated that "it is likely that oral bacteria recovered from blood by culture are probably only part of those present there" (Olsen, 2008). As a result, recently developed methods for the specific detection and identification of microorganisms, particularly polymerase chain reaction

(PCR) techniques, have brought renewed interest to this field, as shown by the studies performed by a number of authors (Kinane et al., 2005; Lockhart et al., 2008; Roberts et al., 2006; Savarrio et al., 2005; Sonbol et al., 2009).

In 2005, Savarrio et al., studying blood cultures taken during root canal treatment, found a lower prevalence of bacteraemia when using PCR analysis than they detected using conventional culture techniques (17% *versus* 30%) (Savarrio et al., 2005). However, Kinane et al., comparing conventional culture methods and PCR analysis, detected the following prevalences of bacteraemia: after ultrasonic scaling (13% by conventional culture and 23% by PCR), periodontal probing (20% and 16%, respectively) and toothbrushing (3% and 13%, respectively) (Kinane et al., 2005). Recently, Castillo et al. assessed the presence of subgingival pathogens (*Porphyromonas gingivalis, Aggregatibacter actinomycetemcomitans, Tannerella forsythia, Eikenella corrodens, Campylobacter rectus* and *Prevotella intermedia*) in peripheral blood samples from patients with periodontitis before and after scaling and root planing; their analysis was based on anaerobic culture and nested PCR. Specific bacterial DNA was detected in 14% of patients before the therapeutic intervention and in 19% after scaling and root planing. Although blood culture rendered higher detection rates immediately after the periodontal intervention, the prevalence fell significantly at subsequent sampling times, whereas detection by nested PCR was more uniform over the sampling period. Those authors therefore concluded that the use of these molecular-based techniques may improve the accuracy of results obtained by blood culture (Castillo et al., 2011).

In 2008, Bahrani-Mougeot et al. compared two different methods for the identification of oral bacteria from blood samples after dental extractions: biochemical analysis and sequence analysis of the 16S ribosomal RNA gene. Of the 58 bacteria isolated in their series, only 17% were identified as the same species by both methods, 55% belonged to the same genus but different species and 28% showed no correlation at all. Those authors stated that DNA sequencing resulted in more accurate identification of a more diverse population of bacteria in bacteraemia following dental extractions (Bahrani-Mougeot et al., 2008). On the other hand, the sensitivity of real-time, quantitative PCR techniques to quantify bacteraemia following dental manipulations has been limited up to now. In a paper published by Lockhart et al., the sensitivity of the method was 25 colony-forming units (CFU) per polymerase chain reaction, which corresponds to 10^3 to 10^4 CFU per millilitre of blood, all samples being below this detection threshold (Lockhart et al., 2008). Nevertheless, it has recently been demonstrated that real-time PCR with pyrosequencing can accurately identify microorganisms directly from positive blood culture bottles with the same sensitivity as culture-based methods (the two techniques were concordant for 97.8% of the bacteria) (Jordan et al., 2009).

The genetic relatedness between isolates from oral cavity and bloodstream samples may be analyzed by PCR techniques. Pérez-Chaparro et al., using a pulsed-field gel electrophoresis technique, recently confirmed the coexistence of the same bacterial clone in samples from the subgingival plaque and from peripheral blood in 16% of patients with bacteraemia following scaling and root planing (Pérez-Chaparro et al., 2008).

Hence, it is imperative that these molecular sequence-based approaches be validated and used in prospective trials to achieve a better understanding of the bacterial characteristics associated with oral bacteraemia.

5. Bacteraemia of oral origin

Numerous authors have studied the development of bacteraemia of oral origin, although the differences detected in the methodology used and in the characteristics of the study groups make it difficult to compare results from different series.

5.1 Baseline bacteraemia

A number of pioneers of the research into the field of bacteraemia of oral origin assumed that there was no bacteraemia at baseline (prior to any dental manipulation) and they therefore performed no pre-manipulation determinations in their studies (Giglio et al., 1992; Lockhart, 1996). However, in 2004, the British Society of Cardiology and the Royal College of Physicians of London were emphatic on this matter: "Those studies of bacteraemia of oral origin that do not to incorporate into their methodology a blood sample taken at baseline should not be considered evaluable" (British Society of Cardiology [BSC] & the Royal College of Physicians [RCP] of London, 2004).

Approximately 70% of the papers on bacteraemia following dental procedures include analysis of a baseline blood culture (Diz et al., 2011). In most of those studies the authors found that there was no bacteraemia rate before the intervention (Heimdahl et al., 1990; Okabe et al., 1995), although some authors reported positive blood cultures in 7% to 11% of cases (Roberts et al., 1998b; Savarrio et al., 2005). In 2005, Kinane et al., using PCR analysis, detected a baseline bacteraemia of 9% (Kinane et al., 2005). Roberts's group from the University of London deserves special mention; this group has repeatedly detected a higher prevalence of baseline bacteraemia in children (varying between 19% and 57%) (Lucas et al., 2002b; Lucas et al., 2007), although their results have not been confirmed by other authors studying paediatric patients. Surprisingly, Fine et al. recently detected a baseline bacteraemia (intensity of 1-2 CFU/ml) in half of adults with mild to moderate gingivitis (Fine et al., 2010). From a review of the literature, we have found that baseline bacteraemia is of very low intensity (median of the majority of series published to date, 0.33 CFU/ml). Although Lucas et al., in another paediatric case series, observed that baseline bacteraemia was mainly staphylococcal in nature (Lucas et al., 2002b; Lucas et al., 2007), Castillo et al., applying PCR analysis, recently detected *Prevotella gingivalis* in all patients with bacteraemia prior to scaling and root planing (Castillo et al., 2011).

To determine the prevalence of bacteraemia of oral origin it is essential to clarify its definition. Up to a few years ago, the detection of a positive post-dental manipulation blood culture was considered to indicate bacteraemia of oral origin. However, in 2004, the BSC and the RCP of London established a new concept of bacteraemia of oral origin defined as "that bacteraemia that is statistically significant with respect to the bacteraemia present at baseline" (BSC & RCP, 2004).

5.2 Bacteraemia following surgical and non-surgical procedures

5.2.1 Prevalence

In 1945, Bender & Pressman (Bender & Pressman, 1945) stated that the practice of dental extractions led to the entry of bacteria into the bloodstream due to the rupture of blood vessels in the gingival sulcus and the pumping effect induced by the manipulation. Over 70% of the literature on bacteraemia following oral surgery focuses on dental extraction as a procedure at risk of producing bacteraemia, probably because of the high frequency of this procedure and the associated bleeding (Diz et al., 2011).

An important aspect is the time at which the blood sample is collected. Roberts et al., in a study of 229 children undergoing dental extractions, determined the prevalence of bacteraemia at different times after completing the procedure (10, 60, 120, 180 and 600 seconds). They demonstrated that the optimum time for drawing the blood sample was 30 seconds after completion of the dental manipulation (Roberts et al., 1992). However, the time of collection of the post-manipulation blood sample varies between studies, ranging from "during" the procedure to 5 minutes after the completing treatment (Baltch et al., 1982; Josefsson et al., 1985; Okabe et al., 1995).

SURGICAL PROCEDURES	**PREVALENCE OF BACTERAEMIA Median[1] (range)**
Dental extractions	Children: 52% (30%-76%) Adults: 76% (58%-100%)
Extraction of third molars	49% (10%-62%)
Maxillofacial surgical techniques	18% (0%-58%)
Removal of osteosynthesis plates	8% (0%-20%)
Incision and drainage of abscesses	12%‡
Removal of oral sutures	10% (5%-16%)
Placement of dental implants	7%[2]
NON-SURGICAL PROCEDURES	**PREVALENCE OF BACTERAEMIA Median[1] (range)**
Conservative procedures	22% (4%-66%)
Orthodontic procedures	22% (7%-57%)
Endodontic procedures	15% (0%-42%)
Local anaesthetic techniques	73% (16%-97%)

[1]Median of the majority of series published to date.
[2]The absence of a prevalence range is due to there being only one paper on this subject in the literature reviewed.

Table 1. Prevalence of bacteraemia following surgical and non-surgical dental manipulations

A review of the literature revealed a prevalence of positive post-extraction blood cultures that varied between 30% and 76% in children and between 58% and 100% in adults.

Surprisingly, these percentages are significantly higher than those obtained after the extraction of impacted or partially erupted third molars (10%-62%) and after more aggressive maxillofacial surgical techniques (0%-58%) (Diz et al., 2011). Recently, Piñeiro et al. showed that even implant placement via a mucoperiosteal flap does not carry a significant risk of producing bacteraemia compared with the baseline percentage (the prevalence was 6.7% at 30 seconds and 3.3% at 15 minutes *versus* 2% at baseline) (Piñeiro et al., 2010) (Table 1). A possible explanation for these results is that the periodontal space is not invaded in these other surgical procedures, a factor which would suggest that this space represents the critical region from which oral bacteria enter the bloodstream (Parahitiyawa et al., 2009).

When evaluating non-surgical dental interventions (Table 1), the prevalence of bacteraemia was similar after conservative dental procedures (4%-66%) and after other orthodontic procedures (7%-57%), and was lower after performing root canal treatment (0%-42%) (Diz et al., 2011). In 1997, Roberts et al. were the first authors to study the prevalence of bacteraemia secondary to 13 different dental manipulations in 735 children undergoing dental treatment under general anaesthesia. Those authors found that matrix band insertion with a wooden wedge and the placement of a rubber dam led to a significant increase in the percentage of positive blood cultures compared to baseline conditions (32% and 29% *versus* 9%). However, low- and high-speed drilling led to positive blood cultures in a very small percentage of cases (4% and 13%, respectively) (Roberts et al., 1997). These findings were corroborated in subsequent studies conducted by the same research group (Roberts et al., 2000). According to Roberts et al., placement of a matrix band with a wooden wedge or placement of a rubber dam produces to changes in local pressures which could facilitate the passage of bacteria from the dental plaque to the gingival tissues (Roberts et al., 1997). In contrast, high- or low-speed drilling did not lead to a high prevalence of post-manipulation bacteraemia, questioning the initial hypothesis that these manoeuvres could break up bacterial plaque into small fragments which could easily penetrate the gingival spaces (Roberts et al., 2000).

In 2002, Lucas et al. used the lysis-filtration technique to analyze bacteraemia after different orthodontic procedures in a series of 142 children. Contrary to previous results (Erverdi et al., 1999; McLaughlin et al., 1996), those authors showed that the manipulation which caused the highest percentage of positive blood cultures was band cementation (44%), followed by the placement of interproximal separators (36%), the taking of alginate impressions (31%) and, finally, changing the archwire (19%). Curiously, despite the high percentage of positive blood cultures detected, the prevalence was not significantly higher than the baseline bacteraemia, which varied between 23% and 36%, so the post-manipulation bacteraemic episodes in that series should theoretically be considered as non-significant bacteraemia (Lucas et al., 2002b).

One of the first studies on the prevalence of bacteraemia secondary to endodontic procedures was performed by Bender et al. in 1960. Those authors stated that manipulation of the root canal involved a small, confined operating field with a significantly lower number of capillaries and blood vessels than are exposed when performing dental extractions or periodontal techniques; in addition, the operating field is usually isolated, avoiding contact with the saliva. These characteristics of endodontic treatment could explain the low prevalence of post-manipulation bacteraemia detected in the different series (Bender et al., 1960).

Regarding methods of local anaesthetic infiltration, Roberts et al. investigated the prevalence of bacteraemia after infiltrative, intraligamental and modified intraligamental techniques in children. The results showed that all three of the anaesthetic techniques caused to the passage of bacteria into the bloodstream, though there was a higher risk of bacteraemia with intraligamental injection (97% of cases) than with the modified intraligamental (50%) or infiltrative techniques (16%) (Roberts et al., 1998a). It has been suggested that bacteria which colonise the surfaces of the teeth at the border of the gingival sulcus are dragged into the sulcus by the tip of the needle and from there enter the blood vessels due to the high pressures generated by the intraligamental anaesthetic technique (Roberts, 1999). On the other hand, Lockhart suggested that injection of a local anaesthetic containing epinephrine could restrict the passage of bacteria into the circulatory system by reducing local blood flow (Lockhart, 1996).

A review of the literature has shown that, except for dental extraction and intraligamental anaesthesia, there are no significant differences in the prevalence of bacteraemia when performing surgical or non-surgical procedures (Diz et al., 2011) thus confirming that visible bleeding is not predictive of bacteraemia secondary to dental manipulations (BSC & RCP, 2004; Roberts, 1999). According to Roberts et al., invasion of the bloodstream by the bacterial inoculum is probably a consequence of the creation of a negative pressure which would lead to an aspiration effect of the bacteria towards the interior of the blood vessels. This pressure would form part of an intermittent positive and negative pressure cycle occurring during any dentogingival manipulation, with the exception of local anaesthetic techniques (which only induce high positive pressures at the time of injection). Microscopic changes occur in the gingival capillaries due to these pressure changes, facilitating bacterial access (Roberts, 1999).

5.2.2 Duration

Using dental extraction as the reference surgical procedure (due to the lack of published data on other surgical manipulations), it has been found that the prevalence of bacteraemia was 39% to 80% in the first 15 minutes after the manipulation, 10% to 40% at 30 to 45 minutes and 5% to 28% at 1 hour (Diz et al., 2011). In a study published by Roberts et al., in 2006 conducted on a group of 500 children undergoing dental extractions, the authors observed that the risk of a positive blood culture after performing an extraction was no longer statistically significant after 15 minutes (Roberts et al., 2006). These findings confirm the premise established by the AHA in the 1960s, that "bacteraemias of oral origin are transient and usually last no more than 15 minutes after completion of the dental manipulation" (AHA, 1960). Under physiological conditions, these bacteria are transferred from the bloodstream into tissues and are rapidly cleared by the reticuloendothelial system.

With regard to the duration of bacteraemia caused by non-surgical dental interventions, the majority of studies evaluated this aspect in the context of endodontic procedures, detecting positive blood cultures in 0% to 17% of patients in the first 10 minutes and 13% at 45 minutes after completion of root canal treatment (Diz et al., 2011). On the basis of the literature reviewed, it appears that the duration of bacteraemia following surgical and non-surgical dental treatments is related to the nature of the procedure and is prolonged after a dental extraction.

5.2.3 Intensity and bacterial diversity

It has been stated that bacteraemia secondary to dental procedures is usually of low intensity and contrasts with the high bacterial load used to induce IE in experimental animals (between 10^6 and 10^7 CFU/ml) (Carmona et al., 2002). The magnitude of bacteraemia caused by a surgical dental procedure varies between 0 and 300 CFU/ml (median of the majority of series published to date, 1.7 CFU/ml). Paradoxically, after relatively non-aggressive manoeuvres, such as an intraligamental injection or placement of a rubber dam, some authors detected bacteraemias in the range 10^3-10^5 CFU/ml (Roberts et al., 1998b; Roberts et al., 2000). However, in general it has been demonstrated that non-surgical dental treatments provoke bacteraemias of very low intensity (median of the majority of series published to date, 0.5 CFU/ml). Accordingly, taking into account the magnitude of bacteraemia at baseline (median of the majority series published to date, 0.33 CFU/ml), many of these episodes should be considered as non-significant bacteraemia (Lucas et al., 2002b; Lucas et al., 2007; Roberts et al., 2000; Sonbol et al., 2009). Nevertheless, conventional microbiological cultures could be providing us with inaccurate information on the true magnitude of the bacteraemia; this aspect may be improved in a near future through the use of quantitative PCR techniques.

Analysis of the literature shows that the bacteria most frequently isolated from blood cultures obtained after surgical dental interventions in adults (mainly dental extractions) were obligate anaerobic bacteria (50%), *Streptococcus* spp. (30%) and *Staphylococcus* spp. (5%) (Diz et al., 2011); however, Lockhart et al., applying PCR techniques, recently detected a high percentage of streptococcal isolates responsible for post-extraction bacteraemia (Lockhart et al., 2008). No data are available from large series on non-surgical interventions (Diz et al., 2011). In children, there was a predominance of *Streptococcus* spp. (55%) in the positive blood cultures taken after both surgical and non-surgical dental procedures; these were followed in frequency by *Staphylococcus* spp. (15%) and, at a much lower frequency, obligate anaerobic bacteria (1%-7%) (Diz et al., 2011). In recent paediatric case series in which patients underwent dental extractions or conservative dental procedures and bacteraemia was evaluated using PCR techniques, the predominant bacterial species identified in the positive post-manipulation blood cultures was *Streptococcus* spp. (Roberts et al., 2006; Sonbol et al., 2009).

5.2.4 Contributing factors

Most of the studies published on bacteraemia following surgical (mainly dental extractions) and non-surgical dental manipulations evaluated the influence of different factors on the development of bacteraemia of oral origin.

A number of paediatric case series published in the 1970s reported a frequency of post-extraction bacteraemia of 30% (Speck et al., 1976), significantly lower than the figures reported for adults (Shanson et al., 1978). Some authors suggested that the differences were due primarily to the small volume of blood drawn from younger patients (Robinson et al., 1950). In the past decade, despite the increased sensitivity of blood culture techniques, the prevalence of post-extraction bacteraemia detected in children is still lower than that reported in adults (Heimdahl et al., 1990; Roberts et al., 1998b). In 2009, Lockhart et al., using a logistic regression model, found that the prevalence of bacteraemia following dental extractions increased significantly with age (Lockhart et al. 2009).

Very few authors have analysed the influence of gender on the prevalence of oral bacteraemia. Okabe et al. reported no statistically significant gender-related differences in the prevalence of bacteraemia following dental extractions (Okabe et al., 1995). However, Tomás et al. detected a significantly higher prevalence of post-extraction bacteraemia at 15 minutes in females (with a higher value also observed at one hour), though no significant differences were observed in the oral health status between females and males (Tomás et al., 2007). It has been suggested that gender could affect the prevalence of certain septic episodes, although a higher susceptibility of one or other gender continues to be a subject of debate (Eachempati et al., 1999; Offner et al., 1999). Many experiments performed in animals have demonstrated that the immune response to bacteraemia could differ between males and females (Yanke et al., 2000) due to the immune modulating properties of the sex hormones on certain cells of the immune system on which specific receptors for these hormones have been identified (Angele et al., 2000).

Many authors have investigated whether the aggressiveness of different dental procedures could affect the prevalence of bacteraemia, although the results have been inconclusive. Elliott & Durban and Peterson & Peacock observed that the extraction of primary teeth caused bacteraemia in a considerable percentage of cases (32% and 36%, respectively), although in both series this was lower than the rate detected after the extraction of permanent teeth (64% and 61%, respectively) (Elliott & Durban, 1968; Peterson & Peacock, 1976). However, these findings have not been confirmed in more recent studies (Onçag et al., 2006). In agreement with the results of previous studies (Bender et al., 1963; Robinson et al., 1950), Okabe et al. found that the frequency of positive blood cultures increased significantly with the number of teeth extracted (65% in cases of one to five extractions compared with 100% in patients with more than 15 extractions) (Okabe et al., 1995). Subsequently, Roberts et al. also detected a higher percentage of bacteraemia (>50%) in children after multiple extractions compared with a single extraction (39%) (Roberts et al., 1997). In contrast, Coulter et al., in a series in children, observed that the number of teeth extracted did not influence the prevalence or intensity of post-extraction bacteraemia (Coulter et al., 1990), and Heimdahl et al. and Lockhart detected bacteraemia in almost 100% of adults after performing a single dental extraction (Heimdahl et al., 1990; Lockhart, 1996). In the series published by Tomás et al., the number of teeth extracted did not influence the prevalence of bacteraemia at 30 seconds, 15 minutes or one hour post-extraction (Tomás et al., 2007)

Some authors demonstrated an association between the severity of haemorrhage secondary to the surgical manipulation and the appearance of bacteraemia (more than 90% of patients with a blood loss exceeding 50 ml developed bacteraemia compared to 67% when the blood loss was less than 10 ml) (Okabe et al., 1995). In contrast, Takai et al. found that the prevalence of bacteraemia associated with various oral and maxillofacial surgical procedures was not affected by blood loss during surgery (Takai et al., 2005). Okabe et al. studied the effect of the duration of surgery and found that when the operation exceeded 100 minutes the frequency of post-extraction bacteraemia was 96% compared to 67% when the surgery was of shorter duration (Okabe et al., 1995); however, other authors have reported conflicting results (Josefsson et al., 1985).

With respect to minor surgical manipulations, Giglio et al. observed that the risk of bacteraemia associated with the removal of sutures was directly related to the number of sutures removed, as positive blood cultures were only obtained from patients in whom five or more sutures were removed (Giglio et al., 1992).

In non-surgical dental procedures, Bender et al. demonstrated that although vitality of the pulp did not affect the prevalence of bacteraemia following endodontic procedures, the percentage of positive blood cultures varied with the depth of the instrumentation. When instrumentation was performed within the limits of the root canal, bacteria did not necessarily reach the general circulation, but with trans-apical instrumentation the bacteria were introduced directly into the interior of the vascular structures (Bender et al., 1960). Debelian et al., despite recognising the statistical limitations of the small size of their sample, reported no significant differences in the prevalence of post-endodontic bacteraemia according to the degree of periapical invasion or the size of the periapical lesion (Debelian et al., 1995).

Few studies have been published on the influence of the anaesthetic modality (local *versus* general anaesthesia) on the development of bacteraemia of oral origin, and the results are not consistent (Baltch et al., 1982; Keosian et al., 1956; Takai et al., 2005). In a paper published in 1956, a higher percentage of positive post-extraction blood cultures was detected after surgery under local anaesthesia than under general anaesthesia (26% *versus* 13%) (Keosian et al., 1956). In 2005, Takai et al. reported a similar prevalence of post-manipulation bacteraemia in patients undergoing extractions under general anaesthesia and under local anaesthesia (57.7% and 58.1%, respectively) (Takai et al., 2005). In contrast, Barbosa et al. found that the prevalence and duration of bacteraemia following dental extractions was higher in patients treated under general anaesthesia than in those treated under local anaesthesia (at 30 seconds, 89% *versus* 53%; at 15 minutes, 64% *versus* 24%; and at one hour, 21% *versus* 4%), suggesting that the practice of dental treatment under general anaesthesia could be a risk factor for bacteraemia. Those authors considered three hypotheses associated with general anaesthesia to explain the results obtained in their series: the appearance of bacteraemia secondary to the manoeuvres of nasotracheal intubation, the transitory changes in blood flow and in the immune response caused by the anaesthetic agents, and other factors such as the administration of contaminated anaesthetic agents (Barbosa et al., 2010).

With regard to oral health status, it appears that the number of teeth present in the mouth, their state of decay, and the existence of periapical abscesses do not alter the risk of post-intervention bacteraemia (Brennan et al., 2007; Coulter et al., 1990; Roberts et al., 1998b; Takai et al., 2005; Tomás et al., 2007). Some paediatric case series have reported significant differences in gingival inflammation scores between children with post-extraction bacteraemia and those with negative blood cultures (Roberts et al., 1998b). In addition, Roberts et al. suggested that the health of gingival tissues not only conditioned the prevalence of post-extraction bacteraemia but also probably its intensity by influencing the size of the bacterial inoculum (Roberts et al., 1998b). However, the majority of the authors consider that the state of gingival and periodontal health is not a determining factor in either surgical or non-surgical interventions (Burden et al., 2004; Lockhart et al., 2009; Lucas et al., 2002b; Roberts et al., 2000; Takai et al., 2005; Tomás et al., 2007), although it has been observed that the prevalence of post-extraction bacteraemia increased in the presence of an acute infectious process affecting the teeth (Okabe et al., 1995; Takai et al., 2005). For example, Takai et al. reported a significant increase in the prevalence of bacteraemia after the extraction of teeth with some type of infection (periodontal or periapical infection or pericoronitis) compared to the prevalence detected after the extraction of uninfected teeth (68% *versus* 23%) (Takai et al., 2005).

5.3 Bacteremia following periodontal procedures

5.3.1 Prevalence

The special interest of periodontal procedures is that they involve manipulation of the critical area through which oral bacteria enter the bloodstream (Fig. 1). Table 2 shows the prevalence of bacteraemia after different periodontal procedures.

The literature shows that surgical periodontal treatments (the most invasive procedures in terms of aggressiveness due to the need for dissection of a mucoperiosteal flap) are associated with a prevalence of bacteraemia of 39% to 60%. Approximately half of the published articles on bacteraemia following periodontal procedures focus on scaling as a procedure at risk of producing bacteraemia, with a reported prevalence that ranged from 8% to 77%. Similar figures have been reported after dental cleaning procedures (15%-60%). Less invasive manoeuvres, such as subgingival irrigation or periodontal probing (which is the introduction of a probe into the periodontal space for diagnostic purposes), can provoke bacteraemia in 0% to 30% and 10% to 40% of cases, respectively (Diz et al., 2011).

In 1973, Lineberger & De Marco studied the prevalence of bacteraemia associated with different periodontal manipulations (gingivectomy, flap surgery and/or osteoplasty) in 20 patients with chronic periodontitis, differentiating between those who had undergone previous periodontal treatment (scaling and routine dental prophylaxis) and those who had not. Although the size of the sample means that the results must be viewed with caution, they detected positive post-periodontal-surgery blood cultures in 50% of patients (Lineberger & De Marco, 1973). In studies in children undergoing dental treatment under general anaesthesia, Roberts et al. found that, after raising a mucoperiosteal flap, bacteraemia was detected in 39% to 43% of cases (Roberts et al., 1997; Roberts et al., 1998b).

Witzenberger et al. observed that 55% of patients with periodontitis developed bacteraemia after scaling and root planing (Witzenberger et al., 1982). Recently Lafaurie et al. and Maestre et al., in studies of adult patients with periodontitis, detected bacteria in the blood in 74% and 76%, respectively, of patients immediately after scaling and root planing (Lafaurie et al., 2007; Maestre et al., 2008). Other authors have shown that almost 30% of children develop bacteraemia secondary to professional cleaning with a rubber cup (De Leo et al., 1974; Roberts et al., 1997). Lucas & Roberts, in a paediatric case series, compared the prevalence of bacteraemia after scaling and after rubber-cup cleaning, finding no statistically significant difference in the number of positive blood samples in the groups studied (40% and 25%, respectively) (Lucas & Roberts, 2000).

In 1997 the AHA advised against the application of antiseptics using gingival irrigators (Dajani et al., 1997), probably assuming that the practice of subgingival irrigation could favour the passage of oral bacteria into the bloodstream. However, few papers have been published on this subject and their results are contradictory. Witzenberger et al. and Lofthus et al. studied bacteraemia secondary to subgingival irrigation in patients with periodontal pockets with a depth equal to or greater than 4 mm and macroscopic bleeding. Witzenberger et al. did not detect any positive post-manipulation blood cultures whereas

Lofthus et al. reported a bacteraemia rate of 30% (6 of 20 patients) at 2 minutes after irrigation (Lofthus et al., 1991; Witzenberger et al., 1982). Daly et al. observed bacteraemia after periodontal probing in 43% of subjects with untreated periodontal disease (Daly et al., 1997), while Kinane et al. recently detected positive post-probing blood cultures in 18% of volunteers with untreated periodontal disease, a prevalence similar to that detected by the same authors after ultrasonic scaling. Those authors suggested that detectable bacteraemia induced by periodontal procedures may be less intense than previously reported. Adult patients with periodontitis could represent a unique patient base whose immune systems are highly primed to cope with periodontal bacteria, such that when bacteraemia is induced it is quickly and efficiently cleared by the patient's reticuloendothelial system (Kinane et al., 2005). Roberts et al. performed a dental examination based on the removal of bacterial plaque close to the gingival margin (without performing probing of the sulcus) in 53 children, detecting positive post-manipulation blood cultures in 17% of cases (Roberts et al., 1997).

In the literature reviewed, there were no significant differences in the prevalence of bacteraemia when performing surgical or non-surgical (mainly scaling and dental cleaning procedures) periodontal interventions; this would indicate that visible bleeding is not a predictive factor for bacteraemia secondary to dental manipulations (Roberts, 1999).

PERIODONTAL PROCEDURES	PREVALENCE OF BACTERAEMIA Median[1] (range)
Periodontal surgery	42% (39%-60%)
Scaling	40% (8%-77%)
Professional cleaning	27% (15%-60%)
Subgingival irrigation	15% (0%-30%)[2]
Periodontal probing	18% (10%-40%)

[1]Median of the majority of series published to date.
[2]Mean has been expressed due to the small number of series published to date

Table 2. Prevalence of bacteraemia following different periodontal procedures

5.3.2 Duration

There are very few references in the literature that have evaluated the duration of bacteraemia following periodontal treatment. In early series, bacteraemic episodes persisted for at least 30 minutes in more than a third of patients undergoing ultrasound scaling (Baltch et al., 1982). Recently, Forner et al. detected bacteraemia in 13% of patients at 10 minutes after performing scaling and in 5% at 30 minutes (Forner et al., 2006). In contrast, Lafaurie et al., after performing scaling and root planing, detected positive blood cultures in 38% at 15 minutes and in 19% at 30 minutes after completion of the periodontal manipulation (Lafaurie et al., 2007).

5.3.3 Intensity and bacterial diversity

Although the authors of some studies in adults have reported that the bacteria most frequently isolated were *Streptococcus* spp., followed by obligate anaerobic bacteria (Daly et al., 1997; Forner et al., 2006), other authors have identified a predominance of obligate anaerobic bacteria in post-scaling bacteraemia, particularly periodontopathogenic bacteria such as *Porphyromonas gingivalis, Micromonas micros, Aggregatibacter actinomycetemcomitans, Prevotella* spp. and *Fusobacterium nucleatum* (Castillo et al., 2011; Lafaurie et al., 2007; Maestre et al., 2008). In a study of children undergoing various periodontal manipulations, the bacteria identified in positive post-manipulation blood cultures were mainly streptococci and staphylococci (Lucas & Roberts, 2000).

5.3.4 Contributing factors

The studies reviewed on bacteraemia following periodontal procedures showed considerable heterogeneity in methodological issues such as periodontal diagnosis, and the small sample size in some of the studies may have affected the statistical significance of the results obtained. Lineberger & De Marco determined the prevalence of bacteraemia associated with different periodontal surgical manipulations in patients with chronic periodontitis, observing no influence of age or sex on the results (Linerberger & De Marco, 1973). Equally, in other series, it has been demonstrated that the magnitude of post-scaling bacteraemia was not affected by age, gender, smoking or the duration of scaling (Forner et al., 2008).

Forner et al. showed that the prevalence and magnitude of bacteraemia after scaling was significantly higher in patients with periodontitis than in patients with gingivitis or healthy controls (Forner et al., 2008). Daly et al. studied the prevalence of positive blood cultures after periodontal probing in adults with untreated periodontitis and compared the results with those obtained in patients with chronic gingivitis. Patients with periodontal disease presented nearly a six-fold increase in the risk of developing bacteraemia compared with patients with gingivitis (Daly et al., 2001). Other authors, however, found no statistical differences in the prevalence or magnitude of post-scaling bacteraemia between patients with chronic periodontitis and those with aggressive periodontitis (Forner et al., 2008; Lafaurie et al., 2007). In children, the percentages of bacteraemia following scaling and rubber-cup cleaning were not affected by the plaque or gingival indices. Nevertheless, it seems that the presence of periodontal disease does condition the development of bacteraemia when performing periodontal treatment.

With regard to the influence of other factors, Reinhardt et al. showed that the use of sterile water *versus* non-sterile water during scaling with ultrasound did not affect the prevalence or intensity of post-manipulation bacteraemia (Reinhardt et al., 1982). Lofthus et al. detected no significant differences in the prevalence of post-irrigation bacteraemia when chlorhexidine or sterile water was used as the irrigating solution (Lofthus et al., 1991).

5.4 Bacteraemia following everyday oral activities

5.4.1 Prevalence

Everyday oral activities such as toothbrushing, dental flossing, use of water irrigation devices or chewing can provoke bacteraemia, possibly because these activities produce small movements of the tooth within the socket, causing intermittent positive and negative pressures that favour the movement of microorganisms into the bloodstream (Roberts, 1999). Specifically, it is estimated that the prevalence of bacteraemia attributable to toothbrushing is of 0% to 62% (median of the majority of series published to date, 22%), the risk with the use of irrigation devices is of 0% to 50% (median of the majority of series published to date, 13%) and the lowest risk is with chewing (median of the majority of series published to date, 3%) (Table 3) (Diz et al., 2011).

EVERYDAY ORAL ACTIVITIES	PREVALENCE OF BACTERAEMIA Median[1] (range)
Toothbrushing	22% (0%-62%)
Supragingival irrigation	13% (0%-50%)
Flossing	19% (0%-41%)
Chewing	3% (0%-17%)

[1]Median of the majority of series published to date.

Table 3. Prevalence of bacteraemia following everyday oral activities

Studies on bacteraemia following everyday oral activities in both adults and children have focused principally on bacteraemia after toothbrushing (Diz et al., 2011). Madsen demonstrated that both toothbrushing and the use of toothpicks produced bacteraemia in 36% of patients with gingival and periodontal alterations (Madsen, 1974). Schlein et al. determined the percentage of positive blood cultures five minutes after completing toothbrushing and found that 25% of subjects had post-activity bacteraemia (Schlein et al., 1991). Roberts et al. and Lucas et al. demonstrated in various studies in children that almost 40% of subjects developed bacteraemia secondary to toothbrushing (Roberts et al., 1997; Lucas et al., 2008), while others authors detected prevalences of up to 62% (Bhanji et al., 2002). In contrast, in recent studies such as those published by Hartzell et al. and Jones et al., the rate of bacteraemia following toothbrushing was zero (Hartzell et al., 2005; Jones et al., 2010). However, it is important to note that the study group in the series published by Jones et al. was formed of mechanically ventilated adults, of whom 87% were receiving empirical antibiotic therapy, which could have affected the results (Jones et al., 2010).

Although some authors were unable to show that supragingival irrigation with water produced a bacteraemic episode (Romans & App, 1971; Tamimi et al, 1969), Felix et al. found that half of the patients with periodontitis who performed this procedure for one minute presented positive post-manipulation blood cultures (Felix et al., 1971). Berger et al. investigated the prevalence of bacteraemia secondary to the use of an oral irrigator for one minute in subjects with no gingival or periodontal disease and, of the 30 individuals evaluated, eight (27%) had positive blood cultures at one minute after completing the irrigation compared to none after simple toothbrushing (Berger et al., 1974). Ramadan et al. found that 18% of patients with advanced periodontitis yielded positive blood cultures after the use of dental floss or Stim-U-Dents, while Crasta et al. recently reported that 40% of subjects presented positive blood cultures after flossing (Crasta et al., 2009; Ramadan et al., 1975).

Although Cobe demonstrated in 1954 that chewing a hard sweet led to bacteraemia in 17% of patients (Cobe, 1954), Degling did not detect positive blood cultures in any patients with fixed orthodontic appliances after chewing gum for five minutes (Degling, 1972). Similarly, Murphy et al. recently showed that chewing did not cause bacteraemia in patients with chronic periodontitis or plaque-induced gingivitis and that this activity may not be a risk factor for IE (Murphy et al., 2006). Schlegel et al. performed an interesting experiment on dogs in which dental implants had been placed nine months earlier; those authors looked for the presence of bacteraemia after inoculating a suspension of *Staphylococcus aureus* into the peri-implant sulcus and allowing the animals to eat for five minutes. They did not detect any positive blood cultures. Together with the histological findings, this allowed the authors to suggest that the epithelium and connective tissue surrounding the implants acted as a barrier as if it were a "physiological pocket" (Schlegel et al., 1978).

Various authors have compared the prevalence of bacteraemia following everyday oral activities, mainly toothbrushing, with that detected after performing certain dental treatments (Forner et al., 2006; Kinane et al., 2005, Lockhart et al., 2008; Lucas & Roberts, 2000). Lineberger & De Marco analysed the frequency of bacteraemia secondary to the use of dental floss and of a gingival stimulator, finding that between 20% and 30% of patients had positive post-manipulation blood cultures, compared to 50% of patients undergoing periodontal surgery (Lineberger & De Marco, 1973). Lockhart et al. detected a significantly lower number of positive cultures in patients performing toothbrushing than in those undergoing dental extractions (19% and 58%, respectively) (Lockhart et al., 2008). Forner et al. studied the prevalence of positive blood cultures after toothbrushing, chewing and scaling, detecting a significantly lower percentage of bacteraemia after toothbrushing (1.6%) and chewing (6.6%) than after scaling (35%) (Forner et al., 2006). In the series by Kinane et al., the prevalences of bacteraemia after the different activities were the following: toothbrushing, 8%; periodontal probing, 18%; and ultrasonic scaling, 18% (Kinane et al., 2005). In contrast, Lucas & Roberts found no significant differences in the prevalence of positive blood cultures between three groups (toothbrushing, 39%; professional cleaning with a rubber cup, 25%; and scaling, 40%) (Lucas & Roberts, 2000).

5.4.2 Duration

Approximately one third of the publications on bacteraemia following everyday oral activities have evaluated the duration of bacteraemia. It has been found that the prevalence of bacteraemia was 0% to 20% in the first 15 minutes after the activity, 0% to 1% at 20 to 40 minutes and of 2% at one hour (Diz et al., 2011). It may therefore be said that bacteraemia following everyday oral activities does not usually persist for more than 15 minutes and that the duration is shorter than is observed after performing dental extractions.

5.4.3 Intensity and bacterial diversity

Bacteraemia following everyday oral activities is generally of low intensity (median of the series published to date, 0.97 CFU/ml; range; 0.01-32 CFU/ml), although its magnitude is significantly higher than the baseline bacteraemia observed in the same series (median of the series published to date, 0.02 CFU/ml; range, 0.01-0.05 CFU/ml). In the study by Forner et al., the intensity of bacteraemia following everyday oral activities (toothbrushing and chewing) was significantly lower than those authors detected after scaling (0.11 CFU/ml and 0.19 CFU/ml *versus* 0.78 CFU/ml) (Forner et al., 2006). In contrast, the results published by Lucas & Roberts revealed that the intensity of bacteraemia was higher after toothbrushing (32.2 ± 231 CFU/ml) than after professional cleaning with a rubber cup or scaling (15.9 ± 83.5 CFU/ml and 2.2 ± 13.2 CFU/ml, respectively) (Lucas & Roberts, 2000). Nevertheless, analysis of the intensity of bacteraemia following everyday oral activities must take into account the constraints of microbiological quantification techniques, given the indirect information provided by conventional culture and the limitations of sensitivity of quantitative-PCR when dealing with a very small bacterial inoculum (Lockhart et al., 2008).

In the literature reviewed, the most frequently isolated bacteria in positive post-toothbrushing blood cultures were *Streptococcus* spp. (45%) followed by obligate anaerobes (19%) and *Staphylococcus* spp. (15%). Lockhart et al., applying a 16S ribosomal RNA sequencing method for bacterial identification, observed that 48% of positive cultures in the toothbrushing group were viridans group streptococci (Lockhart et al., 2008).

5.4.4 Contributing factors

Toothbrushing is the activity of everyday living for which there is most evidence regarding the influence of different factors that may contribute to the prevalence of bacteraemia. Lockhart et al. demonstrated that older age was a predictive factor for developing bacteraemia after toothbrushing (Lockhart et al., 2009). There is also a widely held view that the probability of developing bacteraemia after toothbrushing using an electric toothbrush could be higher than after using a manual toothbrush (Bhanji et al., 2002; Misra et al., 2007).

Lockhart et al. found no significant relationship between the prevalence of bacteraemia after toothbrushing and any measures of caries (presence and depth of caries, presence and size of apical lucency) (Lockhart et al., 2009). In a number of papers on bacteraemia following toothbrushing, various authors found no statistically significant relationship between the state of oral hygiene or the gingival or periodontal status and the prevalence of bacteraemia (Hartzell et al., 2005; Kinane et al., 2005; Madsen, 1974; Schlein et al., 1991; Sconyers et al., 1973). However, in patients with moderate and high plaque indices (PI≥ 1.51) and gingival indices (GI≥ 1.51), Silver et al. detected a prevalence of bacteraemia of 60% and 62%, respectively, after toothbrushing compared to 35% and 25%, respectively, in patients with low PI and GI (scores of 0–1.50). Those authors also demonstrated that positive post-toothbrushing blood cultures with isolation of more than three different bacterial species were significantly more common in patients with a GI equal to or greater than 1.51 than in those with a GI of 0 to 1.50 (28% *versus* 2%)(Silver et al., 1977). Lockhart et al., analysing the influence of a number of clinical parameters, found that a PI equal to or greater than 2 (OR, 3.78), a calculus index (CI) equal to or greater than 2 (OR, 4.43) and the type of bleeding (generalised bleeding) after the activity (OR, 7.96) had a significant effect on the prevalence and duration of post-toothbrushing bacteraemia (Lockhart et al., 2009). One of the authors of the present chapter (Tomás et al., 2011) performed a meta-analysis in order to clarify the influence of oral hygiene and gingival and periodontal status on the development of bacteraemia from everyday oral activities. The results obtained in that meta-analysis showed a significant influence of the plaque and gingival indices (0-1.50 *versus* ≥ 1.51) on the prevalence of bacteraemia following toothbrushing.

With respect to other everyday oral activities, Murphy et al. stated that differing consistencies of the various chewing mediums might contribute to the differences in the reported prevalence of bacteraemia following chewing (Murphy et al., 2006). Cobe showed that chewing hard candy provoked a higher percentage of bacteraemia than did chewing gum (17.4% *versus* 0%) (Cobe, 1954). Few published studies have looked at the influence of oral hygiene and gingival and periodontal status on the prevalence of bacteraemia after performing dental flossing or chewing. In those studies, there was no statistically significant association between the state of oral hygiene or gingival or periodontal status and the prevalence of bacteraemia (Crasta et al., 2006; Fine et al., 2010; Forner et al., 2006; Murphy et al., 2006; Robinson et al., 1950).

5.5 "Cumulative exposure"

Although the potential clinical impact of these episodes of low-level bacteraemia caused by everyday oral activities is unknown, its significance is based on the so-called "cumulative exposure" (Guntheroth, 1984; Roberts, 1999). In 1984, Guntheroth estimated the cumulative exposure to bacteraemia over a period of one month after a tooth extraction and compared this to the results obtained after toothbrushing, during chewing and "in situations of oral sepsis". For this purpose, he multiplied the duration of bacteraemia, expressed in minutes per day, by its prevalence in each situation and calculated that in one month, the cumulative exposure to bacteraemia secondary to two extractions was of only six minutes, whereas this reached 120 minutes after toothbrushing, 510 minutes with chewing and 4,740 minutes with "physiological bacteraemia due to oral sepsis" (Guntheroth, 1984).

In 1999, Roberts repeated the estimation of cumulative exposure to bacteraemia applying a similar methodology to that used by Guntheroth but with certain modifications: to the frequency of positive post-dental-manipulation blood cultures and the duration of the episodes (assuming a mean time of 15 minutes), as applied by Guntheroth, he added the size of the bacterial inoculum and estimated the number of dentogingival procedures that a patient with cardiac pathology would undergo in a period of one year. Roberts calculated the index of cumulative exposure as an expression of the "relative risk" of developing bacteraemia after a certain dental procedure by comparing the results with those obtained after a standard manipulation (extraction of a deciduous molar). In that study, certain conservative dental procedures, such as the placement of a rubber dam, led to a risk of cumulative exposure to bacteraemia 2,110,341 times higher than the extraction of a deciduous molar, and toothbrushing (twice a day) carried a risk 154,219 times higher than the dental extraction. He also attributed a high risk of cumulative exposure to bacteraemia of oral origin to the activities of everyday living in patients with and without oral infection (7,691,707 and 5,640,585 times higher, respectively, than a deciduous tooth extraction) (Roberts, 1999).

Three years later, the Roberts' research group estimated the cumulative exposure to bacteraemia (expressed as the number of CFU/ml/min/year) secondary to various dental procedures in a group of 136 children with cardiac pathology, differentiating between dental manipulations in which the administration of antibiotic prophylaxis was indicated and those in which it was not. According to those authors, the placement of a rubber dam caused the highest value of cumulative exposure (8,849,000 CFU/ml/min/year) and the extraction of a deciduous tooth the lowest (0.059 CFU/ml/min/year). Dental examination produced a cumulative exposure of 1,999 CFU/ml/min/year and rubber-cup dental polishing with prophylactic paste an exposure of 16,410 CFU/ml/min/year (Al-Karaawi et al., 2001).

Despite the above, experts on this subject such as Delahaye & De Gevigney suggested that caution should be observed in the interpretation of this "theoretical analysis", as factors such as the duration of the bacteraemia could vary between patients. According to those authors, a prospective study must be designed in order to analyse all the components of cumulative exposure to bacteraemia individually. The concept of "cumulative exposure" has generated significant controversy in the scientific community (Delahaye & De Gevigney, 2001).

6. Current perspective on the prevention of infective endocarditis of oral origin

The American Heart Association (AHA) published the first protocol for the prevention of IE associated with dental procedures in 1955 (AHA, 1955). Since that time, many expert committees in different countries have drawn up distinct prophylactic regimens, many of which have subsequently been revised and modified based on different types of studies, including those on the prevalence of bacteraemia secondary to dental procedures.

In the latest guidelines published by the British Society for Antimicrobial Chemotherapy, the AHA, the National Institute for Health and Clinical Excellence (NICE) of the United Kingdom, and the European Society of Cardiology (Gould et al., 2006; Habib et al., 2009; Wilson et al., 2007; National Institute for Health and Clinical Excellence [NICE], 2008), the emphasis for the cause of IE has shifted from procedure-related bacteraemia to cumulative bacteraemia due to everyday oral activities. NICE considered that it was "biologically implausible" that a dental procedure could lead to a greater risk of IE than regular toothbrushing (NICE, 2008). Some of those expert committee guidelines concurred with the premise: "Maintenance of optimal oral hygiene and periodontal health may reduce the incidence of bacteraemia following everyday oral activities and is more important than prophylactic antibiotics for a dental procedure to reduce the risk of IE" (NICE, 2008; Wilson et al. 2007). NICE has adopted a drastic stance in this respect, issuing the statement that "antibiotic prophylaxis for IE is not recommended in individuals undergoing dental procedures" (NICE, 2008).

7. Conclusions

Apart from its possible implication in the onset of episodes of IE, there has been increasing interest in bacteraemia of oral origin in the past two decades due to the major role it is considered to play in the progression of atherosclerosis and consequently in the occurrence of chronic diseases.

It is imperative that molecular sequence-based approaches be validated and used in prospective trials to achieve a better understanding of the bacterial characteristics associated with bacteraemia of oral origin.

Dental extraction is the procedure that carries the highest risk of bacteraemia in terms of prevalence, duration and magnitude. There is no conclusive evidence on the contributing factors that predispose to the development of bacteraemia in patients undergoing dental procedures, although it is likely that gingival and periodontal health is relevant to the onset of bacteraemia when performing periodontal interventions.

Activities of everyday living, such as chewing and toothbrushing, can also cause bacteraemia and their clinical importance is based on the concept of "cumulative exposure to bacteraemia". A meta-analysis showed that elevated plaque accumulation and gingival inflammation scores significantly increase the prevalence of bacteraemia following toothbrushing.

Scientific evidence in the field of oral bacteraemia has greatly influenced clinical practice guidelines on prophylaxis against IE of oral origin.

8. Acknowledgement

This work was supported by Xunta de Galicia (Grant PGIDT 08CSA010208PR), Spain.

9. References

Abrahamson, L. (1931). Subacute bacterial endocarditis following removal of septic foci. *British Medical Journal,* Vol.2, No.3678, pp.8-9, ISSN 0007-1447.

Al-Karaawi, ZM., Lucas, VS., Gelbier, M., & Roberts, GJ. (2001). Dental procedures in children with severe congenital heart disease: a theoretical analysis of prophylaxis and non-prophylaxis procedures. *Heart,* Vol.85, No.1, pp.66-68, ISSN 1355-6037.

American Heart Association. (1955). Prevention of rheumatic fever and bacterial endocarditis through control of streptococcal infections. *Circulation,* Vol.11, pp.317-320, ISSN 0009-7322.

American Heart Association. (1960). Prevention of rheumatic fever and bacterial endocarditis through control of streptococcal infections. *Circulation,* Vol.21, pp.151-155, ISSN 0009-7322.

Angele, MK., Schwacha, MG., Ayala, A., & Chaudry, IH. (2000). Effect of gender and sex hormones on immune responses following shock. *Shock: Molecular, Cellular, and Systemic Pathobiological Aspects and Therapeutc Appro,* Vol.14, No.2, pp. 81-90, ISSN 1073-2322.

Bahrani-Mougeot, FK., Paster, BJ., Coleman, S., Ashar, J., Knost, S., Sautter, RL., & Lockhart, PB. (2008). Identification of oral bacteria in blood cultures by conventional *versus* molecular methods. *Oral Surgery, Oral Medicine, Oral Pathology, Oral Radiology, and Endodontics,* Vol.105, No.6, pp.720-724, ISSN 1079-2104.

Baltch, AL., Pressman, HL., Hammer, MC., Sutphen, NC., Smith, RP., & Shayegani, M. (1982). Bacteremia following dental extractions in patients with and without penicillin prophylaxis. *American Journal of the Medical Sciences,* Vol.283, No.3, pp.129-140, ISSN 0002-9629.

Barbosa, M., Carmona, IT., Amaral, B., Limeres, J., Álvarez, M., Cerqueira, C., & Diz, P. (2010). General anesthesia increases the risk of bacteremia following dental extractions. *Oral Surgery, Oral Medicine, Oral Pathology, Oral Radiology, and Endodontics,* Vol.110, No.6, pp.706-712, ISSN 1079-2104.

Beck, J., García, R., Heiss, G., Vokonas, PS., & Offenbacher S. (1996). Periodontal disease and cardiovascular disease. *Journal of Periodontology,* Vol.67, Suppl.10, pp.1123-1137, ISSN 0022-3492.

Bender, IB, & Pressman, RS. (1945). Factors in dental bacteremia. *Journal of the American Dental Association,* Vol.32, No.1, pp.836-853, ISSN 0002-8177.

Bender, IB., Seltzer, S., & Yermish, M. (1960). The incidence of bacteremia in endodontic manipulation: preliminary report. *Oral Surgery, Oral Medicine, and Oral Pathology,* Vol. 13, pp.353-360, ISSN 0030-4220.

Bender, IB., Seltzer, S., Tashman S., & Meloff, G. (1963). Dental procedures in patients with rheumatic heart disease. *Oral Surgery, Oral Medicine and Oral Pathology,* Vol.16, pp.466-473, ISSN 0030-4220.

Berger, SA., Weitzman, S., Edberg, SC., & Casey, JI. (1974). Bacteremia after the use of an oral irrigation device. A controlled study in subjects with normal-appearing gingiva: comparison with use of toothbrush. *Annals of Internal Medicine,* Vol.80, No.4, pp.510-511, ISSN 0003-4819.

Bernstein, M. (1932). Subacute bacterial endocarditis following the extraction of teeth: report of a case. *Annals of Internal Medicine,* Vol.5, No.9, pp.1138-1144, ISSN 0003-4819.

Bhanji, S., Williams, B., Sheller, B., Elwood, T., & Mancl, L. (2002). Transient bacteremia induced by toothbrushing: a comparison of the Sonicare toothbrush with a conventional toothbrush. *Pediatric Dentistry,* Vol.24, No.4, pp.295-299, ISSN 0164-1263.

Billings, F. (1909). Chronic infectious endocarditis. *Archives of Internal Medicine,* Vol.4, No.5, pp.409-431, ISSN 0003-9926.

Billings, F. (1912). Chronic focal infections and their etiologic relations to arthritis and nephritis. *Archives of Internal Medicine,*Vol.9, No.4, pp.484-498, ISSN 0003-9926.

Billings, F. (1916). *Focal infection: The Lane Medical Lectures,* D. Appleton and Company, New York.

Brennan, MT., Kent, ML., Fox, PC., Norton, HJ., & Lockhart, PB. (2007). The impact of oral disease and nonsurgical treatment on bacteremia in children. *Journal of the American Dental Association,* Vol.138, No.1, pp.80-85, ISSN 0002-8177.

Bristish Cardiac Society Clinical Practice Committee & Royal College of Physicians. (2004). Dental aspects of endocarditis prophylaxis: new recommendations from a Working Group of the Bristish Cardiac Society Clinical Practice Committee and Royal College of Physicians Clinical Effectiveness and Evaluation, In: *Bristish Cardiac Society Clinical Practice Committee & Royal College of Physicians,* July 2010, Available from: < http://www.bcs.com/library>.

Brown, HH. (1932). Tooth extraction and chronic infective endocarditis. *British Medical Journal,* Vol.1, No.3721, pp.796-797, ISSN 0007-1447.

Burden, DJ., Coulter, WA., Johnston, CD., Mullally, B., & Stevenson, M. (2004). The prevalence of bacteraemia on removal of fixed orthodontic appliances. *European Journal of Orthodontics,* Vol.26, No.4, pp.443-447, ISSN 0141-5387.

Burket, LW., & Burn CG. (1937). Bacteremias following dental extraction. Demonstration of source of bacteria by means of a non-pathogen (*Serratia marcescens*). *Journal of Dental Research,* Vol.16, pp.521-530, ISSN 0022-0345.

Carmona, IT., Diz-Dios, P., & Scully, C. (2002). An update on the controversies in bacterial endocarditis of oral origin. *Oral Surgery, Oral Medicine, Oral Pathology, Oral Radiology, and Endodontics,* Vol.93, No.6, pp.660-670, ISSN 1079-2104

Castillo, DM., Sánchez-Beltrán, MC., Castellanos, JE., Sanz, I., Mayorga-Fayad, I., Sanz, M., & Lafaurie, GI. (2011). Detection of specific periodontal microorganisms from bacteraemia samples after periodontal therapy using molecular-based diagnostics. *Journal of Clinical Periodontology,* Vol.38, No.5, pp.418-427, ISSN 0303-6979.

Chapin, K., & Lauderdale, TL. (1996). Comparison of Bactec 9240 and Difco ESP blood culture systems for detection of organisms from vials whose entry was delayed. *Journal of Clinical Microbiology,* Vol.34, No.3, pp.543-549, ISSN 0095-1137.

Cobe, HM. (1954). Transitory bacteremia. *Oral Surgery, Oral Medicine, and Oral Pathology,*Vol.7, No.6, pp.609-615, ISSN 0030-4220.

Cohen, DJ., Malave D., Ghidoni, JJ., Lakovidis, P., Everett, MM., You, S., Liu, Y., &, Boyan, BD. (2004). Role of oral bacterial flora in calcific aortic stenosis: an animal model. *The Annals of Thoracic Surgery,* Vol.77, No.2, pp. 537-543, ISSN 0003-4975.

Coulter, WA., Coffey, A., Saunders, ID., & Emmerson, AM. (1990). Bacteremia in children following dental extraction. *Journal of Dental Research,* Vol.69, No.10, pp.1691-1695, ISSN 0022-0345.

Crasta, K., Daly, CG., Mitchell, D., Curtis, B., Stewart, D., & Heitz-Mayfield, LJ. (2009). Bacteraemia due to dental flossing. *Journal of Clinical Periodontology,* Vol.36, No.4, pp.323-332, ISSN 0303-6979.

Dajani, AS., Taubert, KA., Wilson, W., Bolger, AF., Bayer, A., Ferrieri, P., Gewitz, MH., Shulman, ST., Nouri, S., Newburguer, JW., Hutto, C., Pallasch, TJ., Gage, TW., Levison, ME., Peter, G., & Zuccaro, G.Jr. (1997). Prevention of bacterial endocarditis. Recommendations by the American Heart Association. *Journal of the American Medical Association,* Vol.277, No.22, pp.1794-1801, ISSN 0098-7484.

Daly, C., Mitchell, D., Grossberg, D, Highfield, J., Stewart, D. (1997). Bacteraemia caused by periodontal probing. *Australian Dental Journal,* Vol.42, No.2, pp.77-80, ISSN 0045-0421.

De Leo, AA., Schoenknecht, FD., Anderson, MW., & Peterson, JC. (1974). The incidence of bacteremia following oral prophylaxis on pediatric patients. *Oral Surgery, Oral Medicine, and Oral Pathology* Vol.37, No.1; pp.36-45, ISSN 0030-4220.

Debelian, GJ., Olsen, I., & Tronstad, L. (1995). Bacteremia in conjunction with endodontic therapy. *Endodontics & Dental Traumatology,* Vol.11, No.3, pp.142-149, ISSN 0109-2502.

Degling, TE. (1972). Orthodontics, bacteremia, and the heart damaged patient. *The Angle Orthodontists,* Vol.42, No.4, pp. 399-402, ISSN 0003-3219.

Delahaye, F., & De Gevigney, G. (2001). Should we give antibiotic prophylaxis against infective endocarditis in all cardiac patients, whatever the type of dental treatment?. *Heart,* Vol.85, No.1, pp.9-10, ISSN 1355-6037.

DeStefano, F., Anda, RF., Kahn, HS., Williamson, DF., & Russell CM. (1993). Dental disease and risk of coronary heart disease. *British Medical Journal (Clinical Research ed.),* Vol.306, No.6879, pp.688-691, ISSN 0959-535X.

Dietrich, T., Jimenez, M., Krall-Kaye, EA., Vokonas, PS., & Garcia, RI. (2008). Age-dependent associations between chronic periodontitis/edentulism and risk of coronary heart disease. *Circulation,* Vol.117, No.13, pp.1668-1674, ISSN 0009-7322.

Diz, P., Tomás, I., & Limeres, J. (2011). Bacteremias producidas por intervenciones odontológicas, In: *Patología Periodontal y Cardiovascular. Su interrelación e implicaciones para la salud,* Sociedad Española de Periodoncia y Osteointegración and Sociedad Española de Cardiología, pp. 159-167, Editorial Médica Panamericana, ISBN 978-84-9835-313-6, Madrid.

Drangsholt, MT. A new causal model of dental diseases associated with endocarditis (1998). *Annals of Periodontology*; Vol.3, No.1, pp.184-196, ISSN 1553-0841.

Eachempati, SR., Hydo, L., & Barie, PS. (1999). Gender-based differences in outcome in patients with sepsis. *Archives of Surgery*, Vol.134, No.12, pp.1342-1347, ISSN 0004-0010.

Easlick, KA. (1951). An evaluation of the effect of dental foci of infection on health. *Journal of the American Dental Association*, Vol.42, No.6, pp.615-697, ISSN 0002-8177.

Elliott, RH., & Dunbar, JM. (1968). Streptococcal bacteraemia in children following dental extractions. *Archives of Disease in Childhood*, Vol.43, No.230, pp.451-454, ISSN 0003-9888.

Elliott, SD. (1939). Bacteraemia and oral sepsis. *Proceedings of the Royal Society of Medicine*, Vol.32, pp.747-754, ISSN 0035-9157.

Erverdi, N., Kadir, T., Özkan, H., & Acar, A. (1999). Investigation of bacteremia after orthodontic banding. *Amerian Journal of Orthodontics and Dentofacial Orthopedics*, Vol.116, No.6, pp.687-690, ISSN 0889-5406.

Feldman, L., & Trace, IM. (1938). Subacute bacterial endocarditis following the removal of teeth or tonsils. *Annals of Internal Medine*, Vol.11, No.12, pp.2124-2132, ISSN 0003-4819.

Felix, JE., Rosen, S., & App, GR. (1971). Detection of bacteremia after the use of an oral irrigation device in subjects with periodontitis. *Journal of Periodontology*, Vol.42, No.12, pp.785-787, ISSN 0022-3492.

Fine, DH., Furgang, D., McKiernan, M., Tereski-Bischio, D., Ricci-Nittel, D., Zhang, P., & Araujo, MW. (2010). An investigation of the effect of an essential oil mouthrinse on induced bacteraemia: a pilot study. *Journal of Clinical Periodontology*, Vol.37, No.9, pp.840-847, ISSN 0303-6979.

Fish, EW., & Maclean, I. (1936). The distribution of oral streptococci in the tissues. *British Dental Journal*, Vol.61, pp.336-362, ISSN 0007-0610.

Forner, L., Larsen, T., Kilian, M., & Holmstrup, P. (2006). Incidence of bacteremia after chewing, toothbrushing and scaling in individuals with periodontal inflammation. *Journal of Clinical Periodontology*, Vol.33, No.6, pp.401-407, ISSN 0303-6979.

Gaetti-Jardim, E Jr., Marcelino, SL., Feitosa, AC., Romito, GA., & Avila-Campos, MJ. (2009). Quantitative detection of periodontopathic bacteria in atherosclerotic plaques from coronary arteries. *Journal of Medical Microbiology*, Vol.58, No.12, pp.1568-1575, ISSN 0022-2615.

Geiger, AJ. (1942). Relation of fatal subacute bacterial endocarditis to tooth extraction. *Journal of the American Dental Association*, Vol.29, pp.1023-1025, ISSN 0002-8177.

Giglio, JA., Rowland, RW., Dalton, HP., & Laskin, DM. (1992). Suture removal-induced bacteremia: a possible endocarditis risk. *Journal of the American Dental Association*, Vol.123, No.8, pp.65-70, ISSN 0002-8177.

Gould, FK., Elliot, TS., Foweraker, J., Fulford, M., Perry, JD., Roberts, GJ., Sandoe, JA., Watkin, RW., & Working Party of the British Society for Antimicrobial Chemotherapy. (2006). Guidelines for the prevention of endocarditis: report of the Working Party of the British Society for Antimicrobial Chemotherapy. *Journal of Antimicrobial Chemotherapy*, Vol.57, No.6, pp.1035-1042, ISSN 0305-7453.

Guntheroth, WG. (1984). How important are dental procedures as a cause of infective endocarditis?. *The American Journal of Cardiology*, Vol.54, No.7, pp.797-801, ISSN 0002-9149.

Habib, G., Hoen, B., Tornos, P., Thuny, F., Prendergast, B., Vilacosta, I., Moreillon, P., de Jesus Antunes, M., Thilen, U., Lekakis, J., Lengyel, M., Müller, L., Naber, CK., Nihoyannopoulos, P., Moritz, A., Zamorano, JL., ESC Committee for Practice Guidelines., Vahanian, A., Auricchio, A., Bax, J., Ceconi, C., Dean, V., Filippatos, G., Funck-Brentano, C., Hobbs, R., Kearney, P., McDonagh, T., McGregor, K., Popescu, BA., Reiner, Z., Sechtem, U., Sirnes, PA., Tendera, M., Vardas, P., Widimsky, P, Vahanian. A., Aguilar, R., Bongiorni, MG., Borger, M., Butchart, E., Danchin, N., Delahaye, F., Erbel, R., Franzen, D., Gould, K., Hall, R., Hassager, C., Kjeldsen, K., McManus, R., Miró, JM., Mokracek, A., Rosenhek, R., San Román, JA., Seferonic, P., Selton-Suty, C., Sousa, M., Trinchero, R., & van Camp, G. (2009). Guidelines on the prevention, diagnosis, and treatment of infective endocarditis (new version 2009): the Task Force on the Prevention, Diagnosis, and Treatment of Infective Endocarditis of the European Society of Cardiology (ESC). Endorsed by the European Society of Clinical Microbiology and Infectious Disease (ESCMID) and the International Society of Chemotherapy (ISC) for Infection and Cancer. *European Heart Journal*, Vol.30, No.19. pp.2369-2413, ISSN 0195-668X.

Hall, G., Hedström, SA., Heimdahl, A., & Nord, CE. (1993). Prophylactic administration of penicillins for endocarditis does not reduce the incidence of postextraction bacteremia. *Clinical Infectious Disease*, Vol.17, No.2, pp.188-194, ISSN 1058-4838.

Hartzell, JD., Torres, D., Kim, P., & Wortmann, G. (2005). Incidence of bacteraemia after routine tooth brushing. *American Journal of the Medical Sciences*, Vol.329, No.4, pp.178-180, ISSN 0002-9629.

Heimdahl, A., Hall, G., Hedberg, M., Sandberg, H., Söder, PO., Tunér, K., & Nord, CE. (1990). Detection and quantitation by lysis-filtration of bacteremia after different oral surgical procedures. *Journal of Clinical Microbiology*, Vol.28, No.10, pp.2205-2209, ISSN 0095-1137.

Hirsh, HL., Vivino, JJ., Merril, A., & Dowling, HF. (1948). Effect of prophylactically administered penicillin on incidence of bacteremia following extraction of teeth; results in patients with healed rheumatic and bacterial endocarditis. *Archives of Internal Medicine*, Vol.81, No.6, pp.868-878, ISSN 0730-188X.

Holman, WL. (1928). Focal infection and "elective localization". *Archives of Pathology & Laboratory Medicine*, Vol.5, pp.68-136, ISSN 0003-9985.

Hopkins, JA. (1939). *Streptococcus viridans*: bacteremia following extraction of the teeth. *Journal of the American Dental Association*, Vol.26, pp.2002-2008, ISSN 0002-8177.

Hunter, W. (1900). Oral sepsis as a cause of disease. *British Medical Journal*, Vol.2, No.2065, pp. 215-216, ISSN 0007-1447.

Hupp, JR. (1993). Changing methods of preventing infective endocarditis following dental procedures: 1943-1993. *Journal of Oral and Maxillofacial Surgery*, Vol.51, No.6, pp. 616-623, ISSN 0278-2391.

Jones, DJ., Munro, CL., Grap, MJ., Kitten, T., & Edmond, M. (2010). Oral care and bacteremia risk in mechanically ventilated adults. *Heart & Lung: The Journal of Critical Care*, Vol.39, Suppl.6, pp.S57-S65, ISSN 0147-9563.

Jordan, JA., Jones-Laughner, J., & Durso, MB. (2009). Utility of pyrosequencing in identifying bacteria directly from positive blood culture bottles. *Journal of Clinical Microbiology*, Vol.47, No.2, pp.368-372, ISSN 0095-1137.

Josefsson, K., Heimdahl, A., von Konow, L., & Nord, CE. (1985). Effect of phenoxymethylpenicillin and erythromycin prophylaxis on anaerobic bacteraemia after oral surgery. *Journal of Antimicrobial Chemotherapy,* Vol.16, No.2, pp.243-251, ISSN 0305-7453.

Kelson, SR., & White, PD. (1945). Notes on 250 cases of subacute bacterial (streptococcal) endocarditis studied and treated between 1927 and 1939. *Annals of Internal Medicine,*Vol.22, No.1, pp.40-60, ISSN 0003-4819.

Keosian, J., Rafel, S., & Weinman, I. (1956). The effect of aqueous diatomic iodine mouthwashes on the incidence of postextraction bacteremia. *Oral Surgery, Oral Medicine, and Oral Pathology,* Vol.9, No.12, pp.1337-1341, ISSN 0030-4220.

Kinane, DF., Riggio, MP., Walker, KF., MacKenzie, D., & Shearer, B. (2005). Bacteremia following periodontal procedures. *Journal of Clinical Periodontology,* Vol.32, No.7, pp.708-713, ISSN 0303-6979.

Lafaurie, GI., Mayorga-Fayad, I., Torres, MF., Castillo, DM., Aya, MR., Barón, A., & Hurtado, PA. (2007). Periodontopathic microorganisms in peripheric blood after scaling and root planing. *Journal of Clinical Periodontology,* Vol.34, No.10, pp.873-879, ISSN 0303-6979.

Lineberger, LT., & De Marco, TJ. (1973). Evaluation of transient bacteremia following routine periodontal procedures. *Journal of Periodontology,* Vol.44, No.12, pp.757-762, ISSN 0022-3492.

Lockhart, PB., Brennan, MT., Thornhill, M., Michalowicz, BS., Noll, J., Bahrani-Mougeot, FK., & Sasser, HC. (2009) Poor oral hygiene as a risk factor for infective endocarditis-related bacteremia. *Journal of the American Dental Association,* Vol.140, No.10, pp.1238-1244, ISSN 0002-8177.

Lockhart, PB. (1996). An analysis of bacteremias during dental extractions. A doble-blind, placebo-controlled study of chlorhexidine. *Archives of Internal Medicine,* Vol.156, No.5, pp.513-520, ISSN 0003-9926.

Lockhart, PB., Brennan, MT., Sasser, HC., Fox, PC., Paster, BJ., & Bahrani-Mougeot, FK. (2008). Bacteremia associated with toothbrushing and dental extraction. *Circulation,* Vol.117, No.24, pp.3118-3125, ISSN 0009-7322.

Lofthus, JE., Waki, MY., Jolkovsky, DL., Otomo-Corgel, J., Newman, MG., Flemming, T., & Nachnani, S. (1991). Bacteremia following subgingival irrigation and scaling and root planing. *Journal of Periodontology,* Vol.62, No.10, pp. 602-607, ISSN 0022-3492.

Loza Fernández de Bobadilla, E., Planes, A., & Rodríguez, M. (2003). Procedimientos en Microbiología Clínica. Recomendaciones de la Sociedad Española de Enfermedades Infecciosas y Microbiología Clínica. 3a Hemocultivos, In: *Sociedad Española de Enfermedades Infecciosas en Microbiología Clínica,* July 2010, Available from: <http://www.seimc.org/documentos/protocolos/microbiologia/>

Lucas, VS., & Roberts, GJ. (2000). Odontogenic bacteremia following tooth cleaning procedures in children. *Pediatric Dentistry,* Vol.22, No.2, pp.96-100, ISSN 0164-1263.

Lucas, VS., Gafan, G., Dewhurst, S., & Roberts, GJ. (2008). Prevalence, intensity and nature of bacteremia after toothbrushing. *Journal of Dentistry,* Vol.36, No.7, pp.481-487, ISSN 0300-5712.

Lucas, VS., Kyriazidou, A., Gelbier, M., & Roberts, GJ. (2007). Bacteraemia following debanding and gold chain adjustment. *European Journal of Orthodontics,* Vol.29, No.2, pp. 161-165, ISSN 0141-5387.

Lucas, VS., Lytra, V., Hassan, T., Tatham, H., Wilson, M., & Roberts, GJ. (2002a). Comparison of lysis filtration and an automated blood culture system (BACTEC) for detection, quantification, and identification of odontogenic bacteremia in children. *Journal of Clinical Microbiology,* Vol.40, No.9, pp.3416-3420, ISSN 0095-1137.

Lucas, VS., Omar, J., Vieira, A., & Roberts, GJ. (2002b). The relationship between odontogenic bacteraemia and orthodontic treatment procedures. *European Journal of Orthodontics,* Vol.24, No.3, pp.293-301, ISSN 0141-5387.

Madsen, KL. (1974). Effect of chlorhexidine mouthrinse and periodontal treatment upon bacteremia produced by oral hygiene procedures. *Scandinavian Journal of Dental Research,* Vol.82, No.1, pp.1-7, ISSN 0022-0345.

Maestre, JR., Mateo, M., & Sánchez, P. (2008). Bacteremia secundaria a procedimientos odontológicos periodontales. *Revista Española de Quimioterapia,* Vo.21. No.3, pp.153-156, ISSN 0214-3429.

McLaughlin, JO., Coulter, WA., Coffey, A., & Burden DJ. (1996). The incidence of bacteremia after orthodontic banding. *American Journal of Orthodontics and Dentofacial Orthopedics,* Vol.109, pp.639-644, ISSN 0889-5406.

Misra, S., Percival, RS., Devine, DA., & Duggal, MS. (2007). A pilot study to assess bacteremia associated with tooth brushing using conventional, electric or ultrasonic toothbrushes. *European Archives of Paediatric Dentistry,* Vol.8, Suppl.1, pp.42-45, ISSN 1818-6300.

Monteiro, AM., Jardini, MA., Alves, S., Giampaoli, V., Aubin, EC., Figueiredo-Neto, AM., & Gidlund, M. (2009). Cardiovascular disease parameters in periodontitis. *Journal of Periodontology,* Vol.80, No.3, pp.378-388, ISSN 0022-3492.

Murphy, AM., Daly, CG., Mitchell, DH., Stewart, D., & Curtis, BH. (2006). Chewing fails to induce oral bacteraemia in patients with periodontal disease. *Journal of Clinical Periodontology,* Vol.33, No.10, pp.730-736, ISSN 0303-6979.

Murray, M., & Moosnick, BS. (1941). Incidence of bacteremia in patients with dental disease. *Journal of Laboratory and Clinical Medicine,* Vol.26, pp.801-802, ISSN 0022-2143.

Nakano, K., Nemoto, H., Nomura, R., Inaba, H., Yoshioka, H., Taniguchi, K., Amano, A., & Ooshima, T. (2009). Detection of oral bacteria in cardiovascular specimens. *Oral Microbiology and Immunology,* Vol.24, No.1, pp.64-68, ISSN 0902-0055.

National Institute for Health and Clinical Excellence. (2008). Prophylaxis against infective endocarditis, In: *National Institute for Health and Clinical Excellence,* July 2010, Available from: http://www.nice.org.uk/nicemedia/pdf/PIEGuidelines.pdf.

Northrop, PM., & Crowley, MC. (1943). The prophylactic use of sulfathiazole in transient bacteremia following extraction of teeth. *Journal of Oral Surgery,* Vol.1, pp.19-29, ISSN 0022-3255.

Offner, PJ., Moore, EE., & Biffl, WL. (1999). Male gender is a risk factor for major infections after surgery. *Archives of Surgery,* Vol.134, No.9, pp.935-940, ISSN 0004-0010.

Okabe, K., Nakagawa, K., & Yamamoto, E. (1995). Factors affecting the occurrence of bacteremia associated with tooth extraction. *International Journal of Oral and Maxillofacial Surgery,* Vol.24, No.3, pp.239-242, ISSN 0901-5027.

Okell, CC., & Elliott, SD. (1935). Bacteremia and oral sepsis with special reference to the aetiology of subacute endocarditis. *Lancet;* Vol.2, pp.869-872, ISSN 0140-6736.

Olsen, I. (2008). Update on bacteraemia related to dental procedures. *Transfusion and Apheresis Science,* Vol.39, No.2, pp. 173-178, ISSN 1473-0502.

Onçag, O., Aydemir, S., Ersin, N., & Koca, H. (2006). Bacteremia incidence in pediatric patients under dental general anesthesia. *Congenital Heart Disease,* Vol.1, No.5, pp.224-228, ISSN 1747-079X.

Pallasch, TJ. (2003). Antibiotic prophylaxis: problems in paradise. *Dental Clinics of North America,* Vol.47, No.4, pp.665-79, ISSN 0011-8532

Palmer, HD., & Kempf, M. (1939). *Streptococcus viridans* bacteremia following extraction of teeth: a case of multiple mycotic aneurysms in the pulmonary arteries: report of cases and necropsies. *Journal of the American Medical Association,* Vol.113, No.20, pp.1788-1792, ISSN 0098-7484.

Parahitiyawa, NB., Jin, LJ., Leung, WK., Yam, WC., & Samaranayake, P. (2009). Microbiology of odontogenic bacteremia: beyond endocarditis. *Clinical Microbiology Reviews,* Vol.22, No.1, pp. 46-64, ISSN 0893-8512.

Pérez-Chaparro, PJ., Gracieux, P., Lafaurie, GI., Donnio, PY., & Bonnaure-Mallet, M. (2008). Genotypic characterization of *Porphyromonas gingivalis* isolated from subgingival plaque and blood sample in positive bacteremia subjects with periodontitis. *Journal of Clinical Periodontology,* Vol.35, No.9, pp.748-753, ISSN 0303-6979.

Peterson, LJ., & Peacock, R. (1976). The incidence of bacteremia in pediatric patients following tooth extraction. *Circulation,* Vol. 53, No.4, pp.676-679, ISSN 0009-7322.

Piñeiro, A., Tomás, I., Blanco, J., Álvarez, M., Seoane, J., & Diz, P. (2010). Bacteraemia following dental implants' placement. *Clinical Oral Implants Research,* Vol.21, No.9, pp.913-918, ISSN 0905-7161.

Pucar, A., Milasin, J., Lekovic, V., Vukadinovic, M., Ristic, M., Putnik, S., & Kenney, EB. (2007). Correlation between atherosclerosis and periodontal putative pathogenic bacterial infections in coronary and internal mammary arteries. *Journal of Periodontology,* Vol.78, No.4, pp.677-682, ISSN 0022-3492.

Ramadan, AE., Zaki, SA., & Nour, ZM. (1975). A study of transient bacteraemia following the use of dental floss silk and interdental stimulators. *Egyptian Dental Journal,* Vol. 21, No.4, pp.19-28, ISSN 0070-9484.

Reimann, HA., & Havens, WP. (1940). Focal infection and systemic disease: a critical appraisal. The case against indiscriminate removal of teeth and tonsils clinical lecture at St. Louis Session. *Journal of the American Medical Association,* Vol.114, No.1, pp.1-6, ISSN 0098-7484.

Reinhardt, RA., Bolton, RW., & Hlava, G. (1982). Effect of nonsterile *versus* sterile water irrigation with ultrasonic scaling on postoperative bacteremias. *Journal of Periodontology,* Vol.53, No.2, pp.96-100, ISSN 0022-3492.

Rhoads, PS., Schram, WR., & Adair, D. (1950). Bacteremia following tooth extraction: prevention with penicillin and N U 445. *Journal of the American Dental Association,* Vol.41, No.1, pp.55-61, ISSN 0002-8177.

Richards, JH. (1932). Bacteremia following irritation of foci of infection. *Journal of the American Medical Association,* Vol.99, No.18, pp.1496-1497, ISSN 0098-7484.

Roberts, G., Gardner, P., & Simmons, N. (1992). Optimum sampling time for detection of dental bacteraemia in children. *International Journal of Cardiology* Vol.35, No.3; pp.311-315. ISSN 0167-5273

Roberts, GJ. (1999). Dentists are innocent! "Everyday" bacteremia is the real culprit: a review and assessment of the evidence that dental surgical procedures are a principal cause of bacterial endocarditis in children. *Pediatric Cardiology,* Vol.20, No.5, pp.317-325, ISSN 0172-0643.

Roberts, GJ., Gardner, P., Longhurst, P., Black, AE., & Lucas, VS. (2000). Is there a need for antibiotic prophylaxis for some aspects of paediatric conservative dentistry?. *British Dental Journal,* Vol.188, No.2, pp.95-98, ISSN 0007-0610.

Roberts, GJ., Holzel, HS., Sury, MR., Simmons, NA., Gardner, P., & Longhurst, P. (1997). Dental bacteremia in children. *Pediatric Cardiology,* Vol.18, No.1, pp.24-27, ISSN 0172-0643.

Roberts, GJ., Jaffray, EC., Spratt, DA., Petrie, A., Greville, C., Wilson, M., & Lucas, VS. (2006). Duration, prevalence and intensity of bacteraemia after dental extractions in children. *Heart,* Vol.92, No.9, pp.1274-1277, ISSN 1355-6037.

Roberts, GJ., Simmons, NB., Longhurst, P., & Hewitt, PB. (1998a). Bacteraemia following local anaesthetic injections in children. *British Dental Journal,* Vol.185, No.6, pp.295-298, ISSN 0007-0610.

Roberts, GJ., Watts, R., Longhurst, P., & Gardner P. (1998b). Bacteremia of dental origin and antimicrobial sensitivity following oral surgical procedures in children. *Pediatric Dentistry,* Vol.20, No.1, pp.28-36, ISSN 0164-1263.

Robinson, L., Kraus, FW., Lazansky, JP., Wheeler, RE., Gordon, S., & Johnson, V. (1950). Bacteremias of dental origin. II. A study of the factors influencing occurrence and detection. *Oral Surgery, Oral Medicine, and Oral Pathology,* Vol.3, pp.923-926, ISSN 0030-4220.

Romans, AR, & App, GR. (1971). Bacteremia, a result from oral irrigation in subjects with gingivitis. *Journal of Periodontology,* Vol.42, No.12, pp.757-760, ISSN 0022-3492.

Romero, J., Bouza, E., Loza, E., Planes, A., Rodríguez, A. (1993). *Procedimientos en Microbiología Clínica. Recomendaciones de la Sociedad Española de Enfermedades Infecciosas y Microbiología Clínica. 3 Hemocultivos,* In: Sociedad Española de Enfermedades Infecciosas en Microbiología Clínica, July 2010, Available from: <http://www.seimc.org/documentos/protocolos/microbiologia/>

Rosenow, EC. (1914). Transmutations within the *Streptococcus-Pneumococcus* group. *Journal of Infectious Disease,* Vol.14, No.1, pp.1-32, ISSN 0022-1899.

Savarrio, L., Mackenzie, D., Riggio, M., Saunders, WP., & Bagg, J. (2005). Detection of bacteraemias during non-surgical root canal treatment. *Journal of Dentistry,* Vol.33, No.4, pp.293-303, ISSN 0300-5712.

Schlegel, D., Reichart, PA., & Pfaff, U. (1978). Experimental bacteremia to demonstrate the barrier function of epithelium and connective tissue surrounding oral endosseous implants. *International Journal of Oral Surgery,* Vol.7, No.6, pp.569-572, ISSN 0300-9785.

Schlein, RA., Kudlick, EM., Reindorf, CA., Gregory, J., & Royal, GC. (1991). Toothbrushing and transient bacteraemia in patients undergoing orthodontic treatment. *American Journal of Orthodontics and Dentofacial Orthopedics,* Vol.99, No.5, pp.466-472, ISSN 0889-5406.

Sconyers, JR., Crawford, JJ., & Moriarty, JD. (1973). Relationship of bacteremia to toothbrushing in patients with periodontitis. *Journal of the American Dental Association,* Vol.87, No.3, pp.616-622, ISSN 0002-8177.

Seymour, RA., Lowry, R., Whitworth, JM., & Martin, MV. (2000). Infective endocarditis, dentistry and antibiotic prophylaxis; time for a rethink?. *British Dental Journal,* Vol.189, No.11, pp.610-616, ISSN 0007-0610.

Shanson, DC., Cannon, P., & Wilks, M. (1978). Amoxycillin compared with penicillin V for the prophylaxis of dental bacteraemia. *The Journal of the Antimicrobial Chemotherapy,* Vol.4, No.5, pp.431-436, ISSN 0305-7453.

Silver, JG., Martin, AW., & McBride, BC. (1977). Experimental transient bacteraemias in human subjects with varying degrees of plaque accumulation and gingival inflammation. *Journal of Clinical Periodontology,* Vol.4, No.2. pp.92-99, ISSN 0303-6979.

Sonbol, H., Spratt, D., Roberts, GJ., & Lucas, VS. (2009). Prevalence, intensity, and identity of bacteraemia following conservative dental procedures in children. *Oral Microbiology and Immnunology,* Vol.24, No.3, pp.177-182, ISSN 0902-0055.

Speck, WT., Spear, SS., Krongrad, E., Mandel, L., & Gersony, WM. (1976). Transient bacteremia in pediatric patients after dental extraction. *American Journal of Diseases of Children,* Vol.130, No.4, pp.406-407, ISSN 0002-922X.

Stein, JM., Kuch, B., Conrads, G., Fickl, S., Chrobot, J., Schulz, S., Ocklenburg, C., & Smeets, R. (2009). Clinical periodontal and microbiologic parameters in patients with acute myocardial infarction. *Journal of Periodontology,* Vol.80, No.10, pp.1581-1589, ISSN 0022-3492.

Takai, S., Kuriyama, T., Yanagisawa, M., Nakagawa, K., & Karasawa, T. (2005). Incidence and bacteriology of bacteremia associated with various oral and maxillofacial surgical procedures. *Oral Surgery, Oral Medicine, Oral Pathology, Oral Radiology, and Endodontics,* Vol.99, No.3, pp.292-298, ISSN 1079-2104.

Tamimi, HA., Thomassen, PR., & Moser, EH Jr. (1969). Bacteremia study using a water irrigation device. *Journal of Periodontology,* Vol.40, No.7, pp.4-6, ISSN 0022-3492.

Thomas, CB., France, R., & Reichsman F. (1941). Prophylactic use of sulfanilamide. In patients susceptible to rheumatic fever. *Journal of the American Medical Association,* Vol.116, No.7, pp.551-560, ISSN 0098-7484.

Tomás, I., Álvarez, M., Limeres, J., Potel, C., Medina, J., & Diz, P. (2007). Prevalence, duration and aetiology of bacteraemia following dental extractions. *Oral Diseases,* Vol.13, No.1, pp.56-62, ISSN 1354-523X.

Tomás, I., Diz, P., Tobías, A., Scully, C., & Donos N. (2011). Periodontal health status and bacteremia from daily oral activities: systematic review/meta-analysis. *Journal of Clinical Periodontology,* (in press), ISSN 0303-6979.

Wilson, W., Taubert, KA., Gewitz, M., Lockhart, PB., Baddour, LM., Levison, M., Bolger, A., Cabell, CH., Takahashi, M., Baltimore, RS., Newburger, JW., Strom, BL., Tani, LY., Gerber, M., Bonow, RO., Pallasch, T., Shulman, ST., Rowley, AH., Burns, JC., Ferrieri, P., Gardner, T., Goff, D., Durack, DT., American Heart Association Rheumatic Fever, Endocarditis and Kawasaki Disease Committee., American Heart Association and Council on Cardiovascular Disease in the Young., American Heart Association Council on Clinical Cardiology., American Heart Association Council on Cardiovascular Surgery and Anesthesia., & Quality of Care and Outcomes Research Interdisciplinary Working Group. (2007). Prevention of infective endocarditis: guidelines from the American Heart Association: a guideline from the American Heart Association Rheumatic Fever, Endocarditis, and Kawasaki Disease Committee, Council on Cardiovascular Disease in the Young, and the Council on Clinical Cardiology, Council on Cardiovascular Surgery and Anesthesia, and the Quality of Care and Outcomes Research Interdisciplinary Working Group. *Circulation,* Vol.116, No.15, pp.1736-1754, ISSN 0009-7322.

Witzenberger, T., O'Leary, TJ., & Gillette, WB. (1982). Effect of a local germicide on the occurrence of bacteremia during subgingival scaling. *Journal of Periodontology,* Vol.53, No.3, pp.172-179, ISSN 0022-3492.

Yanke, SJ., Olson, ME., Davies, HD., & Hart, DA. (2000). A CD-1 mouse model of infection with *Staphylococcus aureus*: influence of gender on infection with MRSA and MSSA isolates. *Canadian Journal of Microbiology,* Vol.46, No.10, pp.920-926, ISSN 0008-4166.

4

Platelet-Bacterial Interactions as Therapeutic Targets in Infective Endocarditis

Steven W. Kerrigan and Dermot Cox
Royal College of Surgeons in Ireland
Dublin,
Ireland

1. Introduction

Endocarditis is an inflammation of the lining of the heart and valves. It can be due to a non-infectious cause (Asopa et al., 2007) but when the inflammation is associated with an infection, usually bacterial, it is known as infective endocarditis (IE) and is characterized by the development of a large septic thrombus on one of the cardiac valves (Beynon et al., 2006; Moreillon and Que, 2004). As this thrombus grows, it can lead to valve failure or may fragment forming a septic embolus that is associated with high mortality if the target of the embolus is the brain, heart or lung (Homma and Grahame-Clarke, 2003). Untreated the mortality is very high and even with aggressive therapy with antibiotics and valve replacement surgery there is a significant mortality. Primarily the disease is due to the formation of a platelet-bacteria thrombus on a cardiac valve and this review will look at the interaction between bacteria and platelets within the context of endocarditis.

2. Traditional role of platelets in thrombosis

Platelets are anucleate fragments of megakaryocytes and their primary role is in haemostasis. Damage to the endothelium surrounding blood vessels leads to the exposure of the sub-endothelial layer that is rich in collagen and immobilised plasma proteins such as von Willebrand factor (vWf). Platelets bind to the newly exposed collagen and become activated. Many blood vessels, such as the coronary arteries are high shear vessels and the blood is flowing too fast to allow the platelets to bind to the collagen. However, under these high shear conditions immobilised vWf can interact with platelet GPIb, which slows down the platelets allowing them to subsequently interact with collagen. Once activated platelets aggregate to form a thrombus which the damaged blood vessel. GPIIb/IIIa mediates platelet aggregation by binding plasma fibrinogen, which as a divalent protein can bind to two separate GPIIb/IIIa molecules. As a result, activated platelets are cross-linked by fibrinogen, which forms the aggregates that seal the damaged vessel.

Platelets are highly responsive and can be activated by many different agonists. As well as two different collagen receptors ($\alpha2\beta1$ and GPVI) and two ADP receptors P_2X_1 and P_2Y_{12}, a serotonin receptor, an adrenergic receptor and a thromboxane A_2 receptor there are also three thrombin receptors (Protease-activated receptor (PAR)-1, GPIbα and PAR-4). Platelet activation is dependent on the sum of the signals from all of these receptors and not on any specific receptor. Signalling from these receptors is either phospholipase A_2/cyclooxygenase (COX)-mediated, resulting in the generation of thromboxane A_2, or protein kinase C-mediated. In contrast, the generation of intracellular cAmp in response to prostacylin binding to its receptor acts to inhibit platelet activation.

Aside from their ability to adhere to sites of damage and to form aggregates, platelets also secrete their granule contents in response to activation. Platelets contain three different granules: α-granules, dense granules and lysosomes. Dense granules are rich in small molecules especially ATP/ADP and serotonin, α-granules contain numerous plasma proteins typically associated with haemostasis and the lysosomes contain acid hydrolases. These secreted products act to enhance haemostasis as ADP activates other platelets, serotonin causes vasoconstriction and the secreted proteins support platelet aggregation.

3. The role of platelets in innate immunity

The biological role of platelets is not confined to haemostasis as platelets also play an important role in the innate immune system (Cox et al., 2011; Semple and Freedman, 2010). Platelets are ideally suited to this as they are present at very high concentration in the blood and are the first responders to any damage to the vasculature, which is the primary mechanism by which pathogens gain entry to the blood. To facilitate this, platelets contain surface receptors that allow it to respond to pathogens. Platelets contain pattern recognition receptors, especially Toll-like receptors (TLRs). These and other receptors (see below) allow platelets to respond to pathogens. As with other platelet agonists, platelets respond to pathogens by adhering to them and subsequently become activated leading to thrombus formation and secretion. In the context of the innate immune system, secretion is the primary response. Activated platelets secrete anti-microbial peptides that act to kill bacteria (Mercier et al., 2004). They also secrete cytokines such as CD40L and RANTES (Antczak et al., 2010) that act to recruit and activate a variety of immune cells to deal with the invading microorganism. Thus, platelets play a key role in the innate immune system where they directly act to kill bacteria as well as coordinating the response of the immune system to the pathogens.

4. The role of platelets in infective endocarditis

IE arises when the bacteria subvert the platelet response to infection and as a result, platelets become part of the pathogenic process. In IE the platelets interact with the bacteria and become activated. They secrete anti-microbial peptides but the bacteria are resistant. Once activated the platelets aggregate resulting in the formation of a platelet-bacteria aggregate. Not only are the bacteria resistant to the anti-bacterial peptides (Bayer et al., 1998; Fowler et al., 2000), they become surrounded by platelets and are able to evade immune surveillance. To further complicate matters even if the bacteria are susceptible to antibiotics, many antibiotics have poor penetration into the thrombus despite adequate plasma levels making treatment more difficult.

While the list of pathogens that have been known to cause IE is long (Baddour et al., 2005), the vast majority of cases with an identified pathogen are due to Staphylococci (primarily *S. aureus*) or Streptococci (primarily *S. sanguinis and S. oralis*). However, around 25% of IE cases are culture negative with no bacteria isolated from the blood (Naber and Erbel, 2007). There are a number of reasons for the failure to culture any organisms such as commencement of antibiotic therapy prior to obtaining the blood sample, infection with a fastidious bacterium or a non-bacterial (e.g., fungal) endocarditis. In this review we will focus on the mechanism of platelet activation by Staphylococci and Streptococci as not only are they the dominant species involved in IE but they are also the best studied. While even different strains of a bacterial species differ in their ability to interact with platelets some general principles can be seen which is important in devising new treatment strategies.

5. Platelet-bacterial interactions: General observations

There are three different types of interaction between platelets and bacteria. The first is an inherent ability of platelet receptors to recognise bacterial surface components. Alternatively, plasma proteins can bind to bacteria and these proteins can in turn bind to a platelet receptor. Typically these are acute phase reactants such as fibrinogen and complement. A third mechanism for interacting with platelets is the secretion of bacterial products or toxins that interact with platelets. The binding of platelets to bacteria either through a direct interaction or via a bridging protein can mediate platelet adhesion and/or platelet activation. Interactions with bacterial toxins leads to either platelet lysis or platelet activation. Typically bacterial proteins that mediate adhesion are distinct from those that mediate aggregation. Thus, bacteria can support platelet adhesion and/or trigger platelet activation. During sepsis the primary interaction between platelets and bacteria is platelet activation and is mediated by both toxin secretion and a direct interaction with the bacteria. However, infective endocarditis is a focal infection of a damaged heart valve. The initial step is mediated by adhesion to the damaged valve as well as subsequent adhesion of platelets to the immobilised bacteria. This adhesive interaction is important in ensuring that the bacteria and thrombus remain attached to the valve despite the presence of turbulent flow conditions. For IE to develop the initial adhesive interaction must be followed by activation of the platelets leading to platelet recruitment and growth of the thrombus. Most bacteria can interact with platelets through multiple mechanisms making it difficult to identify the roles of the different proteins (both bacterial and platelet) and is further complicated by interactions that are not only species-specific but strain-specific as well.

6. Platelet-bacterial interactions: The Staphylococcus

Regardless of the modern advances in antimicrobial therapy and surgical intervention *Staphylococcus aureus* is still the most frequent etiologic microorganism found in Infective endocarditis (Rasmussen et al., 2011). Its interaction with platelets is well characterised. Much of the investigations to date have focused on two separate but related features of this relationship; 1) toxins and 2) cell wall protein mediators of platelet activation (Table 1).

S. aureus is known to secrete several extracellular toxins. Alpha (α)-toxin is a 34 kDa toxin composed of 293 amino acids (Bernheimer, 1965). It is produced by almost all strains of *S. aureus*. Its expression is accessory-gene regulon (agr)-regulated and is secreted into the extracellular environment as a monomeric water soluble protein (Ikigai and Nakae, 1985). The toxin disrupts the cell membranes by binding to the lipid bilayer, forming an oligomeric structure that forms a water filled transmembrane pore (Valeva et al., 1996). Studies have demonstrated that the toxin has primarily two modes of interaction with host cells. These include binding specifically to the host target at low concentrations and non-specific adsorption to host target cell membranes at higher concentrations (Hildebrand et al., 1991).

Siegel and Cohen were the first to demonstrate that addition of α-toxin to human platelet-rich plasma induced platelets to undergo shape change and aggregation (Siegel and Cohen, 1964). In this study the authors demonstrated that platelets leaked their intracellular ions NAD^+, K^+ and ATP but not protein, into the surrounding environment thus concluding that the platelets were not being lysed. Additional studies demonstrated that when platelets were treated with α-toxin it caused them to swell but there were no clear signs of platelet lysis by electron microscopy (Bernheimer and Schwartz, 1965; Manohar et al., 1967). Further investigations into the molecular mechanism through which platelets became activated, found that pore formation gave rise to an increase in intracellular calcium concentration (Arvand et al., 1990; Baliakina et al., 1999). Arvand et al demonstrated that α-toxin triggers a platelet signal that leads to secretion of intracellular contents including procoagulant mediators, platelet factor 4 and factor V. Secreted factor V in turn associates with the platelet membrane leading to assembly of the prothrombinase complex (Arvand et al., 1990). This explains the major pathway responsible for the procoagulatory effects of α-toxin. Bayer et al. used 2 models to investigate the role of α-toxin on platelets. In the first and consistent with the above observations, the authors demonstrated that α-toxin caused platelet lysis which in turn caused the release of platelet microbial proteins (PMP's). The release of PMPs from platelets was bactericidal to *S. aureus*. Using an animal model of endocarditis the authors demonstrated that different strains of *S. aureus* differed in the expression of functional versus mutant forms of α-toxin. Under these conditions, the *S. aureus* strains producing either minimal or no α-toxin were less virulent in vivo than wild-type strains (Bayer et al., 1997). Wild-type *S. aureus* strains or indeed an isogenic strain engineered to over-express α-toxin were associated with increased release of PMP from platelets. These results suggest that when *S. aureus* releases α-toxin in the vicinity of platelets it triggers them to release of PMP's and therefore forging a protective role for the host by destroying the α-toxin producing *S. aureus*.

Lipoteichoic acid (LTA) is a component of gram positive bacteria (Morath et al., 2005) and is often released from the bacteria upon lysis or after treatment with β-lactam antibiotics (Lotz et al., 2006). It also stimulates a strong immune response through an interaction with toll like receptors expressed on many host cells (Zahringer et al., 2008). Toll like receptor 2 (TLR2) recognises LTA and there are now many reports in the literature demonstrating that TLR2 is expressed and functional on platelets (Blair et al., 2009; Keane et al., 2010b; Kerrigan et al., 2008; Ward et al., 2005) suggesting that platelets can respond to LTA. Early reports demonstrated that *S. aureus* LTA inhibits platelet activation by activating the cyclic AMP pathway (Sheu et al., 2000a; Sheu et al., 2000b).

S. aureus predominantly uses multiple cell wall surface proteins to interact with platelets to trigger their activation. Early studies by Hawiger et al. demonstrated that *S. aureus* cell wall protein A acts as a receptor for specific anti-staphylococcal antibodies which in turn bind FcγRIIa on platelets (Hawiger et al., 1979). This interaction triggers an intracellular signal that leads to granule release and platelet aggregation. While this interaction is important, deletion of protein A failed to abolish *S. aureus* binding to platelets. This observation suggests that other interactions between *S. aureus* and platelets exist.

Clumping factor A (ClfA) is a 97kDa protein has been shown to bind plasma fibrinogen. A mutant of *S. aureus* lacking clumping factor A (ClfA) failed to adhere to platelets, suggesting that ClfA binds fibrinogen which in turn binds the platelet fibrinogen receptor, GPIIbIIIa (Sullam et al., 1996). Further characterisation of this interaction suggested that ClfA also requires IgG in order to trigger platelet aggregation. Addition of fibrinogen and ClfA-specific immunoglobulin to the plasma-free system led to *S. aureus*-induced platelet aggregation. Even though resting GPIIbIIIa has little or no affinity for soluble fibrinogen it can still bind fibrinogen bound to bacteria, however this is not enough to trigger activation. To trigger full platelet activation both fibrinogen and specific immunoglobulin must bind to the A domain on ClfA. There are two distinct sites on ClfA that allows fibrinogen and IgG binding at the same time (Loughman et al., 2005). Once bound fibrinogen molecules can engage resting GPIIbIIIa, aided by bound ClfA specific immunoglobulin, which encourages the clustering of Fc receptor, FcγRIIa. This triggers activation of signal transduction leading to conformational change in GPIIbIIIa and aggregation of platelets.

Deletion of the fibrinogen binding domain (ClfA-PY) but not the IgG binding domain on ClfA led to the discovery of a second pathway S. *aureus* uses to induce platelet aggregation. By removing the fibrinogen binding domain in ClfA *S. aureus* induced platelet aggregation very slowly (between 8-20 minutes compared to 2-4 mins). These results suggest that IgG binding to ClfA alone is not enough to trigger platelet aggregation. Using a series of elimination experiments Loughman et al. demonstrated that complement must assemble on the *S. aureus* surface and then bind to unidentified complement receptors on the platelet. Therefore, in the absence of fibrinogen binding complement and specific immunoglobulin are required for platelet activation to occur (Loughman et al., 2005).

A major limitation in our current understanding of platelet bacterial interactions stems from the fact that the majority of studies cited in the literature to date have been carried out under static conditions (static adhesion assays) or non-physiological stirring conditions (platelet aggregation). Therefore, data obtained using *in vitro* assays may not be relevant to the fluid shear environment that platelets encounter in the vasculature. Indeed many reports suggests that the local fluid environment of the circulation critically affects the molecular pathways of cell-cell interactions (Varki, 1994). All of the early *S. aureus* studies were carried out under static or non-physiological stirring conditions and therefore it is difficult to relate these studies to the disease processes. Studies using a cone and plate viscometer (a device that shears cells at a given flow rate) have demonstrated that protein A, ClfA, SdrC, SdrD and SdrE are important in thrombus formation (George et al., 2007; George et al., 2006; Pawar et al., 2004). However, extremely high shear rates were used in these rheological studies. Using another method of investigating the influence of shear rates on *S. aureus* ability to induce platelet activation, Kerrigan et al. perfused platelets over an immobilised monolayer of *S. aureus* in a parallel flow chamber. This method demonstrated that platelets perfused over *S. aureus* under shear conditions equivalent to arterial pressure led to very strong adhesion followed by rapid aggregate formation (Kerrigan et al., 2008). Deletion of ClfA from *S. aureus*, abolished adhesion and aggregate formation under all shear rates investigated. Using a plasma-free system, fibrinogen led to single platelet adhesion but not aggregate formation. Specific immunoglobulin failed to have any effect on either platelet adhesion or aggregation. However, addition of fibrinogen and specific immunoglobulin to the plasma-free system led to platelet adhesion followed by aggregate formation (Kerrigan et al., 2008) thus highlighting the importance of fibrinogen and IgG in aggregate formation induced by *S. aureus*. No interaction was seen under low shear conditions using a parallel flow chamber.

S. aureus have a wide array of proteins expressed on their surface. This protein expression profile is most likely part of their survival. For example, ClfA is expressed weakly at the exponential phase of growth whereas is expressed strongly at the stationary phase of growth. In contrast to this another major *S. aureus* protein, fibronectin binding protein A (FnBPA) is strongly expressed at the exponential phase of growth and weakly expressed at the stationary phase of growth.

FnBPA is a 112kDa cell wall bound protein which binds plasma fibronectin and immunoglobulin. Fnbp contain a specific immunoglobulin binding domain (A domain) and a separate fibronectin binding domain (BCD). The FnBPA A domain is similar in structure and function to that of the ClfA A domain. FnBPA possesses two different but related mechanisms of engaging and activating platelets (Fitzgerald et al., 2006b). In the first mechanism, fibrinogen can bind to the A domain which crosslinks to GPIIb/IIIa, and specific immunoglobulin must crosslink to FcγRIIa to trigger platelet activation and aggregation (Fitzgerald et al., 2006b). In the second mechanism the fibronectin binding domain, BCD, can independently activate platelets. Fibronectin can bind to *S. aureus* via the FnBPA BCD domain by the tandem β-zipper mechanism (Meenan et al., 2007; Raibaud et al., 2005; Schwarz et al., 2003) and also to platelet GPIIbIIIa through the common integrin recognition motif RGD (Fitzgerald et al., 2006b). The signal to trigger platelet activation/aggregation is complete when specific immunoglobulin binds the A domain of FnBPA and cross links to platelet FcγRIIa.

Clumping factor B is a 98 kDa protein highly expressed on the surface of *S. aureus* during the exponential phase of growth and shares sequence homology with ClfA (McAleese et al., 2001). Similar to ClfA, ClfB can also bind fibrinogen and specific immunoglobulin. Deletion of the fibrinogen binding site on ClfB led to a slower aggregation. Characterization of this slower response suggested that complement assembly was required along with immunoglobulin to trigger aggregation (Miajlovic et al., 2007). Therefore similar to *S. aureus* ClfA and FnBPA, ClfB is also capable of triggering platelet aggregation via 2 specific mechanisms; fibrinogen and immunoglobulin or complement and immunoglobulin. Although the complement receptor on platelets has not yet been definitively identified in these interactions, Nguyen et al. has demonstrated that *S. aureus* protein A is capable of binding to the complement receptor gC1qR/p33 (Nguyen et al., 2000). As gC1qR/p33 is only expressed on platelets upon activation rather than at resting, it suggests that the complement interaction may act as an anchor, as it this interaction occurs after the initial platelet activation response.

Staphylococcal protein A (SpA) is a 55kDa protein expressed on greater than 90% of *S. aureus* strains. SpA is made up of 5 repeat domains (A-E) which have been shown to bind to the A1 domain of the major plasma protein vonWillebrand factor with high affinity (low nM range) (Hartleib et al., 2000; O'Seaghdha et al., 2006). Platelets express a high affinity vonWillebrand factor receptor called GPIbα (Andrews et al., 2003). Under very high shear conditions, Pawar and colleagues demonstrated that deletion of SpA from *S. aureus* significantly reduced its interaction with platelets (Pawar et al., 2004). Furthermore, preincubating platelet rich plasma with a vonWillebrand Factor antibody or indeed blocking the platelet GPIbα receptor with an inhibitory monoclonal antibody partially inhibited the platelet-*S. aureus* interaction (Pawar et al., 2004). Thus highlighting the importance of this platelet specific receptor in recognising *S. aureus*.

Bacteria	Bacterial protein	Platelet receptor	Bridging protein	Response
Staphylococcus aureus	α-toxin	None	None	Aggregation
	Lipoteichoic acid	Not identified	None	Aggregation
	Protein A	FcγRIIa, gC1R/p33, GPIbα	IgG, complement, vonWillebrand factor	Aggregation / adhesion / thrombus formation
	ClfA	GPIIbIIIa, FcγRIIa,	Fibrinogen, IgG & complement	Aggregation / thrombus formation
	SdrC	Not identified	Not identified	Thrombus formation
	SdrD	Not identified	Not identified	Thrombus formation
	SdrE	Not identified	Not identified	Thrombus formation
	FnbpA/B	GPIIbIIIa, FcγRIIa	Fibrinogen, IgG & complement	Aggregation / thrombus formation
	ClfB	GPIIbIIIa, FcγRIIa	Fibrinogen, IgG & complement	
	SraP	Not identified	None	Thrombus formation
	IsdB	GPIIbIIIa	None	Aggregation / adhesion

Table 1. List of molecular interactions between Staphylococci and platelets that contribute to Infective Endocarditis

Serine rich protein SraP is a 227kDa large protein and a member of the highly conserved family of serine rich surface glycoproteins expressed on the cell wall of *S. aureus* (Siboo et al., 2005). A mutant strain of *S. aureus* lacking expression of SraP displayed signs of reduced virulence in a rabbit model of infective endocarditis, implicating its role in the development of a growing thrombus on a cardiac valve. The platelet receptor that SraP binds to is not currently known. SraP shares similarility with a group of cell wall-associated glycoproteins (Ramboarina et al., 2010) found in a number of other organisms including *Streptococcus sanguinis* (Plummer et al., 2005), *Streptococcus gordonii* (Kerrigan et al., 2007) both of which have been have been shown to bind to platelet GPIbα. Interestingly however, SraP does not seem to bind to GPIbα.

In vivo, *S. aureus* has restricted access to iron and as a result express iron regulated surface proteins to capture haem from haemogloblin and transport it into the cell (Skaar and Schneewind, 2004). Iron-regulated surface determinant B (IsdB) is a 70kDa family member that has been shown to bind to the platelet fibrinogen receptor GPIIbIIIa. *S. aureus* grown in iron limited conditions bound to platelets in a plasma free environment, suggesting that a plasma bridge bridge is not necessary for interacting with or inducing platelet activation. Mutants defective in the expression of IsdB were unable to adhere to or aggregate platelets. Using surface plasmon resonance Miajlovic et al demonstrated a direct interaction between purified GPIIbIIIa and recombinant IsdB (Miajlovic et al., 2010).

In addition to *S. aureus* having the ability to interact with platelet either directly or indirectly Youssefian and colleagues reported that platelets were also capable of internalising *S. aureus* (Youssefian et al., 2002). While internalisation corresponded with platelet activation the mechanism through which this occurred is currently not known. Moreover it is also yet to be established whether the *S. aureus* is destroyed once internalised in a manner similar to phagocytosis by immune cells.

7. Platelet-bacterial interactions: The Streptococcus

Viridans streptococci are common commensals of the oral cavity, respiratory tract, and gastrointestinal mucosa. In their respective environment these microorganisms are harmless, however following trauma to the mucous membranes they can enter to the normally sterile environment of the bloodstream. Once inside the bloodstream the viridans streptococci act as pathogens (Baddour et al., 1989) and often colonise heart valves, causing infective endocarditis (Moreillon et al., 2002) or become implanted in atherosclerotic plaques, exacerbating atherosclerosis (Chiu, 1999) mainly through an interaction with platelets (Table 2).

Streptococcus sanguinis is a common oral microorganism that is isolated from patients with infective endocarditis. In fact early studies demonstrated that 60% of *S. sanguinis* strains induced platelet aggregation in vitro (Herzberg and Meyer, 1996). Douglas et al provided strong evidence that there is a relationship between the virulence of the infecting *S. sanguinis* strains and their ability to aggregate platelets *in vitro (Douglas et al., 1990). S. sanguinis* induced platelet aggregation was largely found to be dependent on physiological concentrations of calcium and fibrinogen, and some strains required non-specific antibody. Platelet adhesion to *S. sanguinis* occurred independently of calcium, fibrinogen or non-specific antibody, suggesting that platelet adhesion and platelet aggregation are mediated independently of each other (Kerrigan et al., 2002). These observations led to the early model of platelet bacterial interaction where a class I component mediated adhesion to the platelet, a class II component mediates a calcium dependent activation of the platelet and finally a class III component mediates a calcium and fibrinogen-dependent amplification of the response (Herzberg, 1996).

The initial studies focused on identifying the class I and class II components. Treatment of *S. sanguinis* with L- (tosylamido-2-phenyl) ethyl chloromethyl ketone (TPCK)-trypsin liberated cell free peptides (Herzberg et al., 1983). Purification of these peptides failed to support platelet adhesion or trigger platelet aggregation, however, did inhibit *S. sanguinis* mediated platelet aggregation and adhesion. This studies concluded that that these TPCK-tryptic peptides contained antigenic determinants that recognise platelets thus preventing *S.*

sanguinis from binding. Using immunoaffinity chromatography and ion exchange chromatography, Erickson and colleagues identified a platelet aggregation-associated protein (PAAP) (Erickson and Herzberg, 1990). PAAP is synthesized as a 150 kDa glycoprotein which is 40% carbohydrate and is constitutively expressed on the surface of *S. sanguinis* (Erickson and Herzberg, 1993; Erickson et al., 1992). The peptide sequence pro-gly-glu-gln-gly-pro-lys in the PAAP conforms to a predicted consensus motif common to the platelet interactive domain of collagen, lys-pro-gly-glu-pro-gly-pro-lys (Erickson and Herzberg, 1990). More recently Herzberg and colleagues identified a putative collagen-binding protein containing 2 PAAP sequences (Herzberg et al., 2005). PAAP is environmentally controlled during infection in response to high temperature (fever) or exposed collagen (exposed on damaged blood vessels or damaged heart valves) (Heimdahl et al., 1990). Partial sequence alignment shows homology of PAAP to heat shock proteins of *Mycobacterium tuberculosis* and *E. coli* (Herzberg and Meyer, 1996). The platelet receptor for PAAP is currently unidentified.

Ford et al demonstrated that *S. sanguinis* strain NCTC 7863 induced aggregation of normal platelets suspended in plasma however removal of plasma proteins abolished platelet aggregation (Ford et al., 1996). The long lag time (12-15mins) of *S. sanguinis* strain 7863 was progressively shortened by incubating the bacteria in plasma for increasing lengths of time prior to addition to platelets. This suggested that plasma proteins were essential for platelet aggregation. Subsequent experiments demonstrated that complement assembly on the surface of the bacteria was necessary for aggregation of platelets. Further experiments demonstrated that complement assembly was not enough to trigger platelet aggregation which led to the discovery that IgG and fibrinogen was necessary to complete the aggregation process (Ford et al., 1997). More recently McNicol and colleagues demonstrated that depletion of *S. sanguinis*-specific antibodies from plasma prevented platelet aggregation (McNicol et al., 2006). Following *S. sanguinis* binding, addition of antibodies led to rapid phosphorylation of the platelet antibody receptor, FcγRIIa (Pampolina and McNicol, 2005) and further downstream effector targets such as phospholipase Cγ2, syk and adapter molecule LAT.

In 2002 Kerrigan et al, demonstrated that *S. sanguinis* strain 133-79 bound to the platelet vonWillebrand factor receptor, GPIbα (Kerrigan et al., 2002). There was no requirement for vonWillebrand factor or immunoglobulin binding in this system, suggesting that *S. sanguinis* binds directly to platelet GPIbα. Confirmation for the role of GPIbα was provided when a range of site-specific inhibitory monoclonal antibodies against GPIbα prevented *S. sanguis* binding to the platelet. In addition, enzymatic cleavage of GPIbα using the snake venom from a viper pit localised the binding region within the N-terminal 1-225 portion of GPIbα. Finally, platelets from patients with Bernard Soulier Syndrome (patients who fail to express GPIbα on the surface of their platelets) did not aggregate in response to *S. sanguinis* (Kerrigan et al., 2002). The *S. sanguinis* protein that binds GPIbα was purified from cell wall extracts by chromatography on GPIbα and wheat germ agglutinin affinity matrices (Plummer et al., 2005). This led to the identification of a highly glycosylated serine-rich protein called serine-rich protein A (SrpA). An insertional inactivation mutant lacking the SrpA of *S. sanguinis* showed a significant increase in the lag time to aggregation, implicating this protein in platelet aggregation. In addition, platelet adhesion to the SrpA mutant was significantly reduced, however not abolished, suggesting other factors are involved in supporting platelet adhesion.

Streptococcus gordonii is a close but distinct relative of *S. sanguinis* (Nobbs et al., 2009), however initial reports suggested that *S. gordonii* could not induce platelet aggregation (Douglas et al., 1990). More in depth characterisation has demonstrated that *S. gordonii* is capable of supporting platelet adhesion and inducing platelets aggregation in a strain dependent manner. Glycosylated surface protein B is a large 280kDa protein expressed on the surface of *S. gordonii* strain M99. It is heavily glycosylated with glucose and glucosamine and is transported to the cell surface via an accessory system compromising of the SecA2 and the SecY2 proteins (Bensing and Sullam, 2002; Takahashi et al., 2004). GspB has been shown to be highly homologous to an expanding family of Gram-positive bacterial cell surface proteins that includes *S. aureus* serine rich protein SraP (Siboo et al., 2005) *S. sanguis* serine-rich protein SrpA (Plummer et al., 2005), *S. gordonii* DL1 sialic acid-binding protein Hsa (Takahashi et al., 2002) and the *S. parasanguinis* fimbriae-associated protein Fap1 (Wu et al., 2007). These proteins were originally discovered because of their ability to bind a variety of sialylated glycoproteins. Platelet GPIbα is an example of a sialylated glycoprotein and as a result has been shown to bind *S. gordonii* GspB and Hsa (Bensing et al., 2004). Additional molecular glycan characterisation demonstrated that GspB specifically binds O-linked sialic acid residues on GPIbα (Takamatsu et al., 2005), whereas Hsa specifically binds N-linked sialic acid residues on GPIbα and GPIIbIIIa (Yajima et al., 2005). Interestingly an isogenic mutant lacking the expression of Hsa in *S. gordonii* strain DL1 failed to affect percent platelet aggregation however reduced platelet adhesion by ~ 50%. These more recent functional studies suggest that additional protein interactions are necessary for supporting platelet adhesion (Jakubovics et al., 2005a).

S. gordonii expresses a large protein of ~3500 amino acids with a high molecular weight of 397 kDa designated platelet adherence protein A (PadA) (Petersen et al., 2010). PadA contains a short stretch of amino acid residues which displays weak homology to A1 and C1 domain of the plasma protein, vonWillebrand factor (vWf). These domains in vWf are essential for interactions with platelet GPIb and GPIIb/IIIa, respectively. Disruption of the PadA gene from *S. gordonii* DL1 failed to affect binding to glycocalacin (soluble purified GPIbα), however, ablated binding to purified GPIIb/IIIa. Furthermore, platelet adhesion to *S. gordonii* DL1 was significantly reduced by preincubation of platelets with an integrin recognition RGD-containing peptide or the GPIIb/IIIa inhibitor, abciximab (Petersen et al., 2010). Earlier studies demonstrated that *S. gordonii* DL1 bound specifically to GPIIb but not GPIIIa of the GPIIbIIIa complex (Yajima et al., 2005). Collectively these results suggest that platelet adhesion is a mutlifactorial event where Hsa binds GPIbα and PadA binds GPIIb/IIIa and together they act synergistically to support platelet adhesion.

Platelets are very sensitive to shear and some platelet-substrate interactions only manifest themselves upon exposure to shear. For example, under low shear conditions there is no interaction between platelets and vWf however under high shear conditions platelets roll along the vWf coated surface (Ruggeri, 2009). Perfusing platelets over immobilised *S. sanguinis* or *S. gordonii* in a parallel flow chamber under low shear (veneous shear), platelets interacted with a typical rolling behaviour followed by firm adhesion (Jakubovics et al., 2005a; Plummer et al., 2005). This phenomena is highly characteristic of platelet rolling on damaged endothelium (Ruggeri, 2009). Rolling is mediated by platelet GPIbα where is the fast on-off rate of the receptor allows loss of interaction between GPIbα and the bacteria on one side of the platelet leading to the formation of another GPIbα-bacterial interaction on the other side of the platelet. Deletion of the *S. sanguinis* GPIbα-binding protein SrpA or indeed the *S. gordonii* GPIbα-binding protein Hsa abolished the rolling behaviour, suggesting that these proteins form the initial attachment of platelets with the bacteria under physiological shear conditions. Soluble vWf exists in the plasma in a conformation that is not recognisable by platelet GPIbα. However at the site of injury, vWf binds to extracellular matrix proteins forming a thrombotic surface for the platelet. Typically platelets roll along immobilised vWf under high shear conditions. The high shear induces a conformational change in vWf making it recognisable to GPIbα. As *S. gordonii* Hsa and *S. sanguis* SrpA can support static platelet adhesion, or indeed mediate rolling of platelets under low shear conditions it suggests that Hsa and SrpA exist in a unique conformation that is recognisable by GPIbα, as their receptor conformation is not believed to be altered when subjected to shear. The process of rolling is to slow the platelet down from the high shear force experienced in the vasculature long enough to allow it firmly adhere to the bacteria. Firm adhesion is complete when platelet GPIIb/IIIa interacts with *S. gordonii* PadA.

Once the platelets become firmly adhered to *S. gordonii* by engaging with either GPIbα or GPIIbIIIa, a signal is generated in the platelet that results in the platelet changing shape and spreading out on the bacterial surface. The function of platelet spreading is essential for the platelet to withstand the shear forces experienced in the vasculature. Platelet spreading is a particularly important in the development of thrombotic vegetations in infective endocarditis because the lesions around the lesion on the cardiac valve are often very turbulent. Therefore, platelets require the conversion from a discoid shape to a fully spread cell to withstand turbulent shear force. Keane et al, demonstrated that engagement of either GPIbα or GPIIbIIIa, the ITAM-bearing receptor, FcγRIIa and its downstream effectors syk and phospholipase Cγ2 became tyrosine phosphorylated which suggests that this pathway is essential for platelet spreading (Keane et al., 2010a). In addition tyrosine phosphorylation of the FcγRIIa resulted in platelet degranulation, a step critical for inducing and amplyfing platelet aggregation.

Once platelets become firmly adhered and a signal is generated in the platelet it leads to platelet aggregation. Interestingly, while a mutant *S. gordonii* strain lacking expression of Hsa displayed reduced ability to support platelet adhesion, platelet aggregation remained unaffected. This observation suggests that different proteins expressed on the surface of *S. gordonii* mediate different interactions and subsequent responses in platelets. To address this Kerrigan et al used a proteomic approach to identify differentially expressed proteins on a strain of *S. gordonii* that induces platelet aggregation (*S. gordonii* strain DL1) versus one that does not (*S. gordonii* strain Blackburn). Cell wall proteins from both strains were removed from the cell wall using lysozyme. Recovered proteins were separated by poly-acrylamide gel electrophoresis and 2 bands corresponding to 172 kDa and 164 kDa were shown to be differentially expressed. Mass spectrometry identified these proteins as antigen I/II (Kerrigan et al., 2007). The antigen I/II family of proteins are probably the best characterised proteins on the surface of *S. gordonii*. Originally identified on *Streptococcus mutans*, antigen I/II have now been identified on almost all oral streptococci (Nobbs et al., 2007). In *S. gordonii*, antigen I/II have been designated SspA/B. These proteins are oligospecific adhesins which have been shown to bind to several ligands such as collagen type I (Heddle et al., 2003), β_1 integrins (Nobbs et al., 2007), salivary agglutinin glycoprotein (Prakobphol et al., 2000) as well as other bacteria including *P. gingivalis*, *Candida albicans* and *Actinomyces naeslundii* (Demuth et al., 2001; Egland et al., 2001; Jakubovics et al., 2005b). Deletion of SspA/B from *S. gordonii* DL1 failed to affect either platelet aggregation or platelet adhesion. However, deletion of SspA/B and Hsa together abolished platelet aggregation and reduced platelet adhesion by 50%, similar to the Hsa mutant alone (Kerrigan et al., 2007). Consistent with this over expression of SspA and SspB in the non-platelet reactive surrogate host *Lactococcus lactis* induced platelet aggregation but failed to support platelet adhesion. These results suggest that SspA/B and Hsa must act synergistically when binding to platelets to trigger aggregation and that they are not involved in supporting platelet adhesion. At present the receptor through which SspA/B binds to on the platelets is not current known.

Bacteria	Bacterial protein	Platelet receptor	Bridging protein	Response
S. sanguinis	PAAP	Not identified	None	Aggregation
	Not identified	FcγRIIa	Antibody, fibrinogen & complement	Aggregation
	SrpA	GPIbα	None	Adhesion / aggregation
S. gordonii	GspB	GPIbα	None	Adhesion
	Hsa	GPIbα	None	Adhesion / aggregation
	PadA	GPIIbIIIa	None	Adhesion
	SspA/B	Not identified	None	Adhesion / Aggregation
S. mitis	PblA/B	Not identified	None	Aggregation
	Lysin	GPIIbIIIa	fibrinogen	Aggregation
S. mutans	Rgp	Not identified	IgG	Aggregation
	PAc	Not identified	None	Aggregation
S. oralis	Not identified	Not identified	None	Adhesion / aggregation
S. parasanguinis	FimA	Not identified	None	?
	Fap1	Not identified	None	Adhesion
S. pneumoniae	Not identified	TLR2	None	Aggregation

Table 2. List of molecular interactions between Streptococci and platelets that contribute to Infective Endocarditis

Streptococcus mitis has also been shown to interact with platelets although reports are conflicting. In 1990, Douglas et al, used several strains of *S. mitis* and found that none of these interacted with platelets. Ohkuni and colleagues suggested that *S. mitis* strain Nm-65

released a 66 kDa protein (*S.mitis*-derived human platelet aggregation factor, Sm-PAF) that induced platelet aggregation (Ohkuni et al., 1997). Characterisation of this secreted protein revealed that it was a toxin that lysed platelets rather than induced platelet aggregation. More recent work by Bensing et al, identified two distinct genetic loci of *S. mitis* strain SF100 that contributes to platelet binding (Bensing et al., 2001a). The first locus encodes PblT. The mechanism through which it binds to platelets has not yet been explored. The second locus encodes two cell wall associated proteins; PblA is a 107 kDa protein and PblB which is a 121 kDa protein (Bensing et al., 2001b). These proteins are unique as neither of the proteins expresses homology to any other bacterial adhesins described, however share similarities with structural components of bacteriophages (Mitchell et al., 2007). Bacteria often bind to oligosaccharides on host cells. For example *S. gordonii* GspB binds to α2-3-linked sialic acids on platelets and salivary mucins. Platelets treated with sialidases having different linkage specificities demonstrated that removal of α2-8-linked sialic acids resulted in a reduction in *S. mitis* SF100 binding. Gangliosides are glycosphingolipids rich in sialic acids and are found in abundance in lipid rafts in platelets (Marcus et al., 1972). *S. mitis* strains lacking the expression of PblA and PblB demonstrated significant decrease in platelet binding invitro as well as marked reduction in virulence in an animal model of infective endocarditis (Bensing et al., 2001b; Mitchell et al., 2007). More recent studies have demonstrated that *S. mitis* surface bound lysin can bind both free and platelet bound fibrinogen, through its interaction with the Aa and Bb chains of fibrinogen (Seo et al., 2010). Once *S. mitis* has bound fibrinogen this in turn can bind to the platelet fibrinogen receptor, GPIIbIIIa, initiating thrombus formation.

Although early reports suggest *Streptococcus oralis* is capable of inducing platelet aggregation and supporting platelet adhesion the exact mechanism through which either of these occur is currently unknown.

Streptococcus mutans strain Xc induces platelet aggregation by releasing extracts containing serotype-specific polysaccharides which are composed of rhamnose-glucose polymers. An isogenic mutant lacking synthesis the rhamnose-glucose polymers significantly reduced platelet aggregation (Chia et al., 2004). *S. mutants* failed to induce platelet aggregation in the absence of plasma proteins suggesting that a plasma protein possibly bridges the bacteria to the platelet. Subsequent studies identified that addition of serotype-specific IgG to plasma free platelets restored aggregation. The ability of rhamnose polymers toinduce platelet aggregation has been known for some time. For example, ristocetin is obtained from Amycolatopsis lurida and is well characterised for its ability to induce platelet agglutination. The mechanism of ristocetin induced agglutination of platelets involves vWf binding to platelet GPIbα. Cleavage of the rhamnose tetrasaccharide of ristocetin abolished its ability to induce platelet aggregation (Bardsley et al., 1998). Moreover, *S. sanguinis* expresses a platelet associated aggregating protein (PAAP) which is another rhamnose polymer which is thought to be involved in inducing platelet aggregation. Together these results suggest that rhamnose plays an important role in inducing platelet aggregation. Additional studies by Munro et al, demonstrated that an isogenic mutant of *S. mutans* strain V403 lacking the exopolysaccharides glucan and fructan had decreased infectivity in the rat model of endocarditis compared to the wild-type strain (Munro and Macrina, 1993). Protein antigen C (PAc) is a high molecular weight protein expressed by *S. mutans* that has been shown to interact with an unidentified platelet protein (Matsumoto-Nakano et al., 2009). Clinical strains that do not naturally express PAc failed to induce platelet aggregation.

Although the platelet receptor that recognises PAc was not identified, the authors demonstrated that increasing amounts of anti-PAc serum significantly reduced platelet aggregation, suggesting that antibody recognition may be a critical factor.

Streptococcus parasanguinis expresses a 36kDa surface protein called FimA. A mutant defective on the expression of FimA from *S. parasanguinis* strain FW213 failed to have any effect on supporting platelet adhesion or inducing platelet aggregation however significantly reduced the extent of endocarditis in the rat model (Burnette-Curley et al., 1995). Based on these observations the exact mechanism by which FimA functions as a virulence factor of endocarditis has yet to be determined, however it is possible that FimA plays a role in adherence to fibrin deposits associated with damaged heart valves. Fimbrae-associated protein 1 (Fap1) is a highly glycosylated serine-rich glycoprotein which shares sequence and structural homology with SrpA of *S. sanguinis*, GspB of *S. gordonii* and SraP of *S. aureus*. SrpA of *S. sanguinis* and GspB of *S. gordonii* have both been shown to interact directly with platelet GPIbα to trigger platelet activation (Wu et al., 2007). To date no studies have demonstrated that Fap1 interacts with GPIbα or indeed with platelets directly.

Early studies by Johnson et al, demonstrated that at low concentrations *Streptococcus pneumoniae* pneumolysin had little effect on platelets, however at higher concentrations platelets were lysed presumably by binding to the sterols present in the platelet plasma membrane and forming multimeric transmembrane pores (Johnson et al., 1981). The ability to form these pores may result in lysis of platelets. Lysis occurred in a time-dependent manner where greater than 50% of platelets were lysed. A more recent study demonstrated that a concentrated sample of supernatant from an overnight growth of *S. pneumoniae* that contained pneumolysin failed to induce human platelet aggregation, moreover a pneumolysin-negative strain of *S. pneumoniae* also induced platelet aggregation suggesting that pneumolysin is not involved in inducing platelet aggregation (Keane et al., 2010b). In this report the authors demonstrated that *S. pneumoniae* binds to platelet toll like receptor 2 (TLR2), a pattern recognition receptor which triggered the PI3kinase/RAP1 pathway which leads to activation of the fibrinogen receptor GPIIbIIIa.

8. Platelet-bacterial interactions: Non staphylococcal, non streptococcal

There is no doubt Staphylococcus and Streptococcus species make up the majority of cases of infective endocarditis, however other opportunistic pathogens, while rare, may also play a role (Table 3). For example recent work by Shannon et al. demonstrated that clinical isolates of *Enterococcus faecalis* induced platelet aggregation. The ability of the *E. faecalis* to induce platelet aggregation was dependent on IgG (Rasmussen et al., 2010). *Helicobacter pylori* has also been shown to interact with platelets. When in plasma it binds vonWillebrand factor, which in turn enables it to interact with GPIbα and trigger platelet aggregation. This is a unique interaction as soluble vonWillebrand factor cannot interact with platelet GPIbα. The *H. pylori* protein that binds vonWillebrand factor is currently not identified (Byrne et al., 2003; Corcoran et al., 2007). *Porphyromonas ginigvalis* secretes a protease called gingipains that acts directly on platelet protease activated receptors (Lourbakos et al., 2001). Naito and colleagues also deomstrated that *P. ginigvalis* expresses a protein called Hgp44 which also induces platelet aggregation. Although the platelet receptor has not been definitively identified antibodies against GPIbα abolish the interaction (Naito et al., 2006). Finally, *Escherichia coli* secretes shiga-like toxin which binds to the glycosphingolipid receptors on the surface of the platelet and triggers platelet activation (Cooling et al., 1998), however other groups failed to see the interaction in vivo (Viisoreanu et al., 2000). One explanation for these contradictory results is that in vivo the actions of Shiga toxins are complex and many of its actions on platelets are indirect being mediated through effects on other cells such as monocytes (Guessous et al., 2005) and endothelial cells (Motto et al., 2005).

Bacteria	Bacterial protein	Platelet receptor	Bridging protein	Response
Enterococcus faecalis	Not identified	FcgRIIa	IgG	Aggregation
Helicobacter pylori	Not identified	GPIbα	vonWillebrand Factor	Aggregation
Porphyromonas gingivalis	RgpA/B	PAR1 & PAR4	None	Aggregation
	Hgp44	GPIbα	Not identified	Aggregation
Escherichia coli	Shiga-like toxin	Sphingolipids	None	Aggregation

Table 3. List of molecular interactions between non staphylococcal non streptococcal microorganisms and platelets that may contribute to Infective Endocarditis

9. Current and novel treatment options for infective endocarditis

As infective endocarditis is primarily a bacteria infection, often associated with dental and other medical procedures, prophylactic antibiotic treatment was considered to be normal practice. However, more recently the American Heart Association (AHA) and American College of Cardiology (ACC) released a guidance document on infective endocarditis that significantly changed routine practice (Nishimura et al., 2008). In particular they no longer recommend the prophylactic use of antibiotics for dental or other procedures except for a small group of high-risk patients. This was primarily due to the fact that the risks associated with prophylaxis outweigh the benefits. The review panel felt that the biggest risk for IE is not dental or other procedures but rather bleeding from gums due to poor oral hygiene. Thus, so few cases of IE will be prevented by antibiotic prophylaxis during medical procedures but there will be an increase in antibiotic resistance that the there is little benefit to prophylaxis. They felt that improved oral hygiene would be more effective at preventing the occurrence of IE. The exception was for very high-risk patients, which are basically patients with prosthetic valves or those with a history of IE.

With the increase in antibiotic-resistant strains of pathogenic bacteria researchers have been looking at new strategies to target bacteria. One such approach is to target the host response to the pathogen (Clatworthy et al., 2007). IE is very amenable to this strategy as it basically arises from an ineffective host response to the infection. If the platelet aggregation response can be prevented there would be no thrombus formation.

The obvious strategy would be to use an anti-platelet agent to prevent the thrombus formation. Aspirin is the most widely used anti-platelet agent and acts to inhibit cyclooxygenase but may not be effective in preventing IE (Chan et al., 2003). While aspirin effectively inhibits COX some bacteria can activate platelets in a COX-independent manner. As it is not known prior to the procedure which bacteria are likely to be involved aspirin would not be sufficient. A more effective strategy would be to use a $P2Y_{12}$ antagonist such as clopidogrel. However, its very effectiveness makes it unlikely to be used. The inhibition of platelet function by clopidogrel and other anti-platelet agents cause bleeding and it is unlikely that dentists would be happy to perform extractions and other such procedures when the patient is likely to experience very heavy bleeding. Certainly surgeons will not operate on a patient on clopidogrel and they typically require a reversal of the inhibition before they will consider surgery.

Targeting the bacteria is an approach that is attractive, as it would not interfere with platelet function. However, as we have seen choosing a target is difficult as every species of bacteria interact differently with platelets and even different strains of the same species can interact differently (Fitzgerald et al., 2006a). There is also the problem that bacteria such as *S. aureus* have multiple interactions with platelets and it is not clear which one if any is the critical one during IE. Certainly if it was possible to identify a single bacterial protein that was conserved across many pathogenic strains and was found to be critical in the interaction with platelets it would be possible to produce a vaccine against it (Broughan et al., 2011).

Despite the limitations associated with the use of anti-platelet agents platelets are still a promising target for any potential new drug. This is because so far there are only a few platelet receptors implicated in the response to bacteria primarily GPIIb/IIIa and GPIbα. GPIIb/IIIa plays an important role in *S. aureus*-and *S. gordonii* mediated platelet aggregation but as the fibrinogen receptor it also plays a critical role in platelet aggregation. Because of this important role in platelet function a number of inhibitors of this receptor have been developed. Although only for intravenous use these drugs have been very effective anti-platelet agents (Curtin, 2004). However, they are very potent in their inhibition and will cause a profound inhibition of platelet function along with a prolongation of bleeding time that will not be suitable for prophylaxis during procedures such as dental manipulations.

A second platelet receptor that is important in the platelet response to bacteria is GPIbα, which is the von Willebrand factor receptor. GPIbα is very important in platelet adhesion under shear stress and is a very attractive target in cardiovascular disease. However, despite the efforts of many researchers to discover GPIbα inhibitors none have yet made it to the market (Vanhoorelbeke et al., 2007).

FcγRIIa has been shown to mediate platelet activation by many different bacteria including Staphylococci and Streptococci. It typically acts in conjunction with GPIbα, GPIIb/IIIa or the complement receptor. Unlike receptors such as GPIbα and GPIIb/IIIa FcγRIIa is not involved in thrombosis as its role are primarily involved in the immune function of platelets. Thus, antagonists of FcγRIIa will have little impact on platelet function and will not cause bleeding problems making it an ideal target for prophylactic therapy for IE.

The interaction between platelets and bacteria is the key element of infective endocarditis. While there are many different bacterial proteins that can bind to platelets there are only a few potential receptors on the platelet for these proteins. This makes the platelet a good target for novel strategies to inhibit this interaction. While there is always a risk of causing bleeding problems with anti-platelet agents FcγRIIa has been found to be the critical receptor on platelets for the interaction with bacteria. As this receptor is associated with the innate immune functions of platelets rather than with its role in thrombosis targeting FcγRIIa will have minimal effects on the role of platelets in thrombosis. This strategy would be in line with the recent guidance document on infective endocarditis from AHA/ACC. Prophylactic use of an FcγRIIa antagonist during medical procedures with no risk of developing resistance. Antibiotic therapy could then be reserved for cases of sepsis or confirmed infective endocarditis.

10. References

Andrews, R.K., E.E. Gardiner, Y. Shen, J.C. Whisstock, and M.C. Berndt. 2003. Glycoprotein Ib-IX-V. *Int J Biochem Cell Biol* 35:1170-1174.

Antczak, A.J., N. Singh, S.R. Gay, and R.G. Worth. 2010. IgG-complex stimulated platelets: A source of sCD40L and RANTES in initiation of inflammatory cascade. *Cellular Immunology* 263:129-133.

Arvand, M., S. Bhakdi, B. Dahlback, and K.T. Preissner. 1990. Staphylococcus aureus alpha-toxin attack on human platelets promotes assembly of the prothrombinase complex. *J Biol Chem* 265:14377-14381.

Asopa, S., A. Patel, O.A. Khan, R. Sharma, and S.K. Ohri. 2007. Non-bacterial thrombotic endocarditis. *Eur J Cardiothorac Surg* 32:696-701.

Baddour, L.M., G.D. Christensen, J.H. Lowrance, and W.A. Simpson. 1989. Pathogenesis of experimental endocarditis. *Rev Infect Dis* 11:452-463.

Baddour, L.M., W.R. Wilson, A.S. Bayer, V.G. Fowler, Jr., A.F. Bolger, M.E. Levison, P. Ferrieri, M.A. Gerber, L.Y. Tani, M.H. Gewitz, D.C. Tong, J.M. Steckelberg, R.S. Baltimore, S.T. Shulman, J.C. Burns, D.A. Falace, J.W. Newburger, T.J. Pallasch, M. Takahashi, and K.A. Taubert. 2005. Infective Endocarditis: Diagnosis, Antimicrobial Therapy, and Management of Complications: A Statement for Healthcare Professionals From the Committee on Rheumatic Fever, Endocarditis, and Kawasaki Disease, Council on Cardiovascular Disease in the Young, and the Councils on Clinical Cardiology, Stroke, and Cardiovascular Surgery and Anesthesia, American Heart Association: Endorsed by the Infectious Diseases Society of America. *Circulation* 111:e394-434.

Baliakina, E.V., E.V. Gerasimovskaia, A. Romanov Iu, and E. Atakhanov Sh. 1999. [Role of staphylococcus aureus hemolytic toxin-alpha in pathogenesis of infectious endocarditis: studies in vitro]. *Ter Arkh* 71:28-31.

Bardsley, B., D.H. Williams, and T.P. Baglin. 1998. Cleavage of rhamnose from ristocetin A removes its ability to induce platelet aggregation. *Blood Coagul Fibrinolysis* 9:241-244.

Bayer, A.S., D. Cheng, M.R. Yeaman, G.R. Corey, R.S. McClelland, L.J. Harrel, and V.G. Fowler, Jr. 1998. In vitro resistance to thrombin-induced platelet microbicidal protein among clinical bacteremic isolates of Staphylococcus aureus correlates with an endovascular infectious source. *Antimicrob Agents Chemother* 42:3169-3172.

Bayer, A.S., M.D. Ramos, B.E. Menzies, M.R. Yeaman, A.J. Shen, and A.L. Cheung. 1997. Hyperproduction of alpha-toxin by Staphylococcus aureus results in paradoxically reduced virulence in experimental endocarditis: a host defense role for platelet microbicidal proteins. *Infect Immun* 65:4652-4660.

Bensing, B.A., J.A. Lopez, and P.M. Sullam. 2004. The Streptococcus gordonii surface proteins GspB and Hsa mediate binding to sialylated carbohydrate epitopes on the platelet membrane glycoprotein Ibalpha. *Infect Immun* 72:6528-6537.

Bensing, B.A., C.E. Rubens, and P.M. Sullam. 2001a. Genetic loci of Streptococcus mitis that mediate binding to human platelets. *Infect Immun* 69:1373-1380.

Bensing, B.A., I.R. Siboo, and P.M. Sullam. 2001b. Proteins PblA and PblB of Streptococcus mitis, which promote binding to human platelets, are encoded within a lysogenic bacteriophage. *Infect Immun* 69:6186-6192.

Bensing, B.A., and P.M. Sullam. 2002. An accessory sec locus of Streptococcus gordonii is required for export of the surface protein GspB and for normal levels of binding to human platelets. *Mol Microbiol* 44:1081-1094.

Bernheimer, A.W. 1965. Staphylococcal alpha toxin. *Ann N Y Acad Sci* 128:112-123.

Bernheimer, A.W., and L.L. Schwartz. 1965. Effect of Staphylococcal and Other Bacterial Toxins on Platelets in Vitro. *J Pathol Bacteriol* 89:209-223.

Beynon, R.P., V.K. Bahl, and B.D. Prendergast. 2006. Infective endocarditis. *Br Med J* 333:334-339.

Blair, P., S. Rex, O. Vitseva, L. Beaulieu, K. Tanriverdi, S. Chakrabarti, C. Hayashi, C.A. Genco, M. Iafrati, and J.E. Freedman. 2009. Stimulation of Toll-like receptor 2 in human platelets induces a thromboinflammatory response through activation of phosphoinositide 3-kinase. *Circ Res* 104:346-354.

Broughan, J., R. Anderson, and A.S. Anderson. 2011. Strategies for and advances in the development of Staphylococcus aureus prophylactic vaccines. *Expert Review of Vaccines* 10:695-708.

Burnette-Curley, D., V. Wells, H. Viscount, C.L. Munro, J.C. Fenno, P. Fives-Taylor, and F.L. Macrina. 1995. FimA, a major virulence factor associated with Streptococcus parasanguis endocarditis. *Infect Immun* 63:4669-4674.

Byrne, M.F., S.W. Kerrigan, P.A. Corcoran, J.C. Atherton, F.E. Murray, D.J. Fitzgerald, and D.M. Cox. 2003. Helicobacter pylori binds von Willebrand factor and interacts with GPIb to induce platelet aggregation. *Gastroenterology* 124:1846-1854.

Chan, K., J. Dumesnil, B. Cujec, A. Sanfilippo, J. Jue, M. Turek, T. Robinson, D. Moher, and I.o.t.M.A.S.i.I. Endocarditis. 2003. A randomized trial of aspirin on the risk of embolic events in patients with infective endocarditis. *J Am Coll Cardiol* 42:775-780.

Chia, J.S., Y.L. Lin, H.T. Lien, and J.Y. Chen. 2004. Platelet aggregation induced by serotype polysaccharides from Streptococcus mutans. *Infect Immun* 72:2605-2617.

Chiu, B. 1999. Multiple infections in carotid atherosclerotic plaques. *Am Heart J* 138:S534-536.

Clatworthy, A.E., E. Pierson, and D.T. Hung. 2007. Targeting virulence: a new paradigm for antimicrobial therapy. *Nat Chem Biol* 3:541-548.

Cooling, L.L., K.E. Walker, T. Gille, and T.A. Koerner. 1998. Shiga toxin binds human platelets via globotriaosylceramide (Pk antigen) and a novel platelet glycosphingolipid. *Infect Immun* 66:4355-4366.

Corcoran, P.A., J.C. Atherton, S.W. Kerrigan, T. Wadstrom, F.E. Murray, R.M. Peek, D.J. Fitzgerald, D.M. Cox, and M.F. Byrne. 2007. The effect of different strains of Helicobacter pylori on platelet aggregation. *Can J Gastroenterol* 21:367-370.

Cox, D., S.W. Kerrigan, and S.P. Watson. 2011. Platelets and the innate immune system: mechanisms of bacterial-induced platelet activation. *Journal of Thrombosis and Haemostasis* 9:1097-1107.

Curtin, R. 2004. Intravenous glycoprotein IIb/IIIa antagonists: their benefits, problems and future developments. *Curr Pharm Des* 10:1577-1585.

Demuth, D.R., D.C. Irvine, J.W. Costerton, G.S. Cook, and R.J. Lamont. 2001. Discrete protein determinant directs the species-specific adherence of Porphyromonas gingivalis to oral streptococci. *Infect Immun* 69:5736-5741.

Douglas, C.W., P.R. Brown, and F.E. Preston. 1990. Platelet aggregation by oral streptococci. *FEMS Microbiol Lett* 60:63-67.

Egland, P.G., L.D. Du, and P.E. Kolenbrander. 2001. Identification of independent Streptococcus gordonii SspA and SspB functions in coaggregation with Actinomyces naeslundii. *Infect Immun* 69:7512-7516.

Erickson, P.R., and M.C. Herzberg. 1990. Purification and partial characterization of a 65-kDa platelet aggregation-associated protein antigen from the surface of Streptococcus sanguis. *J Biol Chem* 265:14080-14087.

Erickson, P.R., and M.C. Herzberg. 1993. The Streptococcus sanguis platelet aggregation-associated protein. Identification and characterization of the minimal platelet-interactive domain. *J Biol Chem* 268:1646-1649.

Erickson, P.R., M.C. Herzberg, and G. Tierney. 1992. Cross-reactive immunodeterminants on Streptococcus sanguis and collagen. Predicting a structural motif of platelet-interactive domains. *J Biol Chem* 267:10018-10023.

Fitzgerald, J.R., T.J. Foster, and D. Cox. 2006a. The interaction of bacterial pathogens with platelets. *Nat Rev Microbiol* 4:445-457.

Fitzgerald, J.R., A. Loughman, F. Keane, M. Brennan, M. Knobel, J. Higgins, L. Visai, P. Speziale, D. Cox, and T.J. Foster. 2006b. Fibronectin-binding proteins of Staphylococcus aureus mediate activation of human platelets via fibrinogen and fibronectin bridges to integrin GPIIb/IIIa and IgG binding to the FcgammaRIIa receptor. *Mol Microbiol* 59:212-230.

Ford, I., C.W. Douglas, D. Cox, D.G. Rees, J. Heath, and F.E. Preston. 1997. The role of immunoglobulin G and fibrinogen in platelet aggregation by Streptococcus sanguis. *Br J Haematol* 97:737-746.

Ford, I., C.W. Douglas, J. Heath, C. Rees, and F.E. Preston. 1996. Evidence for the involvement of complement proteins in platelet aggregation by Streptococcus sanguis NCTC 7863. *Br J Haematol* 94:729-739.

Fowler, V.G., Jr., L.M. McIntyre, M.R. Yeaman, G.E. Peterson, L. Barth Reller, G.R. Corey, D. Wray, and A.S. Bayer. 2000. In vitro resistance to thrombin-induced platelet microbicidal protein in isolates of Staphylococcus aureus from endocarditis patients correlates with an intravascular device source. *J Infect Dis* 182:1251-1254.

George, N.P., K. Konstantopoulos, and J.M. Ross. 2007. Differential kinetics and molecular recognition mechanisms involved in early versus late growth phase Staphylococcus aureus cell binding to platelet layers under physiological shear conditions. *J Infect Dis* 196:639-646.

George, N.P., Q. Wei, P.K. Shin, K. Konstantopoulos, and J.M. Ross. 2006. Staphylococcus aureus adhesion via Spa, ClfA, and SdrCDE to immobilized platelets demonstrates shear-dependent behavior. *Arterioscler Thromb Vasc Biol* 26:2394-2400.

Guessous, F., M. Marcinkiewicz, R. Polanowska-Grabowska, T.R. Keepers, T. Obrig, and A.R. Gear. 2005. Shiga toxin 2 and lipopolysaccharide cause monocytic THP-1 cells to release factors which activate platelet function. *Thromb Haemost* 94:1019-1027.

Hartleib, J., N. Kohler, R.B. Dickinson, G.S. Chhatwal, J.J. Sixma, O.M. Hartford, T.J. Foster, G. Peters, B.E. Kehrel, and M. Herrmann. 2000. Protein A is the von Willebrand factor binding protein on Staphylococcus aureus. *Blood* 96:2149-2156.

Hawiger, J., S. Steckley, D. Hammond, C. Cheng, S. Timmons, A.D. Glick, and R.M. Des Prez. 1979. Staphylococci-induced human platelet injury mediated by protein A and immunoglobulin G Fc fragment receptor. *J Clin Invest* 64:931-937.

Heddle, C., A.H. Nobbs, N.S. Jakubovics, M. Gal, J.P. Mansell, D. Dymock, and H.F. Jenkinson. 2003. Host collagen signal induces antigen I/II adhesin and invasin gene expression in oral Streptococcus gordonii. *Mol Microbiol* 50:597-607.

Heimdahl, A., G. Hall, M. Hedberg, H. Sandberg, P.O. Soder, K. Tuner, and C.E. Nord. 1990. Detection and quantitation by lysis-filtration of bacteremia after different oral surgical procedures. *J Clin Microbiol* 28:2205-2209.

Herzberg, M.C. 1996. Platelet-streptococcal interactions in endocarditis. *Crit Rev Oral Biol Med* 7:222-236.

Herzberg, M.C., K.L. Brintzenhofe, and C.C. Clawson. 1983. Cell-free released components of Streptococcus sanguis inhibit human platelet aggregation. *Infect Immun* 42:394-401.

Herzberg, M.C., and M.W. Meyer. 1996. Effects of oral flora on platelets: possible consequences in cardiovascular disease. *J Periodontol* 67:1138-1142.

Herzberg, M.C., A. Nobbs, L. Tao, A. Kilic, E. Beckman, A. Khammanivong, and Y. Zhang. 2005. Oral streptococci and cardiovascular disease: searching for the platelet aggregation-associated protein gene and mechanisms of Streptococcus sanguis-induced thrombosis. *J Periodontol* 76:2101-2105.

Hildebrand, A., M. Pohl, and S. Bhakdi. 1991. Staphylococcus aureus alpha-toxin. Dual mechanism of binding to target cells. *J Biol Chem* 266:17195-17200.

Homma, S., and C. Grahame-Clarke. 2003. Toward reducing embolic complications from endocarditis. *J Am Coll Cardiol* 42:781-783.

Ikigai, H., and T. Nakae. 1985. Conformational alteration in alpha-toxin from Staphylococcus aureus concomitant with the transformation of the water-soluble monomer to the membrane oligomer. *Biochem Biophys Res Commun* 130:175-181.

Jakubovics, N.S., S.W. Kerrigan, A.H. Nobbs, N. Stromberg, C.J. van Dolleweerd, D.M. Cox, C.G. Kelly, and H.F. Jenkinson. 2005a. Functions of cell surface-anchored antigen I/II family and Hsa polypeptides in interactions of Streptococcus gordonii with host receptors. *Infect Immun* 73:6629-6638.

Jakubovics, N.S., N. Stromberg, C.J. van Dolleweerd, C.G. Kelly, and H.F. Jenkinson. 2005b. Differential binding specificities of oral streptococcal antigen I/II family adhesins for human or bacterial ligands. *Mol Microbiol* 55:1591-1605.

Johnson, M.K., D. Boese-Marrazzo, and W.A. Pierce, Jr. 1981. Effects of pneumolysin on human polymorphonuclear leukocytes and platelets. *Infect Immun* 34:171-176.

Keane, C., H. Petersen, K. Reynolds, D.K. Newman, D. Cox, H.F. Jenkinson, P.J. Newman, and S.W. Kerrigan. 2010a. Mechanism of outside-in {alpha}IIb{beta}3-mediated activation of human platelets by the colonizing Bacterium, Streptococcus gordonii. *Arterioscler Thromb Vasc Biol* 30:2408-2415.

Keane, C., D. Tilley, A. Cunningham, A. Smolenski, A. Kadioglu, D. Cox, H.F. Jenkinson, and S.W. Kerrigan. 2010b. Invasive Streptococcus pneumoniae trigger platelet activation via Toll-like receptor 2. *J Thromb Haemost* 8:2757-2765.

Kerrigan, S.W., N. Clarke, A. Loughman, G. Meade, T.J. Foster, and D. Cox. 2008. Molecular basis for Staphylococcus aureus-mediated platelet aggregate formation under arterial shear in vitro. *Arterioscler Thromb Vasc Biol* 28:335-340.

Kerrigan, S.W., I. Douglas, A. Wray, J. Heath, M.F. Byrne, D. Fitzgerald, and D. Cox. 2002. A role for glycoprotein Ib in Streptococcus sanguis-induced platelet aggregation. *Blood* 100:509-516.

Kerrigan, S.W., N.S. Jakubovics, C. Keane, P. Maguire, K. Wynne, H.F. Jenkinson, and D. Cox. 2007. Role of Streptococcus gordonii surface proteins SspA/SspB and Hsa in platelet function. *Infect Immun* 75:5740-5747.

Lotz, S., A. Starke, C. Ziemann, S. Morath, T. Hartung, W. Solbach, and T. Laskay. 2006. Beta-lactam antibiotic-induced release of lipoteichoic acid from Staphylococcus aureus leads to activation of neutrophil granulocytes. *Ann Clin Microbiol Antimicrob* 5:15.

Loughman, A., J.R. Fitzgerald, M.P. Brennan, J. Higgins, R. Downer, D. Cox, and T.J. Foster. 2005. Roles for fibrinogen, immunoglobulin and complement in platelet activation promoted by Staphylococcus aureus clumping factor A. *Mol Microbiol* 57:804-818.

Lourbakos, A., Y.P. Yuan, A.L. Jenkins, J. Travis, P. Andrade-Gordon, R. Santulli, J. Potempa, and R.N. Pike. 2001. Activation of protease-activated receptors by gingipains from Porphyromonas gingivalis leads to platelet aggregation: a new trait in microbial pathogenicity. *Blood* 97:3790-3797.

Manohar, M., S.K. Maheswaran, S.P. Frommes, and R.K. Lindorfer. 1967. Platelet damaging factor, a fifth activity of staphylococcal alpha-toxin. *J Bacteriol* 94:224-231.

Marcus, A.J., H.L. Ullman, and L.B. Safier. 1972. Studies on human platelet gangliosides. *J Clin Invest* 51:2602-2612.

Matsumoto-Nakano, M., M. Tsuji, S. Inagaki, K. Fujita, K. Nagayama, R. Nomura, and T. Ooshima. 2009. Contribution of cell surface protein antigen c of Streptococcus mutans to platelet aggregation. *Oral Microbiol Immunol* 24:427-430.

McAleese, F.M., E.J. Walsh, M. Sieprawska, J. Potempa, and T.J. Foster. 2001. Loss of clumping factor B fibrinogen binding activity by Staphylococcus aureus involves cessation of transcription, shedding and cleavage by metalloprotease. *J Biol Chem* 276:29969-29978.

McNicol, A., R. Zhu, R. Pesun, C. Pampolina, E.C. Jackson, G.H. Bowden, and T. Zelinski. 2006. A role for immunoglobulin G in donor-specific Streptococcus sanguis-induced platelet aggregation. *Thromb Haemost* 95:288-293.

Meenan, N.A., L. Visai, V. Valtulina, U. Schwarz-Linek, N.C. Norris, S. Gurusiddappa, M. Hook, P. Speziale, and J.R. Potts. 2007. The tandem beta-zipper model defines high affinity fibronectin-binding repeats within Staphylococcus aureus FnBPA. *J Biol Chem* 282:25893-25902.

Mercier, R.-C., R.M. Dietz, J.L. Mazzola, A.S. Bayer, and M.R. Yeaman. 2004. Beneficial Influence of Platelets on Antibiotic Efficacy in an In Vitro Model of Staphylococcus aureus-Induced Endocarditis. *Antimicrob. Agents Chemother.* 48:2551-2557.

Miajlovic, H., A. Loughman, M. Brennan, D. Cox, and T.J. Foster. 2007. Both complement- and fibrinogen-dependent mechanisms contribute to platelet aggregation mediated by Staphylococcus aureus clumping factor B. *Infect Immun* 75:3335-3343.

Miajlovic, H., M. Zapotoczna, J.A. Geoghegan, S.W. Kerrigan, P. Speziale, and T.J. Foster. 2010. Direct interaction of iron-regulated surface determinant IsdB of Staphylococcus aureus with the GPIIb/IIIa receptor on platelets. *Microbiology* 156:920-928.

Mitchell, J., I.R. Siboo, D. Takamatsu, H.F. Chambers, and P.M. Sullam. 2007. Mechanism of cell surface expression of the Streptococcus mitis platelet binding proteins PblA and PblB. *Mol Microbiol* 64:844-857.

Morath, S., S. von Aulock, and T. Hartung. 2005. Structure/function relationships of lipoteichoic acids. *J Endotoxin Res* 11:348-356.

Moreillon, P., Y.A. Que, and A.S. Bayer. 2002. Pathogenesis of streptococcal and staphylococcal endocarditis. *Infect Dis Clin North Am* 16:297-318.

Moreillon, P.P., and Y.-A. Que. 2004. Infective endocarditis. *The Lancet* 363:139-149.

Motto, D.G., A.K. Chauhan, G. Zhu, J. Homeister, C.B. Lamb, K.C. Desch, W. Zhang, H.M. Tsai, D.D. Wagner, and D. Ginsburg. 2005. Shigatoxin triggers thrombotic thrombocytopenic purpura in genetically susceptible ADAMTS13-deficient mice. *J Clin Invest* 115:2752-2761.

Munro, C.L., and F.L. Macrina. 1993. Sucrose-derived exopolysaccharides of Streptococcus mutans V403 contribute to infectivity in endocarditis. *Mol Microbiol* 8:133-142.

Naber, C.K., and R. Erbel. 2007. Infective endocarditis with negative blood cultures. *International Journal of Antimicrobial Agents* 30:32-36.

Naito, M., E. Sakai, Y. Shi, H. Ideguchi, M. Shoji, N. Ohara, K. Yamamoto, and K. Nakayama. 2006. Porphyromonas gingivalis-induced platelet aggregation in plasma depends on Hgp44 adhesin but not Rgp proteinase. *Mol Microbiol* 59:152-167.

Nguyen, T., B. Ghebrehiwet, and E.I. Peerschke. 2000. Staphylococcus aureus protein A recognizes platelet gC1qR/p33: a novel mechanism for staphylococcal interactions with platelets. *Infect Immun* 68:2061-2068.

Nishimura, R.A., B.A. Carabello, D.P. Faxon, M.D. Freed, B.W. Lytle, P.T. O'Gara, R.A. O'Rourke, and P.M. Shah. 2008. ACC/AHA 2008 Guideline Update on Valvular Heart Disease: Focused Update on Infective Endocarditis. A Report of the American College of Cardiology/American Heart Association Task Force on Practice Guidelines. *Circulation* CIRCULATIONAHA.108.190377.

Nobbs, A.H., R.J. Lamont, and H.F. Jenkinson. 2009. Streptococcus adherence and colonization. *Microbiol Mol Biol Rev* 73:407-450, Table of Contents.

Nobbs, A.H., B.H. Shearer, M. Drobni, M.A. Jepson, and H.F. Jenkinson. 2007. Adherence and internalization of Streptococcus gordonii by epithelial cells involves beta1 integrin recognition by SspA and SspB (antigen I/II family) polypeptides. *Cell Microbiol* 9:65-83.

O'Seaghdha, M., C.J. van Schooten, S.W. Kerrigan, J. Emsley, G.J. Silverman, D. Cox, P.J. Lenting, and T.J. Foster. 2006. Staphylococcus aureus protein A binding to von Willebrand factor A1 domain is mediated by conserved IgG binding regions. *FEBS J* 273:4831-4841.

Ohkuni, H., Y. Todome, Y. Watanabe, S. Kotani, and Y. Kimura. 1997. Purification and partial characterization of a novel human platelet aggregation factor in the extracellular products of Streptococcus mitis, strain Nm-65. *Adv Exp Med Biol* 418:689-693.

Pampolina, C., and A. McNicol. 2005. Streptococcus sanguis-induced platelet activation involves two waves of tyrosine phosphorylation mediated by FcgammaRIIA and alphaIIbbeta3. *Thromb Haemost* 93:932-939.

Pawar, P., P.K. Shin, S.A. Mousa, J.M. Ross, and K. Konstantopoulos. 2004. Fluid shear regulates the kinetics and receptor specificity of Staphylococcus aureus binding to activated platelets. *J Immunol* 173:1258-1265.

Petersen, H.J., C. Keane, H.F. Jenkinson, M.M. Vickerman, A. Jesionowski, J.C. Waterhouse, D. Cox, and S.W. Kerrigan. 2010. Human platelets recognize a novel surface protein, PadA, on Streptococcus gordonii through a unique interaction involving fibrinogen receptor GPIIbIIIa. *Infect Immun* 78:413-422.

Plummer, C., H. Wu, S.W. Kerrigan, G. Meade, D. Cox, and C.W. Ian Douglas. 2005. A serine-rich glycoprotein of Streptococcus sanguis mediates adhesion to platelets via GPIb. *Br J Haematol* 129:101-109.

Prakobphol, A., F. Xu, V.M. Hoang, T. Larsson, J. Bergstrom, I. Johansson, L. Frangsmyr, U. Holmskov, H. Leffler, C. Nilsson, T. Boren, J.R. Wright, N. Stromberg, and S.J. Fisher. 2000. Salivary agglutinin, which binds Streptococcus mutans and Helicobacter pylori, is the lung scavenger receptor cysteine-rich protein gp-340. *J Biol Chem* 275:39860-39866.

Raibaud, S., U. Schwarz-Linek, J.H. Kim, H.T. Jenkins, E.R. Baines, S. Gurusiddappa, M. Hook, and J.R. Potts. 2005. Borrelia burgdorferi binds fibronectin through a tandem beta-zipper, a common mechanism of fibronectin binding in staphylococci, streptococci, and spirochetes. *J Biol Chem* 280:18803-18809.

Ramboarina, S., J.A. Garnett, M. Zhou, Y. Li, Z. Peng, J.D. Taylor, W.C. Lee, A. Bodey, J.W. Murray, Y. Alguel, J. Bergeron, B. Bardiaux, E. Sawyer, R. Isaacson, C. Tagliaferri, E. Cota, M. Nilges, P. Simpson, T. Ruiz, H. Wu, and S. Matthews. 2010. Structural insights into serine-rich fimbriae from Gram-positive bacteria. *J Biol Chem* 285:32446-32457.

Rasmussen, M., D. Johansson, S.K. Sobirk, M. Morgelin, and O. Shannon. 2010. Clinical isolates of Enterococcus faecalis aggregate human platelets. *Microbes Infect* 12:295-301.

Rasmussen, R.V., U. Host, M. Arpi, C. Hassager, H.K. Johansen, E. Korup, H.C. Schonheyder, J. Berning, S. Gill, F.S. Rosenvinge, V.G. Fowler, Jr., J.E. Moller, R.L. Skov, C.T. Larsen, T.F. Hansen, S. Mard, J. Smit, P.S. Andersen, and N.E. Bruun. 2011. Prevalence of infective endocarditis in patients with Staphylococcus aureus bacteraemia: the value of screening with echocardiography. *Eur J Echocardiogr* 12:414-420.

Ruggeri, Z.M. 2009. Platelet adhesion under flow. *Microcirculation* 16:58-83.

Schwarz, S., A. Bottner, H.M. Hafez, C. Kehrenberg, M. Kietzmann, D. Klarmann, G. Klein, P. Krabisch, T. Kuhn, G. Luhofer, A. Richter, W. Traeder, K.H. Waldmann, J. Wallmann, and C. Werckenthin. 2003. [Antimicrobial susceptibility testing of bacteria isolated from animals: methods for in-vitro susceptibility testing and their suitability with regard to the generation of the most useful data for therapeutic applications]. *Berl Munch Tierarztl Wochenschr* 116:353-361.

Semple, J., and J. Freedman. 2010. Platelets and innate immunity. *Cellular and Molecular Life Sciences* 67:499-511.

Seo, H.S., Y.Q. Xiong, J. Mitchell, R. Seepersaud, A.S. Bayer, and P.M. Sullam. 2010. Bacteriophage lysin mediates the binding of streptococcus mitis to human platelets through interaction with fibrinogen. *PLoS Pathog* 6:

Sheu, J.R., G. Hsiao, C. Lee, W. Chang, L.W. Lee, C.H. Su, and C.H. Lin. 2000a. Antiplatelet activity of Staphylococcus aureus lipoteichoic acid is mediated through a cyclic AMP pathway. *Thromb Res* 99:249-258.

Sheu, J.R., C.R. Lee, C.H. Lin, G. Hsiao, W.C. Ko, Y.C. Chen, and M.H. Yen. 2000b. Mechanisms involved in the antiplatelet activity of Staphylococcus aureus lipoteichoic acid in human platelets. *Thromb Haemost* 83:777-784.

Siboo, I.R., H.F. Chambers, and P.M. Sullam. 2005. Role of SraP, a Serine-Rich Surface Protein of Staphylococcus aureus, in binding to human platelets. *Infect Immun* 73:2273-2280.

Siegel, I., and S. Cohen. 1964. Action of Staphylococcal Toxin on Human Platelets. *J Infect Dis* 114:488-502.

Skaar, E.P., and O. Schneewind. 2004. Iron-regulated surface determinants (Isd) of Staphylococcus aureus: stealing iron from heme. *Microbes Infect* 6:390-397.

Sullam, P.M., A.S. Bayer, W.M. Foss, and A.L. Cheung. 1996. Diminished platelet binding in vitro by Staphylococcus aureus is associated with reduced virulence in a rabbit model of infective endocarditis. *Infect Immun* 64:4915-4921.

Takahashi, Y., K. Konishi, J.O. Cisar, and M. Yoshikawa. 2002. Identification and characterization of hsa, the gene encoding the sialic acid-binding adhesin of Streptococcus gordonii DL1. *Infect Immun* 70:1209-1218.

Takahashi, Y., A. Yajima, J.O. Cisar, and K. Konishi. 2004. Functional analysis of the Streptococcus gordonii DL1 sialic acid-binding adhesin and its essential role in bacterial binding to platelets. *Infect Immun* 72:3876-3882.

Takamatsu, D., B.A. Bensing, H. Cheng, G.A. Jarvis, I.R. Siboo, J.A. Lopez, J.M. Griffiss, and P.M. Sullam. 2005. Binding of the Streptococcus gordonii surface glycoproteins GspB and Hsa to specific carbohydrate structures on platelet membrane glycoprotein Ibalpha. *Mol Microbiol* 58:380-392.

Valeva, A., A. Weisser, B. Walker, M. Kehoe, H. Bayley, S. Bhakdi, and M. Palmer. 1996. Molecular architecture of a toxin pore: a 15-residue sequence lines the transmembrane channel of staphylococcal alpha-toxin. *EMBO J* 15:1857-1864.

Vanhoorelbeke, K., H. Ulrichts, G. Van de Walle, A. Fontayne, and H. Deckmyn. 2007. Inhibition of platelet glycoprotein Ib and its antithrombotic potential. *Curr Pharm Des* 13:2684-2697.

Varki, A. 1994. Selectin ligands. *Proc Natl Acad Sci U S A* 91:7390-7397.

Viisoreanu, D., R. Polanowska-Grabowska, S. Suttitanamongkol, T.G. Obrig, and A.R. Gear. 2000. Human platelet aggregation is not altered by Shiga toxins 1 or 2. *Thromb Res* 98:403-410.

Ward, J.R., L. Bingle, H.M. Judge, S.B. Brown, R.F. Storey, M.K. Whyte, S.K. Dower, D.J. Buttle, and I. Sabroe. 2005. Agonists of toll-like receptor (TLR)2 and TLR4 are unable to modulate platelet activation by adenosine diphosphate and platelet activating factor. *Thromb Haemost* 94:831-838.

Wu, H., M. Zeng, and P. Fives-Taylor. 2007. The glycan moieties and the N-terminal polypeptide backbone of a fimbria-associated adhesin, Fap1, play distinct roles in the biofilm development of Streptococcus parasanguinis. *Infect Immun* 75:2181-2188.

Yajima, A., Y. Takahashi, and K. Konishi. 2005. Identification of platelet receptors for the Streptococcus gordonii DL1 sialic acid-binding adhesin. *Microbiol Immunol* 49:795-800.

Youssefian, T., A. Drouin, J.M. Masse, J. Guichard, and E.M. Cramer. 2002. Host defense role of platelets: engulfment of HIV and Staphylococcus aureus occurs in a specific subcellular compartment and is enhanced by platelet activation. *Blood* 99:4021-4029.

Zahringer, U., B. Lindner, S. Inamura, H. Heine, and C. Alexander. 2008. TLR2 - promiscuous or specific? A critical re-evaluation of a receptor expressing apparent broad specificity. *Immunobiology* 213:205-224.

5

NVS and Staphylococci in the Oral Cavity – A Cause of Infective Endocarditis

Yuko Ohara-Nemoto[1], Shigenobu Kimura[2] and Takayuki K. Nemoto[1]
[1]*Department of Oral Molecular Biology, Course of Medical and Dental Sciences, Nagasaki University Graduate School of Biomedical Sciences*
[2]*Division of Molecular Microbiology, Department of Microbiology, Iwate Medical University*
Japan

1. Introduction

Oral streptococci including viridans streptococci and nutritionally-variant streptococci (NVS) along with *Staphylococcus* species including *Staphylococcus aureus* and coagulase negative staphylococci (CoNS) are two main bacterial groups known to be causative of infective endocarditis (IE). These bacteria are not pathogenic in principal for healthy individuals, and streptococci are regular commensal occupants of the oral microflora as well as the gastrointestinal tract and female genital tract. *Staphylococcus* species also comprise normal human microflora of the skin, nasal cavity, and gastrointestinal tract. The infectious routes for these pathogenic bacteria entering the bloodstream are not identified in half of examined IE patients. In addition to oral streptococci, *staphylococcus* species are generally isolated from dental plaque and saliva (Smith et al., 2001; Ohara-Nemoto et al., 2008a), thus the oral cavity is considered to be a common habitat for the two main pathogenic bacteria of IE. These findings suggest that peroral bacterial transmission to the bloodstream should be examined as a cause of IE, while systematic studies of the relationships between IE and oral conditions, such as extent of periodontal disease, dentate state (dentate, edentulous, denture wearing), and oral hygiene, are also needed to elucidate the causative role of oral bacteria. From the point of disease due to peroral bacteremia, it is of interest that a substantial part of staphylococcal arthritis is considered to originate from the oral cavity (Jackson et al., 1999). This review focuses on causative bacteria of IE that mainly colonize the oral cavity and their pathogenicity.

2. Causative bacteria of infective endocarditis

IE, an infection of the endocardium of the heart, is an uncommon but life-threatening disease with a high mortality rate ranging from 10-24% (Ferreiros et al., 2006; Yoshinaga et al., 2008; Murdoch et al., 2009). The overall incidence rate has been found to range from 4.4 to 11.6 cases per 100,000 person-years (Berlin et al., 1995; Tleyjeh et al., 2005; Fedeli et al., 2011). Cardiac valvular abnormalities that cause eddy- or jet-type vascular flow are strong risk factors (Strom et al., 1998; Nakatani et al., 2003). Abnormal vascular flow around valves causes clotting deposits, and bacteria which enter the bloodstream and become attached to clots then grow by forming biofilm. According to the most recent surveillance data (848 IE cases reported in 2000 and 2001), the characteristics of IE in Japan include mean age of 55±18 years, with most patients aged from 50 to 70 years, with 82% of IE patients complicated with underlying diseases, such as valvular heart disease (65%), congenital heart disease (9%), or particular implantation (3%), whereas in 18% cases IE occurred without any predisposing cardiac diseases (Nakatani et al., 2003). Noticeably, a route of infection was not identified in 53.9% of those cases. Also, patients with etiologically unidentified IE had no prior infectious disease causing bacteremia, such as urinary tract infection, pneumonia, or cellulitis, and no history of invasive procedure or intravenous drug administration. Thus, it is considered especially important to identify the infectious routes of etiologically unidentified IE in Japan.

The second most common etiology in Japanese IE cases was found to be post-dental procedures and oral hygiene-related conditions in those with viridans streptococci infection (35.7%). Viridans streptococci, indigenous bacteria in the oral cavity, are most frequently identified as pathogenic bacteria of IE and in Guidelines presented in 2003 by the Japanese Circulation Society it was noted that dental procedures may cause IE. This medical background in Japan may be different from Western countries, because no link between IE and dental treatment was shown in a population-based case-control study performed in the United States (Strom et al., 1998).

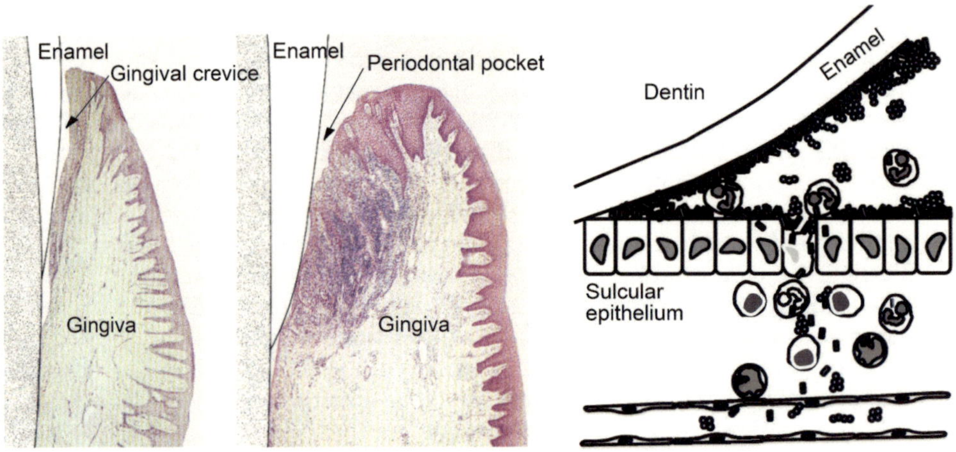

(A) (B) (C)

Fig. 1. Histological observation of (A) healthy and (B) diseased periodontal regions. (C) Scheme of dentogingival junction. The periodontal crevice is bathed in the gingival crevicular fluid. In periodontal disease, a crevice becomes a pocket. Polymorphonuclear neutrophils migrate to the crevice, and lymphocytes and monocytes are shown in a connective tissue. Oral microorganisms are expected to enter into the bloodstream through gingival sulcular epithelium and connective tissue

Until recently, viridans streptococci have been considered as the most common causative microorganisms of IE and detected at a range from 30% to 50% (Strom et al., 1998; Nakatani et al., 2003; Murdoch et al., 2004; Tleyjeh et al., 2005; Alshammary et al., 2008). Viridans streptococci are composed of a total of 21 species, including *S. mitis*, *S. anginosus*, *S. salivalius*, and *S. bovis* (Kawamura et al., 1995). Because of their non-pathogenicity in principal and phenotypical characteristic resemblance, clinical isolates of viridans streptococci obtained from patients with various diseases are usually not identified at the bacterial species level, but rather registered as '*Streptococcus viridans*' or viridans streptococci. For these, though *S. sanguinis* and *S. oralis* are considered to be the most common agents of streptococcal IE, information is limited and molecular based-species identification is needed to clarify their pathogenicity.

In addition to frequent isolation of viridans streptococci, a finding that edentulous state decreased IE risk (Strom et al., 2000) suggests that the opportunity for transmission and amount of transmitting bacteria through the dentogingival interface are functionally important issues in regard to onset of the disease (Okell et al., 1935; Carmona et al., 2002; Ohara-Nemoto et al., 2008a).

Following the incidence rate of IE by viridans streptococci, infection by *Staphylococcus aureus* is significant and ranges from 17% to 43%, while that in combination with CoNS ranges from 9% to 13%. The changing spectrum from streptococci to staphylococci has been reported in recent epidemiological studies performed in many countries (Sandre & Shafran, 1996; Hoen et al., 2002; Cecchi et al., 2004, Ferreiros et al., 2006; Alshammary et al., 2008; Fedeli et al., 2011). *S. aureus* has also been identified as a leading cause of death cases (Alshammary, et al., 2008; Yoshinaga et al., 2008). Etiologic *Staphylococcus* spp. causing IE are assumed to be acquired via a percutaneous route from skin flora, especially in nosocomial infection cases and intravenous drug abusers. However, its infectious route is often not described in cases in Japan (Niwa et al., 2005) and France (Di Filippo et al., 2006). With this in mind, it is reasonable to speculate that a part of staphylococcal IE is caused by peroral infection as in IE cases with viridans streptococci, because the occurrence of oral staphylococci is significantly higher than generally accepted. For example, the prevalence rate of *Staphylococcus* species was found to be 73% in dental plaque and 84% in saliva (Ohara-Nemoto et al., 2008a). In accordance with the existence of oral staphylococci, Etienne et al. (1986) reported cases of staphylococcal IE resulting from dental extraction.

Microorganisms are not found in approximately 15% of the IE cases in Japan, a part of which might be related to NVS, because NVS organisms scarcely grow in ordinary growth media, and require an L-cysteine or pyridoxal supplement. *Abiotrophia defectiva*, formerly *Streptococcus defectiva*, was first described as a new type of viridans group of streptococci 50 years ago (Frenkel & Hirsch, 1961). Later, according to 16S rRNA sequence findings, the genus *Abiotrophia* as well as genus *Granulicatella* was taxonomically established from NVS (Collins & Lawson, 2000). The genus *Abiotrophia* is composed of one species of *A. defectiva*, while the genus *Granulicatella* is composed of *G. adiacens* and *G. elegans*, which are isolated from humans, and *G. balaenopterae* from minke whales. Most clinical strains of NVS reported were isolated as agents of subacute IE and accounted for more than 4% of streptococcal IE (Bouvet, 1995). NVS are also constituents of the normal flora of the oral cavity and upper respiratory tract (George, 1974, Ruoff, 1991, Ohara-Nemoto et al., 1997), thus the infection route for NVS causing IE is likely peroral.

3. NVS

3.1 Occurrence and molecular identification of NVS in saliva and dental plaque specimens

NVS do not grow on Trypticase soy agar with 5% sheep blood, which can support growth of viridans streptococci, whereas they usually grow on either chocolate or Burucella agar with 5% horse blood (Ruoff, 2007), or in nutritionally rich broth supplemented with L-cysteine or pyridoxal (Fenkel & Hirsch, 1961). Furthermore, NVS generally grow well in medium from a commercially available culture bottle system for anaerobic bacteria, such as BACTEC PLUS Anaerobic/F culture bottles at 37°C under anaerobic conditions (Ohara-Nemoto et al., 2005).

To isolate NVS from oral or combined infection specimens, a culture method for monitoring the bacteriolytic activity of NVS may be useful. This activity toward *Micrococcus luteus* was demonstrated only with NVS species and not with other viridans streptococci isolated from IE cases or oral bacteria (Pompei et al., 1990). Using this method, we isolated NVS from saliva and dental plaque specimens (Ohara-Nemoto et al., 1997). Briefly, after appropriate dilutions with phosphate-buffered saline, oral specimens were inoculated onto a double-layer nutrient agar plate with a top layer containing heat-killed *M. luteus* ATCC 9341 and cultured overnight. Use of an anaerobic condition raised the growth rate of NVS as compared with the aerobic condition. Isolates exhibiting bacteriolytic activity, shown as a colony surrounded with a clear halo, were NVS. These isolates also demonstrated satellitism with a streak of *S. aureus* on a Todd-Hewitt agar plate. For species identification, molecular based methods, i.e., 16S rRNA sequencing or 16S rRNA PCR followed by restriction fragment length polymorphism analysis (PCR-RFLP) (Ohara-Nemoto et al., 1997; Ohara-Nemoto et al., 2005), were successfully applied. When 92 oral NVS strains were examined, the PCR-RFLP patterns of *G. adiacens* and *A. defectiva* were readily distinguished from each other, as well as from those of other streptococcal and enterococcal species (Fig. 2).

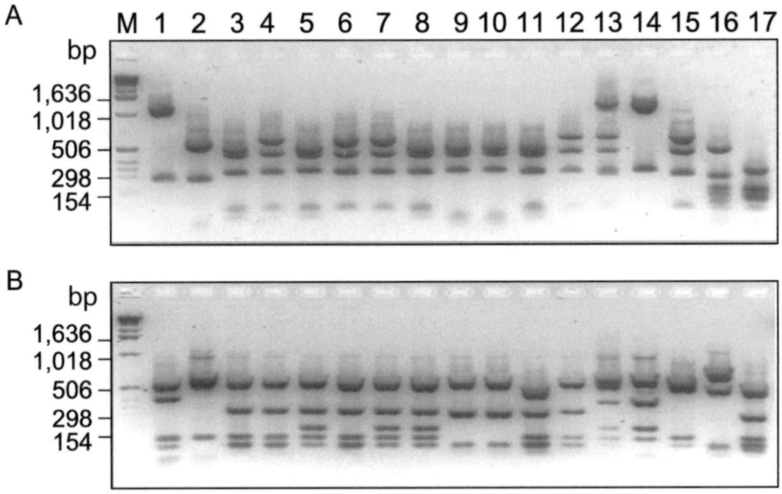

Fig. 2. 16S rDNA PCR-RFLP of *G. adiacens, A. defectiva*, and viridans streptococci. The 16S rRNA gene (1.5 kb) was amplified by PCR using a set of universal primers for eubacteria, then cleaved with (A) *Hae*III or (B) *Msp*I. Lanes: M, size marker; 1, *G. adiacens;* 2, *A. defectiva;* 3, *sanguinis;* 4, *S. oralis;* 5, *S. gordonii;* 6, *S. mitis;* 7, *S. salivarius;* 8, *S. bovis;* 9, *S. mutans;* 10, *S. sobrinus;* 11, *S. pyogenes;* 12, *S. pneumoniae;* 13, *S. aureus;* 14, *S. epidermidis;* 15, *Enterococcus faecalis;* 16, *Haemophilus influenzae;* 17, *Escherichia coli*

Species identification performed by PCR-RFLP completely matched that obtained by phenotypic characteristics. Consequently, it was found that the occurrence of NVS in dental plaque and saliva specimens from healthy dental students was relatively high, as 97.8%

(91/93) of the subjects harbored either one of the two bacterial species. In addition, the prevalence of *G. adiacens* was 87.1% and that of *A. defectiva* was 11.8%, which were comparable or even higher than those of viridans streptococci (Kimura & Ohara-Nemoto, 2007). Interestingly, except for one subject carrying both species, all carried only one, suggesting that these two species may be incompatible with each other.

Recently, Shimoyama et al. (2011) developed a rapid and highly sensitive 16S rRNA PCR identification method for NVS using species-specific sets of primers. With this method, *G. adiacens* (including *G. para-adjacens*) was detected in most healthy adult subjects, followed by *A. defectiva* and *G. elegans* (unpublished results). The high level of occurrence of NVS in the oral cavity demonstrated by this and previous reports (Ohara-Nemoto et al., 1997; Sato et al., 1999) is in good agreement with recent results of normal oral flora examined from 5 subjects ranging in age from 23 to 55 years old (Aas et al., 2005). A culture-independent 16S rRNA gene cloning and sequencing method demonstrated that *S. mitis* and related species were most commonly found in all sites of the oral cavity, followed by the two *Granulicatella* species. *G. adiacens* and *G. elegans* were commonly detected in most areas, such as the buccal, vestibule, tongue dorsum, tongue lateral, hard palate, soft palate, tonsils, tooth surface, and subgingival sites in a wide range of ages. Although the detection rate of *A. defectiva* was somewhat lower than that of *Granulicatella* species, this bacterium was also among the top 21 of commonly observed bacteria of 141 predominant species in the oral cavity. Therefore, with the high occurrence of NVS in the oral cavity in mind, a relatively high incidence of NVS-related IE (more than 4% of streptococcal IE) may be reasonable. Elucidation of the prevalence rates and amounts of NVS in the oral cavity, especially in elderly subjects whose incidence rate for IE is remarkably high, may contribute to better understanding of the pathological process of NVS-related IE. Non-culture methods targeting 16S rRNA (Goldenberger et al., 1997; Shimoyama et al., 2011) are convenient and practical for this purpose.

3.2 Cases of IE caused by NVS

Most clinical NVS isolates reported were derived from culturing blood obtained from IE patients and up to 100 cases of NVS IE have been presented to date. We treated an IE case with severe mitral and aortic valves insufficiencies caused by *G. elegans* derived from the oral cavity (Ohara-Nemoto et al., 2005). A 53-year-old previously healthy female without anamnesis had undergone a dental procedure at a local clinic two months before consulting with us. The patient had a slight fever and cough, and was diagnosed with chronic heart failure and transferred to an outside facility, where IE associated with aortic and mitral valve vegetation was noted in echocardiography findings. Four consecutive arterial and venous blood cultures were successively performed at other and our facilities with BACTEK PLUS Anaerobic/F culture bottles and Brucella HK agar plates under anaerobic conditions. Two sets of cultures were positive and yielded gram-positive coccoides in short chains. At our hospital, the patient received antibiotic treatment with intravenous benzylpenicillin (1.2 million units per day) and gentamicin (60 mg per day), then cardiac surgery was performed 7 days after admission. The left coronary cups of the aortic valve showed perforation and ulceration with multiple vegetation sites, and the mitral valve anterior leaflets were perforated with large amounts of vegetation. The patient was released from the hospital without a fever after 27 days.

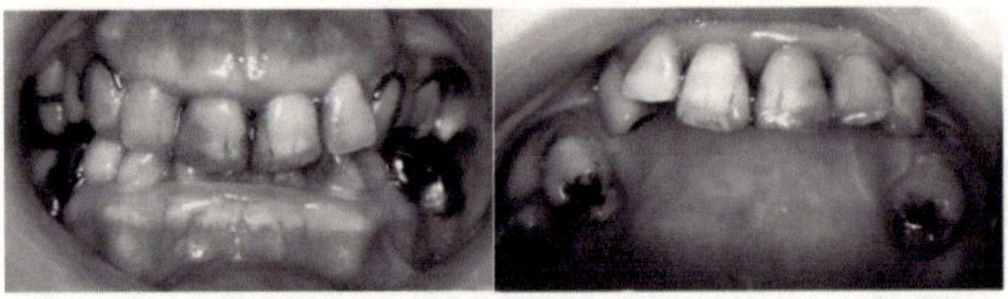

Fig. 3. Oral findings of a patient with IE caused by *G. elegans*. Dental plaque was collected from right upper |34 (Ohara-Nemoto et al., 2005)

Bacterial isolates from the patient were identified as *G. elegans* (IMU02b01) by microbiological characteristics and 16S rRNA gene sequencing. An oral examination of the patient one week after surgery showed widespread redness of the gingiva, dental caries, and deposition of a large amount of dental plaque (Fig. 3). The oral state of the patient suggested a risk of bacteremia due to increased dentogingival surface area, with oral *G. elegans* the suspected agent in this case.

Characteristic	Result for *G. elegans* strain[a]:		
	IMU02b01	IMU02p18	CCUG 26024
Enzyme production	+	+	+
Pyrrolidonyl aminopeptidase	-	-	-
Alkaline phosphatase	-	-	-
Urease	+	+	+
Arginine dihydrolase	-	-	-
α-Galactosidase	-	-	-
β-Galactosidase	-	-	-
β-Glucuronidase	+	+	+
α-Glucosidase	-	-	-
β-Glucosidase	+	+	+
Hippurate hydrolysis	-	-	-
Acetoin production	-	-	-
Acidification of:			
Trehalose	-	-	-
Lactose	-	-	-
Raffinose	-	-	-
Sucrose	+	+	+
Melibiose	-	-	-
Arabinose	-	-	-
Sorbitol	-	-	-
Mannitol	-	-	-
Growth in THB supplemented with:			
L-Cysteine HCL (0.01%)	+	+	+
Pyridoxal HCL (0.001%)	-	-	-

[a] +, positive result; -, negative result

Table 1. Biochemical characteristics of blood- and oral cavity-derived *G. elegans* isolates from an IE patient

To confirm our speculation, a *G. elegans* strain was isolated from a dental plaque specimen obtained from the patient using a selective culture method. As a result, strain IMU03p18 was obtained, which exhibited the same basic phenotypic characteristics as strains IMU02b01 and *G. elegans* CCUG 26024 (Table 1) (Roggenkamp et al., 1998). Among these characteristics, urease production, acidification of raffinose and sucrose, and hydrolysis of hippurate have been reported to be strain dependent (Roggenkamp et al., 1998; Sato et al., 1999; Collins et al., 2000).

We found that both IMU02p18 and IMU02b01 were negative for urease, positive for hippurate hydrolysis, and fermented sucrose but not raffinose. In addition, their antimicrobial susceptibility tendencies were identical, as they were highly susceptible to penicillin and other β-lactams, whereas they were intermediate to amikacin and resistant to arbekacin (Table 2). These properties were in accordance with other *G. elegans* isolates from IE patients (Ruoff, 1991; Tuohy et al., 2000). In accordance with observed in vitro antibiotic susceptibility, combination treatment with benzylpenicillin and gentamicin was effective in this case. Pulsed-field gel electrophoresis (PFGE) and arbitrarily primed PCR also demonstrated that the genotypes of the two strains isolated from blood and dental plaque samples obtained from the patient were indistinguishable from each other (Fig. 4). These phenotypical and molecular-based characteristics clearly indicated that they were derived from an identical clone. Thus, our findings suggested peroral infection of *G. elegans* in this case of IE.

Agent	MIC (μg/ml) [a]		
	IMU02b01	IMU02p18	CCUG 26024
Penicillin	≤0.06	≤0.06	≤0.06
Ampicillin	≤0.25	≤0.25	≤0.25
Cefazolin	≤0.5	≤0.5	≤0.5
Ceftazidime	≤0.5	≤0.5	≤0.5
Cefozopran	≤0.5	≤0.5	≤0.5
Cefdinir	≤0.12	≤0.12	≤0.12
Cefepime	≤0.12	≤0.12	≤0.12
Imipenem	≤0.12	≤0.12	≤0.12
Gentamicin	≤4	≤4	≤4
Amikacin	32	32	≤16
Arbekacin	>16	>16	≤4
Erythromycin	≤0.25	≤0.25	≤0.25
Clarithromycin	≤0.25	≤0.25	≤0.25
Clindamycin	≤0.25	≤0.25	≤0.25
Minocycline	≤2	≤2	≤2
Vancomycin	1	1	≤0.5
Teicoplanin	≤1	≤1	≤1
Fosfomycin	16	16	16
Levofloxacin	≤2	≤2	≤2
Sulfamethoxazole-Trimethoprim	40	40	40

Table 2. Antimicrobial susceptibility of blood- and oral cavity-derived *G. elegans* isolated from an IE patient. [a]MICs were determined using a micro-dilution method developed by the National Committee for Clinical Laboratory Standards

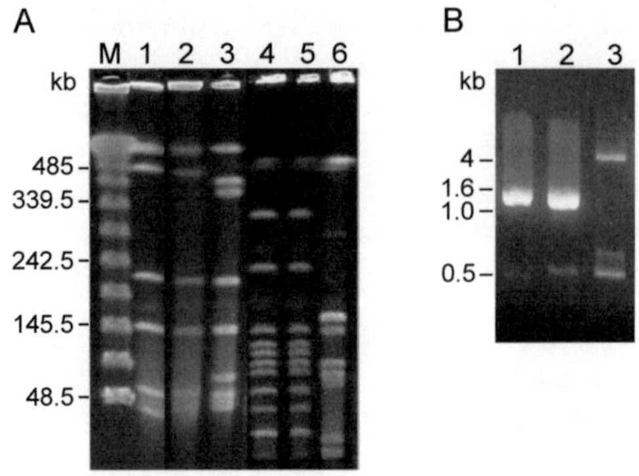

Fig. 4. Molecular based identification of *G. elegans* isolates from blood culture and dental plaque of the IE patient. (A) PFGE was performed after digestion with *Sma*I (lanes 1 to 3) and *Apa*I (lanes 4 to 6). Lanes: M, DNA markers; 1 and 4, IMU02b01; 2 and 5, IMU02p18; 3 and 6, *G. elegans* CCUG 26024. (B) Arbitrarily primed-PCR. Lanes: 1, IMU02b01; 2, IMU02p18; 3, *G. elegans* CCUG 26024

4. Staphylococci

4.1 Occurrence of staphylococci in the oral cavity

Staphylococcus species involving *S. aureus* are considered to be transient bacteria in the oral cavity and the amounts of these organisms in oral specimens (10^2-10^4 cfu/ml in saliva, 10^3-10^5 cfu/g in dental plaque) are quite low as compared to those of viridans streptococci (10^4-10^6 cfu/ml in saliva, 10^7-10^9 cfu/g in dental plaque). However, it is evident that *Staphylococcus* species, especially *S. epidermidis* and *S. aureus*, are frequently isolated from the oral cavity (Reviewed by Smith et al., 2001; El-Solh et al., 2004; Murdoch et al., 2004; Ohara-Nemoto et al., 2008a). Interestingly, oral staphylococcal possession in adults aged from 20 to over 80 years old ranges from 60% to 88%, with the highest prevalence (88% in saliva) observed with elderly subjects aged from 60 to 79 years (Percival et al., 1991). Furthermore, the prevalence of staphylococci at sites of periodontal disease (59%) was found to be significantly higher than that of healthy subgingival sites: 54% in diseased sites and 29% in periodontally healthy control sites (Murdoch et al., 2004).

In addition to dental interest, oral staphylococci have been suggested to be an infectious source of rheumatoid arthritis. Staphylococci are the most common causes of bacterial arthritis in adults, among which *S. aureus* is the primary agent (Goldenberg, 1998; Ryan et al., 1997). Similar to etiologically unidentified cases of IE, etiological sources are not identified in up to 30% of bacterial arthritis cases (Kaandorp et al., 1997). Thus, it is speculated that oral microflora plays a role in the reservoir of agents related to staphylococcal arthritis. According to the report by Jackson et al. (1999), the occurrence of oral staphylococci was 94% in healthy adults (mean 32 years old) and that in healthy elderly subjects (mean 82 years old) was 100%, with 36% of those elderly subjects found to be colonized by *S. aureus*. Furthermore, in rheumatoid arthritis patients (mean 60 years old), staphylococci were isolated from 96% and the proportion of subjects with oral *S. aureus* was 56%, which was significantly higher than that of the healthy subjects (24%). Jacobson et al. (1997) also demonstrated a higher prevalence of *S. aureus* isolated from the oral cavity of patients with rheumatoid arthritis. These findings are of particular interest when considering cases of etiologically unidentified staphylococcal IE.

Our previous study of the occurrence of oral staphylococci also aimed to identify a potential peroral route of staphylococcal IE (Ohara-Nemoto et al., 2008a). *Staphylococcus species* were isolated from saliva and supragingival dental plaque specimens obtained from systemically and dentally healthy adults (n=56, mean 27.1±5.3 years old) using a culture method. Consequently, along with 99 *S. aureus* isolates and 235 isolates of *S. intermedius* and CoNS species, at least 9 of 15 *Staphylococcus* species known to colonize in humans were observed in the oral cavity (Table 3). The isolation frequencies of staphylococci were 83.9% in saliva and 73.2% in dental plaque. Furthermore, *S. epidermidis* (60.7%) and *S. aureus* (46.4%) were the species most frequently isolated from plaque and saliva, respectively, followed in order by *S. hominis, S. warneri, S. intermedius, S. capitis,* and *S. haemolyticus* (12.5-7.1%) from both locations. In contrast, *S. gallinarum* and *S. lugdunensis* were rarely isolated (1/56, 1.8% of all cases) (Table 3). The prevalence tendency of oral staphylococci was similar to that of specimens obtained from the nasal cavity. Staphylococci-positive subjects (n=47) harbored from 1 to 5 species (mean 2.3±1.0) (a portion of those results is shown in Table 4). In addition to *S. aureus* and *S. epidermidis, S. capitis, S. hominis, S. lugdunensis,* and *S. warneri* have been implicated in IE.

Species	No. of positive subjects (% isolation frequency)		
	Saliva[a]	Plaque[a]	Nasal swab[b]
S. aureus	26 (46.4)	19 (33.9)	8 (44.4)
S. capitis	5 (8.9)	5 (8.9)	3 (16.7)
S. epidermidis	23 (41.1)	34 (60.7)	13 (72.2)
S. gallinarum	1 (1.8)	0 (0)	0 (0)
S. haemolyticus	4 (7.1)	3 (5.4)	1 (5.6)
S. hominis	7 (12.5)	7 (12.5)	4 (22.2)
S. intermedius	5 (8.9)	5 (8.9)	1 (5.6)
S. lugdunensis	1 (1.8)	0 (0)	0 (0)
S. warneri	6 (10.7)	5 (8.9)	3 (16.7)
Total staphylococci	47 (83.9)	41 (73.2)	17 (94.4)

Table 3. Occurrence of staphylococci in saliva, dental plaque, and nasal samples. [a]None of the subjects had received antibiotic medication within the previous 3 months (n=56, aged 22-43 years old, 27.1±5.3 years; 37 males, 19 females). [b]Nasal swab samples were taken from 18 (32.7±2.6 years: 12 males, 6 females) of 47 oral staphylococci-positive subjects

The genetic relatedness of these staphylococcal isolates was examined by PFGE and the results revealed nasal-oral trafficking of *Staphylococcus* species (Fig. 5), as PFGE patterns indicated that clinical staphylococcal isolates from each subject were identical clones or close relatives. Furthermore, a longitudinal examination over a 2-month period demonstrated that a single identical or same combination of *Staphylococcus* species was continuously isolated. Thus, *Staphylococcus* species found in the oral cavity are regular residential composers of oral microflora or may be continuously provided from the nasal cavity.

Subject no.	Saliva	Plaque	Nasal
1	***S. aureus***	***S. aureus***	***S. aureus***, *S. epidermidis*, *S. hominis*
2	***S. aureus***, *S. epidermidis*, *S. hominis*	***S. aureus***, *S. epidermidis*, *S. hominis*	***S. aureus***
3	***S. aureus***, *S. intermedius*	***S. aureus***	***S. aureus***, *S. warneri*
4	***S. aureus***, *S. warneri*	***S. aureus***, ***S. epidermidis***	***S. aureus***, *S. capitis*, ***S. epidermidis***
5	***S. aureus***, ***S. epidermidis***	*S. intermedius*	***S. aureus***, ***S. epidermidis***
6	***S. epidermidis***	***S. aureus***, ***S. epidermidis***	***S. aureus***, ***S. epidermidis***, *S. hominis*
7	*S. aureus*, ***S. epidermidis***	***S. epidermidis***	***S. epidermidis***
8	***S. epidermidis***	***S. epidermidis***	***S. epidermidis***
9	***S. epidermidis***	***S. epidermidis***, *S. capitis*, *S. haemolyticus*	***S. epidermidis***
10	***S. epidermidis***, *S. hominis*, *S. warneri*	***S. epidermidis***, *S. intermedius*	***S. epidermidis***, *S. capitis*, *S. hominis*
11	*S. aureus*, ***S. lugdunensis***	*S. aureus*, ***S. epidermidis***, *S. warneri*	***S. epidermidis***, ***S. lugdunensis***
12	*S. aureus*, *S. warneri*	***S. epidermidis***	***S. epidermidis***
13	*S. capitis*	***S. hominis***	***S. hominis***, *S. warneri*
14	*S. epidermidis*	*S. epidermidis*	*S. capitis*, *S. hominis*
15	*S. capitis*	ND	*S. aureus*, *S. epidermidis*, *S. warneri*
16	*S. epidermidis*	*S. epidermidis*	ND
17	*S. intermedius*, *S. warneri*	*S. warneri*	*S. aureus*, *S. epidermidis*
18	*S. intermedius*	ND	*S. epidermidis*

Table 4. Staphylococcal species isolated from oral and nasal cavities. Genetic relatedness of the isolates in bold was confirmed by PFGE. ND, not detected

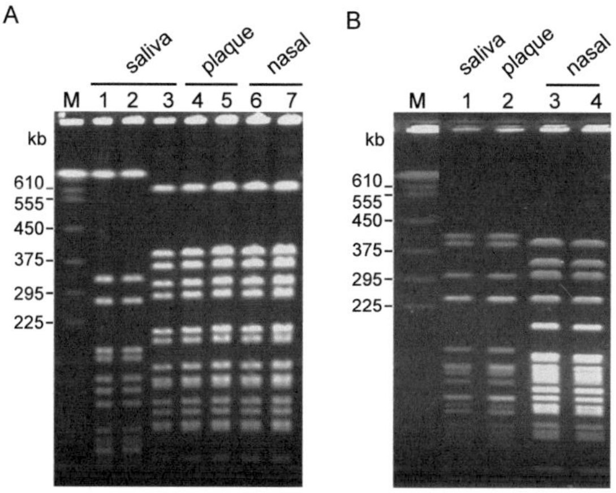

Fig. 5. Genetic relatedness of oral and nasal *S. aureus* (A) or *S. epidermidis* (B) isolates obtained from subjects No. 1 and No. 7 in Table 4, respectively Chromosomal DNA of isolates from oral and nasal specimens was digested with *Sma*I, then separated using PFGE. The relative coefficients of the strains examined were 100% (A, lanes 3-7) and 82.7% (B, lanes 1-4)

Although the composition and proportions of oral microflora in adults are rather stable over long periods, it is notable that occurrence rates of staphylococci, mainly *S. aureus*, tend to increase with age, which is possibly associated with xerostomia (decrease in saliva flow) and denture wearing. The occurrence of staphylococci (88%) was found to be significantly high in denture plaque (Marsh & Martin, 2009), presumably because of their capability of adherence to prosthetic materials. Similarly, *S. aureus* and *S. epidermidis* are the most common pathogens isolated from disease sites of late prosthetic joint infections (Maderazo et al., 1988). On the other hand, the occurrence rates of *S. mutans* and other viridans streptococci are consistent over time after tooth eruption (Percival et al., 1991). This event may be explained by the finding that *S. mutans* colonizes the tongue coat of elderly individuals after loss of teeth, while the prevalence of *Porphyromonas gingivalis*, a major agent of chronic periodontitis, was shown to be closely related to the presence of teeth with periodontal pockets (Kishi et al., 2010). Therefore, when considering that IE as well as rheumatoid arthritis is age-related disease, we speculate that microflora of dental plaque and possibly denture plaque serve to harbor *Staphylococcus* species that cause these diseases. Oral staphylococci are more important for high-risk IE subjects when they are dentate (presence of dentogingival interface) and have poor oral hygiene. Furthermore, periodontal diseases may increase the risk of staphylococcal bacteremia due to increases in dentogingival surface area and bacterial numbers of *S. aureus*. Notably, a recent study also reported a correlation between staphylococci from the oral cavity and developments of atherosclerosis and cardiovascular diseases (Koren et al., 2011).

4.2 Pathogenicity factors of staphylococci

4.2.1 Biofilm formation

A biofilm is a multi-layered membranous aggregate of microorganisms attached to a biotic or abiotic surface. Oral bacteria that colonize on tooth surfaces and soft epithelial tissues are considered to grow primarily based on their ability to form biofilm, as this attachment system is necessary to prevent evacuation by host swallowing. *Staphylococcus* and *Streptococcus* species including NVS form biofilms. For all these except *S. aureus*, which produces potent virulence factors, their ability of biofilm formation plays a role as a major virulence factor of IE. Biofilm components include self-produced polymeric matrix and adhesins, which mediate the primary attachment of bacteria to endocardium and heart valve surfaces, followed by intercellular adhesion. Bacteria in biofilm resist host defenses and antibiotic treatment. Numerous studies have demonstrated that biofilms consist of 4 principal factors; teichoic acids, polysaccharide intercellular adhesins such as PIA from *S. epidermidis* or PNAG from *S. aureus*, extracellular DNA (ecDNA), and proteinaceous adhesins.

Teichoic acid is a cell wall component of gram-positive bacteria, and recently found to be an essential constituent of staphylococcal biofilms (Gross et al., 2001; Sadovskaya et al., 2005). Cell wall and extracellular teichoic acids are a mixture of two kinds of polymers, $\alpha(1\rightarrow5)$-linked poly(ribitol phosphate), substituted at the 4-position of ribitol residues with β-GlucNAc, and $(1\rightarrow3)$-linked poly(glycerol phosphate), partially substituted with D-Ala at the 2-position of glycerol residue (Vinogradov et al., 2006). Since a large fraction of teichoic acid is located in the 'fluffy'-layer region beyond the cell wall, it is considered that it functions in primary adhesion of bacteria to attached surfaces.

The glucosamine-based extracellular polysaccharides PIA and PNAG (PIA/PNAG) is an identical chemical compound, poly-β(1,6)-*N*-acetyl-D-glucosamine, which is responsible for cell-cell attachment (Mack et al., 1996; Cramton et al., 1999). PIA/PNAG is synthesized by enzymes encoded by the *icaADBC* (intercellular adhesin) operon (Heilmann et al., 1996; Götz, 2002) and *icaADBC* mutants of *S. epidermidis* RP62A were shown not to form biofilm (Gerke et al., 1998). However, it has also been demonstrated with many clinical isolates that PIA/PNAG-negative *S. epidermidis* and *S. aureus* exhibit a strong biofilm phenotype (Rohde et al., 2007; Hennig et al., 2007; Boles et al., 2010). Rohde et al. (2007) reported that 27% of biofilm-positive *S. epidermidis* isolates produced PIA-independent biofilms, some of which were possibly mediated by the proteinaceous adhesin Aap, an accumulation-associated protein (Hussain et al., 1997). In addition, other proteins, such as the cell wall lytic enzyme AtlE (Heilmann et al., 1996), biofilm-associated protein Bap (Cucarella et al., 2001), and others are involved in attachment to the polymer surface or host matrix proteins, and related to cell-cell adhesion (Frank & Patel, 2007; Otto, 2009).

It was recently shown that AtlE is responsible for autolysis of *S. epidermidis*, resulting in release of ecDNA, and that ecDNA is a structural component of biofilms formed by *S. epidermidis* and *S. aureus* (Qin et al., 2007; Rice et al., 2007). The ratios of these 3 factors, PIA/PNAG, proteinous, and ecDNA, in biofilm formation seem to be varied for each strain, and become altered by various environmental or culture conditions. The ratios were conveniently semi-quantified *in vitro* by measuring amounts of biofilms formed on polymeric surfaces after incubation with or without dispersin B, trypsin, and DNaseI (Izano et al., 2008). We observed that production of the major extracellular protease GluSE was enhanced under specific culture conditions that also increased biofilm formation (Fig. 6) (Ohara-Nemoto et al., 2002). This observation is quite interesting with considering the relationship to a recent finding that protein-dependent biofilm formation by *S. aureus* was inhibited by expressions of extracellular proteases (Martí et al., 2010). The involvement of proteases in staphylococcal and streptococcal biofilm formation remains to be clarified.

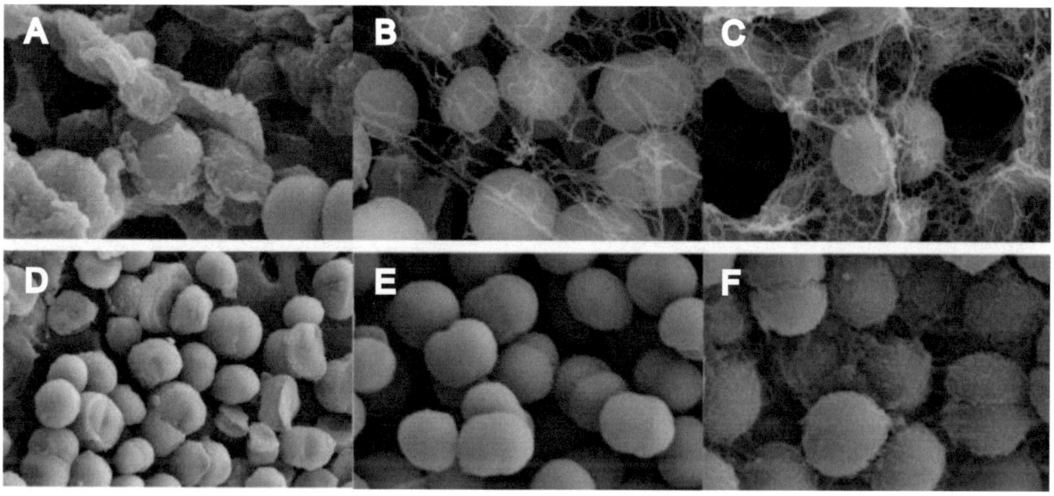

Fig. 6. Culture condition-dependent biofilm formation by *S. epidermidis*. Scanning electron micrographs of 'biofilm-negative' *S. epidermidis* ATCC 12228 (A and D) and 14990 (B and E), and 'biofilm-positive' ATCC 35984 (C and F). Bacteria were cultured in Todd-Hewitt broth (THB) agar (A-C) or THB (D-F). Biofilm formation was clearly demonstrated with strains 12228 and 14990 cultured on THB agar, while it was not evident when these were cultured in THB

4.2.2 Staphylococcal glutamic acid-specific protease

Glutamic acid-specific staphylococcal GluV8-family proteases belong to a serine protease family that possesses a catalytic triad composed of Ser, Asp, and His, forming a competent electron relay. GluV8 from *S. aureus*, first reported by Drapeau et al. (1972) as V8 protease, is related to its bacterial growth *in vivo* and pathogenicity (Coulter et al., 1998). GluV8 processes adhesion molecules that are expressed on the bacterial cell surface and destroy the extracellular matrix of host cells (Karlsson & Arvidson, 2002). GluSE was found as an *S. epidermidis* GluV8 homolog, which is the most abundant extracellular protein (Sasaki et al., 1998), and efficiently degrades host proteins such as elastin, fibronectin, collagen, complement protein C5, and immunoglobulin (Dubin et al., 2001; Moon et al., 2001; Ohara-Nemoto et al., 2002). The gene encoding GluSE is ubiquitously distributed on the chromosome and the protein is expressed in most clinical isolates under *in vitro* culture conditions (Fig. 7). Production frequency was comparable between isolates from patients suffering from IE,

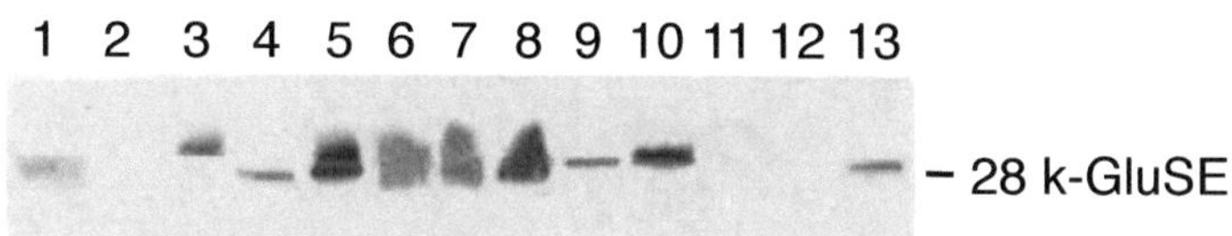

Fig. 7. GluSE production in *S. epidermidis* clinical isolates. Extracellular soluble fractions were subjected to SDS-polyacrylamide gel electrophoresis, followed by immunoblotting with anti-GluSE Ig. Lanes 1-6, isolates from patients: lanes 7-12, isolates from saliva of healthy individuals: 13, purified GluSE

bacteremia, and wound infection (7/10, 70%), as well as in saliva from healthy subjects (44/59, 74.6%) (Ikeda et al., 2004).

As demonstrated by 2D-PAGE followed by protein identification with MALDI TOF-MS and immunoblotting, 28-kDa mature GluSE was observed as the major extracellular protein constituent (Fig. 8A), while another Glu-specific cysteine proteinase, Ecp, was moderately expressed (Ohara-Nemoto et al., 2008b). In a cell wall fraction, limited amounts of 32-, 30-, and 29-kDa proforms of GluSE were observed (Fig. 8B and C), whereas no pro- or matureforms of GluSE were detected in bacterial cytoplasm. These findings indicated that GluSE is immediately secreted after protein synthesis and maturation through cleavage at the Ser_{-1}-Val_1 bond.

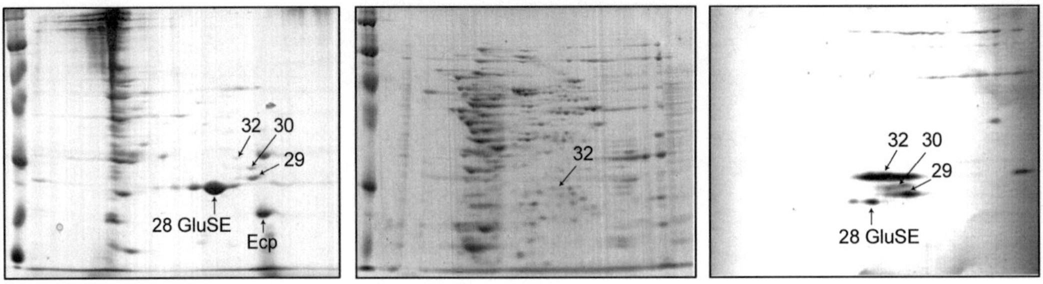

(A) (B) (C)

Fig. 8. 2D-PAGE shows GluSE in extracellular and cell wall fractions. The extracellular fraction of *S. epidermidis* (A) and cell wall fractions (B and C) were separated by 2D-PAGE, and developed with Coomassie brilliant blue staining (A and B) or immunoblotting with anti-GluSE Ig (C). Numbers indicate relative molecular weights (kDa)

Genes encoding GluV8 homologs were recently cloned from other CoNS species, and their proteolytic activities and biochemical characteristics were determined (Nemoto et al., 2008; Ono et al., 2010): They are GluSW from *S. warneri*, GluScp from *S. caprae*, and GluScoh from *S. cohnii*, and the order of specific activity was found to be GluV8>>GluScp>GluSW>GluSE. These GluV8 family proteases may be associated with the survival and spreading of bacteria *in vivo* by cleavage of proteinous molecules involved in host defense. GluV8 degrades α_1-protease inhibitor, which is the major inhibitor of elastase. Inactivation of α_1-protease inhibitor then causes activation of elastase released from activated neutrophilic granulocytes, resulting in damage to host tissues (Arvidson, 2006).

In a comparison of amino acid sequence and proteolytic activity, the following essential amino acid residues in the GluV8-protease family were determined. Val_1 is required to exert proper maturation mediated by cleavage between the Xaa-Val bond and for proteolytic activity itself, with Trp_{185}, Val_{188} and Pro_{189} also involved in proteolytic activity (Fig. 9) (Nemoto et al., 2009). The K_m value of native GluSE harboring a combination of $Tyr_{185}Val_{188}Asp_{189}$ was larger than that of GluV8 with $Trp_{185}Val_{188}Pro_{189}$. Amino acid substitutions in these three residues decreased K_m with a constant k_{cat} value (Table 5). These residues can be involved in substrate affinity, which implicates the mechanism of alteration in proteolytic activity among the members of this family.

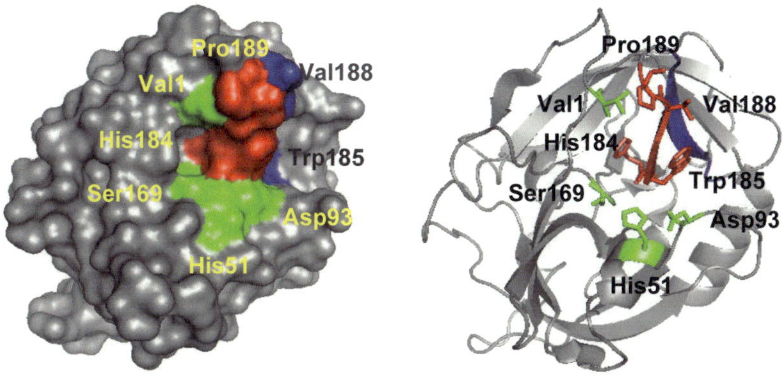

Fig. 9. Amino acid residues involved in proteolytic activity of GluV8 are shown in a three-dimensional structure. The catalytic triad and Val_1 are shown in green, and His_{184} to Pro_{189} and Glu_{191} to Phe_{198}, which form an anti-parallel β-sheet, are shown in red and blue, respectively

Protease	K_m (mM)	k_{cat} (s^{-1})
GluV8 ($W_{185}V_{188}P_{189}$)	0.30±0.08	6147±1117
GluSE ($W_{185}V_{188}P_{189}$)	0.35±0.13	7695±1200
GluSE ($W_{185}V_{188}D_{189}$)	2.84±1.49	8863±1765
GluSE ($Y_{185}V_{188}P_{189}$)	4.15±1.58	7681±3069
GluSE ($W_{185}A_{188}P_{189}$)	1.32±0.10	9059±4205

Table 5. Kinetic parameters of recombinant GluV8 and GluSE with amino acid substitutions at positions 185, 188, and 189

Recently, Iwase et al. (2010) reported that biofilm formation by *S. aureus* was inhibited by GluSE, which also destroyed pre-existing *S. aureus* biofilms. Accordingly, GluSE enhanced the susceptibility of *S. aureus* colonizing the nasal cavity to host immune system components. These observations suggest the existence of bacterial interference among *Staphylococcus* species mediated by GluV8-family proteases in normal microflora. At present, the molecular mechanism remains unclear. It is not easy to speculate how bacterial proteases harbouring the same substrate specificity degrade opponent factors without affecting the corresponding self-factors. Therefore, investigations on the production regulation of GluV8-family proteases and their target molecules are important. Production of GluV8 together with other virulence factors, such as hemolysins and toxins, is regulated by the well-studied system of the accessory gene regulator (*arg*) locus (Ji et al., 1997; Novick 2003). Recent reports have raised the possibility that the *arg* system as well as GluV8 or other extracellular proteases is involved in biofilm detachment (Yarwood et al., 2004; Boles & Horswill, 2008; Martí et al., 2010). Thus, regulation of the biosynthesis of proteinous factors, especially GluV8-family proteases in *Staphylococcus* species, and their relationship with bacterial interference must be elucidated to better understand the molecular mechanism of onset of staphylococcal IE.

5. Acknowledgments

This research was supported by grants-in-aid for scientific research from the Ministry of Education, Science, Sports, and Culture of Japan.

6. References

Aas, J. A., Paster, B. J., Stokes, L. N., Olsen, I. & Dewhirst, F. E. (2005) Defining the normal bacterial flora of the oral cavity. *J. Clin. Microbiol.* vol. 43, pp. 5721-5732, 0095-1137

Alshammary, A., Hervas-Malo, M. & Robinson, J. L. (2008) Pediatric infective endocarditis: Has *Staphylococcus aureus* overtaken viridans group streptococci as the predominant etiological agent? *Can. J. Infect. Des. Med. Microbiol.* vol. 19, pp. 63-68, 1712-9532

Arvidson, S. (2006) Extracellular enzymes, *In*: *Gram-positive pathogens* (2nd ed.), Eds. Fischetti, V. A., Novick, R. P., Ferretti, J. J., Portnoy, D. A. & Rood, J. I., pp. 478-485, ASM Press, 1-55581-343-7, Washington, D.C.

Berlin, J.A., Abrutyn, E., Strom, B.L., Kinman, J.L., Levison, M.E., Korzeniowski, O.M., Feldman, R.S., Kaye, D. (1995) Incidence of infective endocarditis in the Delaware Valley, 1988-1990. *Am. J. Cardiol.* vol. 76, pp. 933-936, 0002-9149

Boles, B. R. & Horswill, A. R. (2008) *agr*-Mediated dispersal of *Staphylococcus aureus* biofilms. *PLoS Pathog.* vol. 4, e1000052, 1553-7366

Boles, B. R., Thoendel, M., Roth, A. J. & Horswill, A. R. (2010) Identification of genes involved in polysaccharide-independent *Staphylococcus aureus* biofilm formation. *PLoS One* vol. 5, e10146, 1932-6203

Bouvet, A. (1995) Human endocarditis due to nutritionally variant streptococci: *Streptococcus adjacens* and *Streptococcus defectivus*. *Eur. Heart J.* vol. 16, Suppl B, pp. 24-27, 0195-668x

Carmona, I. T., Dios, P. D., Posse, J. L., Quintela, A. G., Vázquez, C. M. & Iglesias A. C. (2002) An update on infective endocarditis of dental origin. *J. Dent.* vol. 30, 37-40, 0300-5712

Cecchi, E., Forno, D., Imazio, M., Migliardi, A., Gnavi, R., Dal Conte, I., Trinchero, R.; Piemonte Infective Endocarditis Study Group. (2004) New trends in the epidemiological and clinical features of infective endocarditis: results of a multicenter prospective study. *Ital. Heart J.* vol. 5, pp. 249-256, 1129-4728

Collins, M. D. & Lawson, P. A. (2000) The genus *Abiotrophia* (Kawamura *et al.*) is not monophyletic: proposal of *Granulicatella* gen. nov., *Granulicatella adiacens* comb. nov. and *Granulicatella balaenopterae* comb. nov. *Int. J. Syst. Evol. Microbiol.* vol. 50, pp. 365-369, 1466-5026

Coulter, S. N., Schwan, W. R., Ng, E. Y. W., Langhorne, M. H., Ritchie, H. D., Westbrock-Wadman, S., Hufnagle, W. O., Folger, K. R., Bayer, A. S. & Stover, C. K. (1998) *Staphylococcus aureus* genetic loci impacting growth and survival in multiple infection environment. *Mol. Microbiol.* vol. 30, pp.393-404, 0950-382x

Cramton, S. E., Gerke, C., Schnell, N. F., Nichols, W. W. & Götz, F. (1999) The intercellular adhesion (*ica*) locus is present in *Staphylococcus aureus* and is required for biofilm formation. *Infect. Immun.* vol. 67, pp. 5427-5433, 0019-9567

Cucarella, C., Solano, C., Valle, J., Amorena, B., Lasa, Í. & Penadés, J. R. (2001) Bap, a *Staphylococcus aureus* surface protein involved in biofilm formation. *J. Bacteriol.* vol. 183, pp. 2888–2896, 0021-9193

Di Filippo, S., Delahaye, F., Semiond, B., Celard, M., Henaine, R., Ninet, J., Sassolas, F. & Bozio, A. (2006) Current patterns of infective endocarditis in congenital heart disease. *Heart* vol. 92, pp. 1490-1495, 1355-6037

Drapeau, G. R., Boily, Y. & Houmard, J. (1972) Purification and properties of an extracellular protease of *Staphylococcus aureus*. *J. Biol. Chem.* vol. 247, pp. 6720-6726, 0021-9258

Dubin, G., Chmiel, D., Mak, P., Rakwalska, M., Rzychon, M. & Dubin, A. (2001) Molecular cloning and biochemical characterisation of proteases from *Staphylococcus epidermidis*. *Biol. Chem.* vol. 382, pp. 1575-1582, 1431-6730

El-Solh, A. A., Pletrantoni, C., Bhat A., Okada, M., Zambon, J., Aquilina, A. & Berbary, E. (2004) Colonization of dental plaques: A reservoir of respiratory pathogens for hospital-acquired pneumonia in institutionalized elders. *Chest* vol. 126, pp. 1575-1582, 0012-3692

Etienne, J., Fleurette, J., Ninet, J. F., Favet, P. & Gruer, L. D. (1986) Staphylococcal endocarditis after dental extraction. *Lancet* vol. 2, pp. 511-512, 0140-6736

Fedeli, U., Schievano, E., Buonfrate, D., Pellizzer, G. & Spolaore, P. (2011) Increasing incidence and mortality of infective endocarditis: a population-based study through a record-linkage system. *BMI Infect. Dis.* vol. 11:48, doi:10.1186/1471-2334-11-48

Ferreiros, E., Nacinovich, F., Casabé, J. H., Modenesi, J. C., Swieszkowski, S., Cortes, C., Hernan, C. A., Kazelian, L. &Varini, S.; Eira-2 Investigators. (2006) Epidemiologic, clinical, and microbiologic profile of infective endocarditis in Argentina: a national survey. *Am. Heart J.* vol. 151, pp. 545-552, 0002-8703

Frank, K. L. & Patel, R. (2007) Poly-*N*-acetylglucosamine is not a major component of the extacellular matrix in biofilms formed by *icaADBC*-positive *Staphylococcus lugdunensis* isolates. *Infect. Immun.* vol. 75, pp. 4728-4742, 0019-9567

Frenkel, A. & Hirsch, W. (1961) Spontaneous development of L forms of streptococci requiring secretions of other bacteria or sulphydryl compounds for normal growth. *Nature* vol. 191, pp. 728-730, 0028-0836

George, R. H. (1974) The isolation of symbiotic streptococci. *J. Med. Microbiol.* vol. 7, pp. 77-83, 0022-2615

Gerke, C., Kraft, A., Süssmuth, R., Schweitzer, O. & Götz, F. (1998) Characterization of the N-acetylglucosaminyltransferase activity involved in the biosynthesis of the *Staphylococcus epidermidis* polysaccharide intercellular adhesin. *J. Biol. Chem.* vol. 273, pp. 18586-18593, 0021-9258

Goldenberger, D., Künzle, A., Vogt, P., Zbinden, R. & Altwegg, M. (1997) Molecular diagnosis of bacterial endocarditis by broad-range PCR amplification and direct sequencing. *J. Clin. Microbiol.* vol. 35, pp. 2733-2739, 0095-1137

Goldenberg, D. L. (1998) Septic arthritis. *Lancet* vol. 351, pp. 197-202, 0140-6736

Götz, F. (2002) *Staphylococcus* and biofilms. *Mol. Microbiol.* vol. 43, pp. 1367-1378, 0950-382x

Gross, M., Cramton, S. E., Götz, F. & Peschel, A. (2001) Key role of teichoic acid net charge in *Staphylococcus aureus* colonization of artificial surfaces. *Infect. Immun.* vol. 69, pp. 3423-3426, 0019-9567

Guidelines for the prevention and treatment of infective endocarditis (JCS 2003) (2003) *Circ. J.* vol. 67, *Suppl. IV* pp. 1039-1082, 1346-9843 (in Japanese)

Heilmann, Schweitzer, O., Gerke, C., Vanittanakom, N., Mack, D. & Götz, F. (1996) Molecular basis of intercellular adhesion in the biofilm-forming *Staphylococcus epidermidis*. *Mol. Microbiol.* vol. 20, pp. 1083-1091, 0950-382x

Hennig, S., Wai, S. N. & Ziebuhr, W. (2007) Spontaneous switch to PIA-independent biofilm formation in an *ica*-positive *Staphylococcus epidermidis* isolate. *Int. J. Med. Microbiol.* vol. 297, pp. 117-122, 1438-4221

Hoen, B., Alla, F., Béguinot, I., *et al.* (2002) Changing profile of infective endocarditis: Results of a 1-year survey in France. *JAMA* vol. 288, pp. 75-81, 0098-7484

Hussain, M., Herrmann, M., von Eiff, C., Perdreau-Remington, F. & Peters, G. (1997) A 140-kilodalton extracellular protein is essential for the accumulation of *Staphylococcus epidermidis* strains on surfaces. *Infect. Immun.* vol. 65, pp. 519–524, 0019-9567

Ikeda, Y., Ohara-Nemoto, Y., Kimura, S., Ishibashi, K. & Kaneko, K. (2004) PCR-based identification of *Staphylococcus epidermidis* targeting *gseA* encoding the glutamic-acid- specific protease. *Can. J. Microbiol.* vol. 50, pp. 493-498, 0008-4166

Iwase, T., Uehara, Y., Shinji, H., Tajima, A., Seo, H., Takada, K., Agata, T. & Mizunoe, Y. (2010) *Staphylococcus epidermidis* Esp inhibits *Staphylococcus aureus* biofilm formation and nasal colonization. *Nature* vol. 465, pp. 346-349, 0028-0836

Izano, E. A., Amarante, M. A., Kher, W. B. & Kaplan, J. B. (2008) Differential roles of poly-*N*-acetylglucosamine surface polysaccharide and extracellular DNA in *Staphylococcus aureus* and *Staphylococcus epidermidis* biofilms. *Appl. Environ. Microbiol.* Vol. 74, pp. 470-476, 0099-2240

Jackson, M. S., Bagg, J., Gupta, M. N. & Sturrock, R. D. (1999) Oral carrige of staphylococci in patients with rheumatoid arthritis. *Rheumatology* vol 38, pp. 572-575, 1462-0324

Jacobson, J. J., Patel, B., Asher, G., Woolliscroft, J. O. & Schaberg, D. (1997) Oral staphyloccus in older subjects with rheumatoid arthritis. *J. Am. Geriatr. Soc.* vol. 45, pp. 590-593, 0002-8614

Ji, G., Beavis, R. & Novick, R. P. (1997) Bacterial interference caused by autoinducing peptide variants. *Science* vol. 276, pp. 2027-2030, 0036-8075

Kaandorp, C. J. E., Dinant, H. J., van de Laar, M. A. F. J., Moens, H. J. B., Prins, A. P. A. & Dijkmans, B. A. C. (1997) Incidence and source of native and prosthetic joint infection: a community based prospective survey. *Ann. Rheum. Dis.* vol. 56, 470-475, 0003-4967

Karlsson, A. & Arvidson, S. (2002) Variation in extracellular protease production among clinical isolates of *Staphylococcus aureus* due to different levels of expression of the protease repressor *sarA*. *Infect. Immun.* vol. 70, pp. 4239-4246, 0019-9567

Kawamura, Y., Hou, X. G., Sultana, F., Miura, H. & Ezaki, T. (1995) Determination of 16S rRNA sequences of *Streptococcus mitis* and *Streptococcus gordonii* and phylogenetic relationships among members of the genus *Streptococcus*. *Int. J. Syst. Bacteriol.* vol. 45, pp. 406-408, 0020-7713

Kimura, S. & Ohara-Nemoto, Y. (2007) Early childhood caries and childhood periodontal diseases. In: *Pediatric Infectious Diseases Revisited*, Schroten, H. & Wirth, S. (eds), pp. 177-197, Birkhäuser Verlag, Basel, 3-7643-8099-3

Kishi, M., Ohara-Nemoto, Y., Takahashi, M., Kishi, K., Kimura, S. & Yonemitsu, M. (2010) Relationship between oral status and prevalence of periodontopathic bacteria on the tongues of elderly individuals. *J. Med. Microbiol.* vol. 59, pp. 1354-1359, 0022-2615

Koren, O., Spor, A., Felin, J., Fåk, F., Stombaugh, J., Tremaroli, V., Behre, C. J., Knight, R., Fagerberg, B., Ley, R. E. & Bäckhed, F. (2011) Human oral, gut, and plaque microbiota in patients with atherosclerosis. *Proc. Nat. Acad. Sci. USA* vol. 108, pp. 4592-4598, 0027-8424

Mack, D., Fischer, W., Krokotsch, A., Leopold, K., Hartmann, R., Egge, H. & Laufs, R. (1996) The intercellular adhesin involved in biofilm accumulation of *Staphylococcus epidermidis* is a linear β-1,6-linked glucosaminoglycan: purification and structural analysis. *J. Bacteriol.* vol. 178, pp. 175-183, 0021-9193

Maderazo, E. G., Judson, S. & Pasternak, H. (1988) Late infections of total joint prostheses: a review and recommendation for prevention. *Clin. Orthop. Relat. Res.* vol. 229, pp. 131-142, 0009-921x

Marsh, P. D. & Martin, M. V. (2009) *Oral Microbiology* (5th ed.), Churchill Livingstone Elsevier, 978-0-443-10144-1, London

Martí, M., Trotonda, M. P., Tormo-Más, M. Á., Vergara-Irigaray, M., Cheung, A. L., Lasa, I. & Penadés, J. R. (2010) Extracellular proteases inhibit protein-dependent biofilm formation in *Staphylococcus aureus*. *Microbes. Infect.* vol. 12, pp. 55-64, 1286-4579

Moon, J. L., Banbula, A., Oleksy, A., Mayo, J. A. & Travis, J. (2001) Isolation and characterization of a highly specific serine endopeptidase from an oral strain of *Staphylococcus epidermidis*. *Biol. Chem.* vol. 382, pp. 1095-1099, 1431-6730

Murdoch, F. E., Sammons, R. L. & Chapple, I. L. (2004) Isolation and characterization of subgingival staphylococci from periodontitis patients and controls. *Oral Dis.* vol. 10, pp. 155-162, 1354-523X

Murdoch, D.R., Corey, G. R., Hoen, B., et al. (2009) Clinical presentation, etiology, and outcome of infective endocarditis in the 21st century: the International Collaboration on Endocarditis-Prospective Cohort Study. *Arch. Intern. Med.* vol. 169, pp. 463-473, 0003-9926

Nakatani, S., Misutake, K., Hozumi, T., et al. (2003) Current characteristics of infective endocarditis in Japan. An analysis of 848 cases in 2000 and 2001. *Circ. J.* vol. 67, pp. 901-905, 1346-9843

Nemoto, T. K., Ohara-Nemoto, Y., Ono, Y., Kobayakawa, T., Shimoyama, Y., Kimura, S. & Takagi, T. (2008) Characterization of the glutamyl endopeptidase from *Staphylococcus aureus* expressed in *Escherichia coli*. *FEBS J.* vol. 275, pp. 573-587, 1742-464x

Nemoto, T. K., Ono, T., Shimoyama, Y., Kimura, S. & Ohara-Nemoto, Y. (2009) Determination of three amino acids causing alteration of proteolytic activities of staphylococcal glutamyl endopeptidases. *Biol. Chem.* vol. 390, pp. 277-285, 1431-6730

Niwa, K., Nakazawa, M., Tateno, S., Yoshinaga, M. & Terai, M. (2005) Infective endocarditis in congenital heart disease: Japanese national collaboration study. *Heart* vol. 91, pp. 795-800, 1355-6037

Novick, R. P. (2003) Autoinduction and signal transduction in the regulation of staphylococcal virulence. *Mol. Microbiol.* vol. 48, pp. 1429-1449, 0950-382x

Ohara-Nemoto, Y., Tajika, S., Sasaki, M. & Kaneko, M. (1997) Identification of *Abiotrophia adiacens* and *Abiotrophia defectiva* by 16S rRNA gene PCR and restriction fragment length polymorphism analysis. *J. Clin. Microbiol.* vol. 35, pp. 2458-2463, 0095-1137

Ohara-Nemoto, Y., Ikeda, Y., Kobayashi, M., Sasaki, M., Tajika, S. & Kimura, S. (2002) Characterization and molecular coloning of a glutamyl endopeptidases from *Staphylococcus epidermidis. Microb. Pathog.* vol. 33, pp. 33-41, 0882-4010

Ohara-Nemoto, Y., Kishi, K., Satho, M., Tajika, S., Sasaki, M., Namioka, A. & Kimura, S. (2005) Infective endocarditis caused by *Granulicatella elegans* originating in the oral cavity. *J. Clin. Microbiol.* vol. 43, pp. 1405-1407, 0095-1137

Ohara-Nemoto, Y., Haraga, H., Kimura, S. & Nemoto, T. K. (2008a) Occurrence of staphylococci in the oral cavities of healthy adults and nasal-oral trafficking of the bacteria. *J. Med. Microbiol.* vol. 57, pp. 95-99, 0022-2615

Ohara-Nemoto, Y., Ono, T., Shimoyama, Y., Kimura, S. & Nemoto, T. K. (2008b) Homologous and heterologous expression and maturation processing of extracellular glutamyl endopeptidases of *Staphylococcus epidermidis. Biol. Chem.* vol. 389, pp. 1209-1217, 1431-6730

Okell, C. C., Okell, C. C. & Elliott, S.D. (1935) Bacteriaemia and oral sepsis with special reference to the etiology of subacute endocarditis. *Lancet* vol. 2, pp. 869-872, 0140-6736

Ono, T., Ohara-Nemoto, Y., Shimoyama, Y., Okawara, H., Kobayakawa, T., Baba, T.T., Kimura, S. & Nemoto, T. K. (2010) Amino acid residues modulating the activities of staphylococcal glutamyl endopeptidases. *Biol. Chem.* vol. 391, pp. 1221-1232, 1431-6730

Otto, M. (2009) *Staphylococcus epidermidis* – the 'accidental' pathogen. *Nature Rev. Microbiol.* vol. 7, 555-567, 1740-1526

Percival, R. S., Challacombe, S. J. & Marsh, P. D. (1991) Age-related microbiological changes in the salivary and plaque microflora of healthy adults. *J. Med. Microbiol.* vol. 35, pp. 5-11, 0022-2615

Pompei, R., Caredda, E., Piras, V., Serra, C. & Pintus, L. (1990) Production of bacteriolytic activity in the oral cavity by nutritionally variant streptococci. *J. Clin. Microbiol.* vol. 28, pp. 1623-1627, 0095-1137

Qin, Z., Ou, Y., Yang, L., Zhu, Y., Tolker-Nielsen, T., Molin, S. & Qu, D. (2007) Role of autolysin-mediated DNA release in biofilm formation of *Staphylococcus epidermidis. Microbiology* vol. 153, pp. 2083–2092, 1350-0872

Rice, K. C., Mann, E. E., Endres, J. L., Weiss, E. C., Cassat, J. E., Smeltzer, M. S. & Bayles, K. W. (2007) The *cidA* murein hydrolase regulator contributes to DNA release and biofilm development in *Staphylococcus aureus. Proc. Natl. Acad. Sci. USA* vol. 104, pp. 8113-8118, 0027-8424

Roggenkamp, A., Abele-Horn, M., Trebesius, K.-H., Tretter, U., Autenrieth, I. B. & Heesemann, J. (1998) *Abiotrophia elegans* sp. nov., a possible pathogen in patients with culture-negative endocarditis. *J. Clin. Microbiol.* vol. 36, pp. 100–104, 0095-1137

Rohde, H., Burandt, E. C., Siemssen, N., Frommelt, L., Burdelski, C., Wurster, S., Scherpe, S., Davies, A. P., Harris, L. G., Horstkotte, M. A., Knobloch, J. K., Ragunath, C.,

Kaplan, J. B. & Mack, D. (2007) Polysaccharide intercellular adhesin or protein factors in biofilm accumulation of *Staphylococcus epidermidis* and *Staphylococcus aureus* isolated from prosthetic hip and knee joint infections. *Biomaterials* vol. 28, pp. 1711-1720, 0142-9612

Ruoff, K. L. (1991) Nutritionally variant streptococci. *Clin. Microbiol. Rev.* vol. 4, pp. 184-190, 0893-8512

Ruoff, K. L. (2007) *Aerococcus, Abiotrophia,* and other aerobic catalase-negative, gram-positive cocci. *In Manual of Clinical Microbiology,* (9th ed.) Eds. Murray, P. R. *et al.* ASM Press, pp. 443-454, 1-55581-371-2, Washington, D.C.

Ryan, M. J., Kavanagh, R., Wall, P. G. & Hazleman, B. L. (1997) Bacterial joint infections in England and Wales: analysis of bacterial isolates over a four year period. *Br. J. Rheumatol.* vol 36, pp. 370-373, 0263-7103

Sadovskaya, I., Vinogradov, E., Flahaut, S., Kogan, G. & Jabbouri, S. (2005) Extracellular carbohydrate-containing polymers of a model biofilm-producing strain, *Staphylococcus epidermidis* RP62A. *Infect. Immun.* vol. 73, pp. 3007–3017, 0019-9567

Sandre, R. M. & Shafran, S. D. (1996) Infective endocarditis: review of 135 cases over 9 years. *Clin. Infect. Dis.* vol. 22, pp. 276-286, 1058-4838

Sasaki, M., Ohara-Nemoto, Y., Tajika, S., Kobayashi, M., Ikeda, Y., Kaneko, M. & Takagi, T. (1998) Purification and characterization of glutamic acid-specific protease from *Staphylococcus epidermidis*. *Jpn. J. Oral Biol.* vol. 40, pp. 542-548, 0385-0137

Sato, S., Kanamoto, T. & Inoue, M. (1999) *Abiotrophia elegans* strains comprise 8% of the nutritionally variant streptococci isolated from the human mouse. *J. Clin. Microbiol.* vol. 37, pp. 2553-2556, 0095-1137

Shimoyama, Y., Sasaki, M., Ohara-Nemoto, Y., Nemoto, T. K., Ishikawa, T. & Kimura, S. (in press) Rapid identification of *Abiotrophia/Granulicatella* species using by 16S rRNA PCR and RFLP. *Interface Oral Health Science 2010*

Smith, A. J., Jackson, M. S. & Bagg, J. (2001) The ecology of *Staphylococcus* species in the oral cavity. *J. Med. Microbiol.* vol. 50, pp. 940-946, 0022-2615

Strom, B. L., Abrutyn, E., Berlin, J. A., Kinman, J. L., Feldman, R. S., Stolley, P. D., Levison, M. E., Korzeniowski, O. M. & Kaye, D. (1998) Dental and cardiac risk factors for infective endocarditis: a population-based case-control study. *Ann. Intern. Med.* vol. 129, pp. 761–769, 0003-4819

Strom, B. L., Abrutyn, E., Berlin, J. A., Kinman, J. L., Feldman, R. S., Stolley, P. D., Levison, M. E., Korzeniowski, O. M. & Kaye, D. (2000) Risk factors for infective endocarditis. Oral hygiene and nondental exposures. *Circulation* vol. 102, pp. 2842-2848, 0009-7322

Tleyjeh, I. M., Steckelberg, J. M., Murad, H. S., Anavekar, N. S., Ghomrawi, H. M., Mirzoyev, Z., Houstafa, S. E., Hoskin, T. L., Mandrekar, J. N., Wilson, W. R. & Baddour, L. M. (2005) Temporal trends in infective endocarditis. A population-based study in Olmsted County, Minnesota. *JAMA* vol. 293, pp. 3022-3028, 0098-7484

Tuohy, M. J., Procop, G. W. & Washington, J. A. (2000) Antimicrobial susceptibility of *Abiotrophia adiacens* and *Abiotrophia defectiva*. *Diagn. Microbiol. Infect. Dis.* vol. 38, pp. 189-191, 0732-8893

Vinogradov, E., Sadovskaya, I., Li, J. & Jabbouri, S. (2006) Structural elucidation of the extracellular and cell-wall teichoic acids of *Staphylococcus aureus* MN8m, a biofilm forming strain. *Carbohydr. Res.* vol. 341, pp. 738–743, 0008-6215

Yarwood, J. M., Bartels, D. J., Volper, E. M. & Greenberg, E. P. (2004) Qurum sensing in *Staphylococcus aureus* biofilms. *J. Bacteriol.* vol. 186, pp. 1838-1850, 0021-9193

Yoshinaga, M., Niwa, K., Niwa, A., Ishiwada, N., Takahashi, H., Echigo, S., Nakazawa, M., & Japanese Society of Pediatric Cardiology and Cardiac Surgery. (2008) Risk factors for in-hospital mortality during infective endocarditis in patients with congenital heart disease. *Am. J. Cardiol.* vol. 101, pp. 114-118, 0002-9149

6

Antibiotics Against Endocarditis – Past, Present and Future (Experimental Data)

Cédric Jacqueline, Gilles Amador, Eric Batard,
Virginie Le Mabecque, Gilles Potel and Jocelyne Caillon
Université de Nantes, Faculté de Médecine, UPRES EA 3826, Nantes
France

1. Introduction

"Bacterial infections are becoming increasingly resistant to existing antibiotics, and as the number of patients who have succumbed to these infections rises, the number of new antibiotics being developed continues to plummet." This extract from a letter addressed to President Barack Obama by the president of Infectious Diseases Society of America (IDSA) attests to the urgent need for new therapeutic options to fight multidrug-resistant (MDR) bacteria. Drug-resistant infections and related morbidity and mortality are on the rise in the United States and around the world. Despite the growing antibiotic resistance among Gram-positive and Gram-negative pathogens causing severe infections in hospital and community settings, the number of new antibacterial drugs approved for marketing in the United States continues to decrease. In addition to this worrying situation, only a few novel therapeutics for drug-resistant infections are in the drug development pipeline (Boucher et al., 2009; European Centre for Disease Prevention and Control, 2009). Reports of bacterial isolates resistant to almost all available antibiotics highlight the crucial need for new antibiotic therapies, especially for Gram-negative infections (Maltezou, 2009). Recently, IDSA and United States authorities have developed creative incentives to stimulate new antibacterial research and development (Infectious Diseases Society of America, 2010).

In vivo assessment is recognized as an essential link between in vitro data such as susceptibility testing and clinical studies. As indicated in 1999 in the introduction to the Handbook of Animal Models of Infection (Zak et al., 1999), it is hardly conceivable that a new antibiotic could move into clinical use without thorough verification of its antimicrobial efficacy in animal models of infection at an early stage. To facilitate the extrapolation of animal model data to humans, especially for determination of efficacy, animal models mimicking human disease are required. Pharmacokinetic (PK) and pharmacodynamic (PD) features of new antibacterial agents must be considered and differences between PK of antibiotics in animals and human should be limited using methods for obtaining human-like PK profiles in animals. Animal models mimicking human infections are considered discriminative models and are designed to assess the potent therapeutic effects of antibiotics against pathogens, and in some cases to extend or delimit the indications advisable for humans.

Animal models of endocarditis are used extensively to test the in vivo activities of new drugs or new regimens, and are particularly suitable for PK and PD analysis and optimization of therapeutic efficacy. Experimental endocarditis studies played a major role in the exploration and assessment of new antistaphylococcal drugs beginning with the oxazolidinone, linezolid, in the early 2000s, and were critical to the recent approval of the promising anti-MRSA cephalosporin ceftaroline by the United States Food and Drug Administration (FDA). The endocarditis model is referenced in approximately 100 PubMed publications, most of which are assessments of the in vivo activity of new therapeutic options against *Staphylococcus aureus* such as linezolid (Jacqueline et al., 2002), quinupristin-dalfopristin (Batard et al., 2002), moxifloxacin (Entenza et al., 2001), daptomycin (Sakoulas et al., 2003), tigecycline (Murphy et al., 2000; Jacqueline et al., 2011), ceftobiprole (Tattevin et al., 2010) and ceftaroline (Jacqueline et al., 2007). *Staphylococcus aureus* is the most common cause of endocarditis worldwide and methicillin-susceptible *Staphylococcus aureus* (MSSA) is detected in up to two-thirds of cases (Fowler et al., 2005). High rates of clinical failure have been reported with vancomycin therapy for MRSA endocarditis. The emergence of glycopeptide-intermediate *Staphylococcus aureus* (GISA) strains further highlights the need for new therapeutic options for treatment of infections by *S. aureus* strains that are resistant to methicillin and glycopeptides.

Ideally, clinicians should be able to use clinical trial data to support evidence-based medicine for the treatment of infectious diseases. However, difficulty in performing clinical trials in severe types of infection such as endocarditis has resulted in a lack of clinical information regarding use of new antibiotics in treating severe infections. Experimental animal models are one method used to assess the in vivo activity of new antimicrobials in the treatment of severe infections.

2. Experimental model of endocarditis: How to?

Although experimental rodent endocarditis models are sometimes used, white New Zealand female (weighing 2-2.5 kg) are most commonly used in experimental studies involving evaluation of antimicrobial agents. This model is based on the description by Garrison and Freedman in 1970 (Garrison & Freedman, 1970) modified by Durack and Beeson in 1972 (Durack & Beeson, 1972).

The rabbit model, as currently used, is based on the insertion of a polyethylene catheter via the right carotid artery into the left ventricle under general anaesthesia. The catheter is left in place throughout the experiment (until the euthanasia of the animal). After catherization for 24 hours, each animal is inoculated i.v. (using the marginal ear vein) with 1 mL of a bacterial suspension of the test pathogen. The inoculum is usually prepared from an overnight culture (broth), centrifuged and calibrated in saline to the appropriate dilution (range, 10^5 to 10^9 CFU/mL). Bacterial concentration of the inoculum (CFUs) is controlled by quantitative culture. Then, animals are randomly assigned to the different therapeutic regimens, including a control group (infected, no drug). The treatment is usually initiated 18 to 24 hours after bacterial challenge given that the time between i.v. inoculation of the bacteria and start of antimicrobial therapy is critical. As observed in other animal experimental models, this factor can influence the efficacy of tested drugs. Administration of antibiotics is widely realized by the intramuscular (thigh) or i.v. (marginal ear vein) routes. The animals are euthanized by using an i.v. bolus of thiopental at the beginning of the treatment period (controls) or at the end of therapeutic regimen (range, 1 to 5 days). Aortic valve vegetations are excised; immediately placed on ice; and then weighed, homogenized in saline buffer, and plated on agar plates for surviving bacteria counts. Dilutions are used to eliminate potential carryover. Viable counts after 24 h to 48 h of incubation at 37°C are expressed as the mean ± standard deviation log_{10}CFU per gram of vegetation (most reliable judgement criteria). To determine whether antibiotic regimens could induce the selection of in vivo resistant variants, undiluted vegetation homogenates are spread on agar plates containing antibiotic at concentrations corresponding to two- and fourfold the MIC.

The experimental model of endocarditis has demonstrated to be highly valuable in assessing in vivo efficacy of antimicrobial agents by providing endpoints relevant in the evaluation of antibiotics (Lefort & Fantin, 1999):

- Surviving bacteria (expressed as number of CFU per gram of vegetation)
- Blood cultures (positive/negative)
- Ease of removing blood samples (PK assessment)
- Detection of the emergence of resistant variants during therapy
- Mortality
- Incidence of relapse after therapy discontinuation.

3. Linezolid, the first drug issued from the oxazolidinones, a novel class of synthetic antimicrobials

First marketed as oxazolidinone in the early 2000's, linezolid was approved by the United States FDA for the treatment of adults with nosocomial pneumonia, infections due to vancomycin-resistant *Enterococcus faecium*, complicated and uncomplicated skin and skin-structure infections, and community-acquired pneumonia (Zyvox [package insert], 2000). This new drug was considered a promising new option against MRSA in a context of increasing numbers of infections caused by resistant gram-positive bacteria and the emergence of MRSA strains with reduced susceptibility to glycopeptides (Hiramatsu et al., 1997).

3.1 *In vitro* antibacterial activity of linezolid alone and in combination with other antibacterial agents

Oxazolidinones are bacterial protein synthesis inhibitors: linezolid binds to a site on the bacterial 23S ribosomal RNA of the 50S subunit and prevents the formation of a functional 70S initiation complex (Aoki et al., 2002). This mechanism of action is specific to this class, and no cross-resistance with other antimicrobial agents has been observed. As with most protein synthesis inhibitors, linezolid displays nonbactericidal, time-dependent activity in vitro against staphylococci (Kaatz & Seo, 1996) (Figure 1). The bacteriostatic and time-dependent activity did not work in linezolid's favor for clinical use, especially for treatment of severe infections, where most clinicians are convinced that bactericidal drugs are required. Consequently, many studies examined the in vitro activity of linezolid in combination with partner drugs (Table 1), including vancomycin (Grohs et al., 2003; Jacqueline et al., 2003; Soriano et al., 2005; Sahuquillo Arce et al., 2006; Singh et al., 2009), gentamicin (Grohs et al., 2003; Jacqueline et al., 2003), rifampicin (Grohs et al., 2003; Jacqueline et al., 2003; Soriano et al., 2005; Sahuquillo Arce et al., 2006), carbapenems (Jacqueline, 2005, 2006), fosfomycin (Sahuquillo Arce et al., 2006), doxycycline (Sahuquillo Arce et al., 2006), ciprofloxacin (Grohs et al., 2003), levofloxacin (Soriano et al., 2005;

Sahuquillo Arce et al., 2006), and fusidic acid (Grohs et al., 2003). Although indifference is often observed for linezolid combinations against *S. aureus* (including methicillin-resistant strains), some cases of antagonism and synergism were reported and studied in vivo using the experimental model of endocarditis.

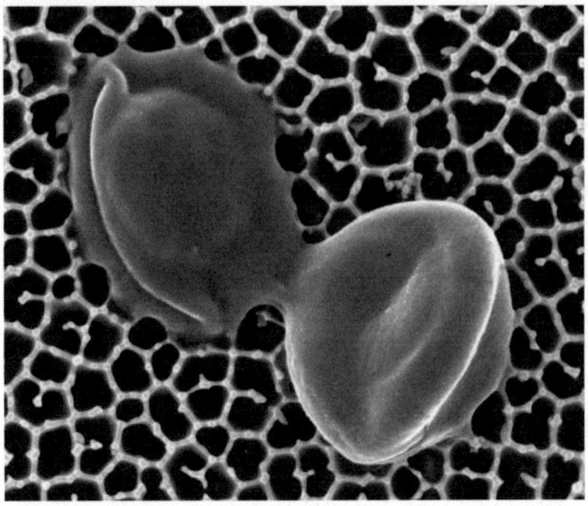

Fig. 1. Scanning electron micrographs of *S. aureus* exposed to linezolid (LNZ) at 8 times the minimum inhibitory concentration (MIC; magnification, ×50,000)

Partner drugs	Class of antibiotics	Interaction	Reference(s)
Vancomycin	Glycopeptides	Antagonism	Grohs et al., 2003; Jacqueline et al., 2003; Soriano et al., 2005; Sahuquillo Arce et al., 2006; Singh et al., 2009;
Gentamicin	Aminoglycosides	Antagonism (inhibition of the early bactericidal activity)	Grohs et al., 2003; Jacqueline et al., 2003
Rifampicin	Rifamycins	Indifference	Grohs et al., 2003; Jacqueline et al., 2003; Soriano et al., 2005; Sahuquillo Arce et al., 2006
Doxycycline	Tetracyclines	Addition	Sahuquillo Arce et al., 2006
Ciprofloxacin	Quinolones	Indifference or Antagonism	Grohs et al., 2003
Levofloxacin			Soriano et al., 2005; Sahuquillo Arce et al., 2006
Acid fusidic	-		Grohs et al., 2003
Fosfomycin	-	Synergy	Sahuquillo Arce et al., 2006
Imipenem	Carbapenems	Synergy	Jacqueline et al., 2005
Ertapenem			Jacqueline et al., 2006

Table 1. In vitro activity of linezolid in combination with partner drugs

3.2 *In vivo* antibacterial activity of linezolid alone and in combination in the experimental model of infective endocarditis

3.2.1 *In vivo* experimental assessment of linezolid activity: Bacteriostatic agent *in vivo*?

First reports of linezolid in vivo activity used oral administration (p.o.) of the drug. Given that linezolid can be administered intravenously (i.v.) or orally, and no dose adjustment is necessary when switching from the i.v. to the oral route of administration in humans (Zyvox [package insert], 2000). Infective endocarditis is considered to require maintenance of bactericidal levels of antibacterial agents for prolonged periods of time to result in eradication of the pathogen. For this reason, it was of special interest to assess the activity of the oxazolidinone in this model of endocarditis. Dailey et al investigated the activity of linezolid at three different p.o. dosages (25, 50, and 75 mg/kg) against MRSA in rabbits with experimental aortic-valve endocarditis (Dailey et al., 2001). After 5 days of treatment, linezolid displayed a stepwise decrease in the mean bacterial counts from the valve vegetation with a significant decrease for both 50 and 75 mg/kg. Showing a 4- to 5-log reduction in valvular bacterial counts, linezolid acted as a bactericidal drug in this study (Dailey et al., 2001).

Based on these results, the authors suggested that linezolid levels at or above the MIC in plasma combined with a minimum number of treatment days was required for the therapeutic efficacy of linezolid in this model. Further studies were then necessary to address the predictive pharmacokinetic and pharmacodynamic (PK/PD) parameters of linezolid.

The extrapolation of results obtained in animal experimental models to human therapy is always a difficult task. Owing to the very short spontaneous half-life of linezolid in rabbits (30 min; unpublished data) and to the difference in bioavailability of orally administered linezolid (approximately 30% bioavailability in rabbits compared to almost 100% in humans (Dailey et al., 2001)), the use of simulation of human pharmacokinetics was required to reach conclusions relevant to human applications. Simulation is particularly suitable for pharmacokinetic and pharmacodynamic analysis, and for the optimization of therapeutic efficacy. Computer-controlled simulation (Bugnon et al., 1998) of human kinetic profiles of linezolid in rabbits was used in the following study to improve the analysis (Jacqueline et al., 2002). The use of a computer-controlled pump allowing an adequate flow of antibiotics to be infused into rabbits enabled us to simulate the in vivo human pharmacokinetics of the antibiotics. The flow can be adjusted to a profile mathematically defined in time (Bugnon et al., 1998). Using this method, the serum linezolid levels obtained after administration of a dose simulating a 10-mg/kg dose in humans are shown in Figure 2. The corresponding mean peak concentration, area under the curve, and half-life were 11.9±1.1 mg/L, 76.3±5.9 mg.h/L, and 2.7±0.1 h, respectively, after administration of the first dose and 21.5±1.3 mg/L, 152.1±9.2 mg.h/L, and 3.4±0.7 h, respectively, at day 5. The increase of linezolid concentrations in plasma at day 5 compared to day 1 suggested drug accumulation as previously shown by Dailey (Dailey et al., 2001) using the same experimental model.

Using the computer-controlled simulation, linezolid significantly decreased the bacterial counts in aortic valve vegetations from rabbits, but failed to exhibit bactericidal activity, despite 5 days of treatment (Figure 3). The comparison with vancomycin administered as a constant-rate intravenous infusion (to obtain a serum steady-state concentration of approximately 20 to 25 mg/L) was in favor of the glycopeptide with at least a 5-log_{10} colony-forming unit (CFU)/g of vegetation decrease (Figure 3). The oxazolidinone is a time-dependent antibiotic and for these drugs, the time above the MIC (T>MIC) is usually considered a critical parameter in the assessment of therapeutic efficacy (Carbon, 1990). In general, the maximal activity of continuous infusion was obtained at a steady-state concentration in serum equal to a multiple of the MIC, as previously demonstrated for ceftazidime (Cappelletty et al., 1995). To confirm this, continuous infusion of linezolid was used by Jacqueline et al (Jacqueline et al., 2002) to investigate whether it improves in vivo activity. A switch from intermittent dosing to continuous infusion (using the same total daily dose) improved the in vivo activity of linezolid against two strains of MRSA. By increasing the time above the MIC (T>MIC of 100%), linezolid continuous infusion achieved bactericidal activity in vivo with a >3-log_{10}-decrease as compared to the control animals (Figure 4).

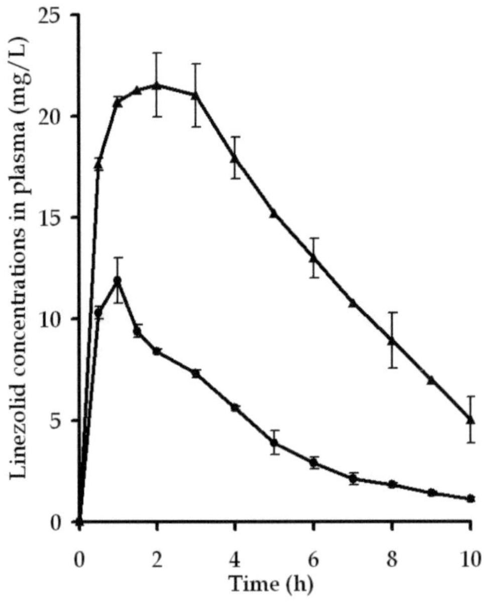

Fig. 2. Linezolid concentrations in plasma after simulation of a dose corresponding to a 10 mg/kg dose in humans (i.e., 600 mg). Circles, concentrations obtained after administration of the first dose; Triangles, concentrations obtained at day 5. Error bars represent standard deviations (adapted from Jacqueline et al., 2002)

Further studies are needed to investigate the potential clinical benefit of continuous infusion, which could be an appropriate alternative to the use of glycopeptides for the treatment of severe MRSA infections. Although no superiority of continuous infusion vs. intermittent dosing was demonstrated in a clinical study with critically ill septic patients (Adembri et al., 2008), Adembri et al showed that the continuous infusion modality has a theoretical advantage over intermittent infusion in the treatment of infection in these patients. Finally, there is a clear need for more powerful clinical trials to demonstrate the potent clinical benefit and the safety of this administration modality.

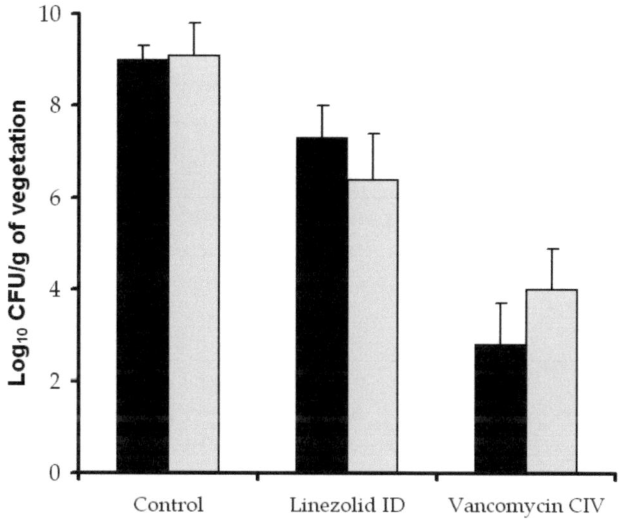

Fig. 3. In vivo activity of linezolid (human-equivalent of 600 mg q12hr, intermittent dosing, ID) and vancomycin (continuous infusion, CIV) against MRSA 1 (black) and MRSA 2 (grey) strains after a 5-day treatment. Error bars represent standard deviations (adapted from Jacqueline et al., 2002)

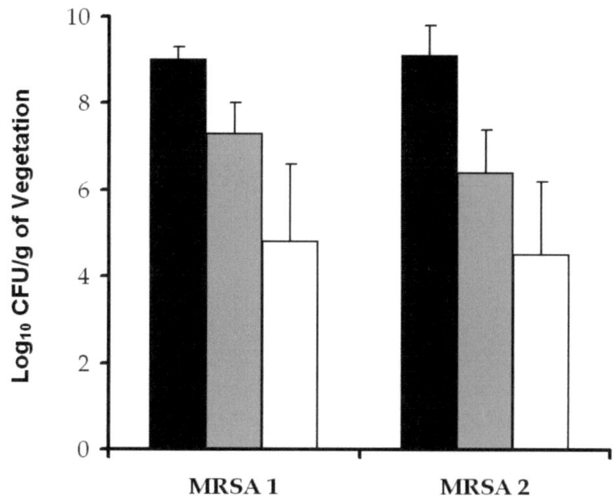

Fig. 4. Impact of the administration mode (intermittent dosing, ID vs. continuous infusion, CIV) on the in vivo activity of linezolid. Control animals (black); Linezolid ID (grey); Linezolid CIV (white). Error bars represent standard deviations (adapted from Jacqueline et al., 2002)

3.2.2 Improvement of the in vivo activity of linezolid by adding a partner drug: What is the good choice?

Infective endocarditis is considered to require bactericidal drugs to achieve clinical efficacy and/or microbiological eradication. Like most protein synthesis inhibitors, oxazolidinones are bacteriostatic agents. Clinicians need to combine linezolid with another drug to (i) increase the bactericidal activity of therapy, (ii) prevent the emergence of drug-resistant subpopulations, and (iii) provide a complementary antibacterial spectrum. Moreover, the use of synergistic antibiotic combinations is appealing as a way to optimize therapy for infective endocarditis, especially when the causative pathogen is resistant (such as MRSA). Although in vitro interactions between linezolid and agents are well-documented (Table 1), the presence of in vitro synergism or antagonism and in vivo correlation or enhanced clinical outcome is not easy to highlight. In addition, the in vitro-in vivo correlation of either positive or negative interactions between two drugs can be difficult to assess and discrepancies occur.

3.2.2.1 Linezolid plus vancomycin

Although the combination of linezolid with vancomycin is not the most obvious choice, many papers have investigated the in vitro activity of this combination and have concluded they are antagonistic. Using the endocarditis model, Chiang et al have tested this association against an MRSA strain and they demonstrated that vancomycin alone was more effective than either linezolid alone or the combination of linezolid and vancomycin (Figure 5) (Chiang & Climo, 2003). This study is in line with in vitro reports (Grohs et al., 2003; Jacqueline et al., 2003) and the combination of linezolid plus vancomycin should be avoided in clinical practice.

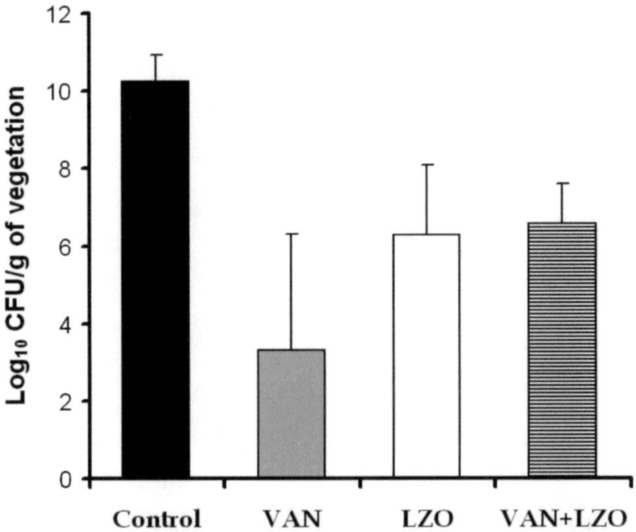

Fig. 5. Outcome of 5-day treatment of experimental MRSA endocarditis. (adapted from Chiang & Climo, 2003)

3.2.2.2 Linezolid plus gentamicin

Linezolid, when added to gentamicin, seemed to inhibit the early in vitro bactericidal activity of gentamicin, particularly over the first 6 h (Jacqueline et al., 2003). During this interval, inhibition of the bactericidal activity of gentamicin was dependent on the linezolid concentration. Aminoglycosides are bactericidal, concentration-dependent antibiotics that act by creating fissures in the outer membrane of the bacterial cell (Gonzalez & Spencer, 1998). A combination of these agents with linezolid could be useful to increase the bactericidal activity of the therapy, especially during the first days of treatment.

Given that the presence of in vitro antagonism is not always correlated with in vivo failure, Jacqueline et al assessed the combination of linezolid plus gentamicin in the endocarditis model against two clinical strains of MRSA exhibiting MICs of 0.125 and 0.5 mg/L (Jacqueline et al., 2004). Using a human-like pharmacokinetic simulation for linezolid and gentamicin, the combination demonstrated a bactericidal activity against the two strains with a decrease of at least 4 log_{10} CFU/g of vegetation compared with controls. PK/PD aspects could probably explain the difference observed between the in vitro and in vivo activities. Contrary to constant concentrations in time-kill curves experiments, the concentrations of linezolid and gentamicin added to the vegetation changed over time. Although previous in vitro results suggest an antagonism, linezolid combined with gentamicin could be of clinical interest for the treatment of severe MRSA infections requiring combination antimicrobial therapy.

3.2.2.3 Linezolid plus rifampicin

Rifampicin is an RNA polymerase inhibitor that blocks bacterial transcription. Rifampicin is used clinically only as a part of combination regimens because development of resistance is rapid (Heep et al., 2000). In addition to its use against *Mycobacterium tuberculosis*, rifampicin is very useful in the management of bone and joint infections due to MRSA. Indifference was the main interaction observed in vitro between linezolid and rifampicin (Grohs et al., 2003; Jacqueline et al., 2003, Soriano et al., 2005; Sahuquillo Arce et al., 2006). The addition of linezolid prevented the selection of rifampicin resistant mutants after 24 h of incubation at 37°C. Consequently, a synergistic interaction can be considered by inhibition of the emergence of the resistance development.

By evaluating the bactericidal activity, synergy, and emergence of antimicrobial resistance, Dailey et al assessed the potent activity of linezolid plus rifampicin in the endocarditis model against a MSSA strain (rifampicin MIC<= 0.12 mg/L) (Dailey et al., 2003). After a 5-day treatment, the combination showed no in vivo antagonism between the drugs. As with in vitro tests, indifference was observed and the combination inhibited the emergence of rifampicin resistance. These data support a clinical interest in the treatment of infections due to *S. aureus*. A similar study was performed against an MRSA strain (rifampicin MIC= 2 mg/L) and indifference between linezolid and rifampicin was observed (Tsaganos et al., 2008). Moreover, this work demonstrated that (i) linezolid limited bacterial growth in the secondary foci of endocarditis, and (ii) that the combination favored the suppression of bacterial growth in the lung.

3.2.2.4 Linezolid plus carbapenems

Beta-lactam antibiotics act by inhibiting penicillin-binding proteins (PBPs) that are involved in peptidoglycan synthesis. Penicillin-binding protein 2A (PBP2A) is the protein responsible for the methicillin resistance mechanism in *S. aureus*. Methicillin resistance confers resistance to all the beta-lactams, including cephalosporins and carbapenems; however, many studies have reported a potent efficacy of imipenem against *S. aureus* when used in combination with other antimicrobial agents, including fosfomycin (Nakazawa et al., 2003), vancomycin

(Totsuka K et al., 1999; Benquan et al., 2002; Rochon-Edouard et al., 2000), and cephalosporins (Uete & Matsuo et al., 1995).

In vitro synergy between linezolid and carbapenems can be difficult to achieve; sub-inhibitory concentrations of the carbapenem must be used with linezolid to achieve synergy and higher concentrations can lead to an antagonism (Jacqueline, 2005, 2006). The infective endocarditis model was very useful to assess in vivo interaction. Continuous infusion of imipenem alone, the first carbapenem tested in this model, showed no activity against MRSA after 5 days of treatment (Jacqueline et al., 2005). The aim of using continuous imipenem infusion was to obtain an in vivo steady-state concentration that mimics the in vitro conditions so that synergy was observed as soon as possible (i.e., to achieve a target concentration of 1/32 the MIC for each strain). Using these conditions, linezolid plus imipenem exhibited bactericidal and synergistic activities against two MRSA strains, with at least a 4-$\log_{10}$ CFU/g decrease compared to the counts for the controls. Subsequent to that study, the carbapenem ertapenem was investigated in combination with linezolid using the same experimental model (Jacqueline et al., 2006). Ertapenem is a parenteral carbapenem antibiotic with a broad antibacterial spectrum and once-a-day dosing that is supported by clinical studies and an extended half-life (Zhanel et al., 2005). In this study, animals were randomly assigned to receive either no treatment (controls), a linezolid regimen mimicking the human dose of 10 mg/kg/12 h, an ertapenem regimen mimicking the human dose of 1 g/day, or a combination of both regimens. As previously observed with imipenem and confirming the in vitro data, linezolid and ertapenem exhibited a highly bactericidal and synergistic activity in vivo against three MRSA strains after 4 days of treatment (Figure 6). Due to the once-daily dosing of ertapenem and availability of an oral form for linezolid, this combination opens new therapeutic avenues in the field of severe Gram-positive bacterial infections, including an option for outpatient parenteral antimicrobial therapy.

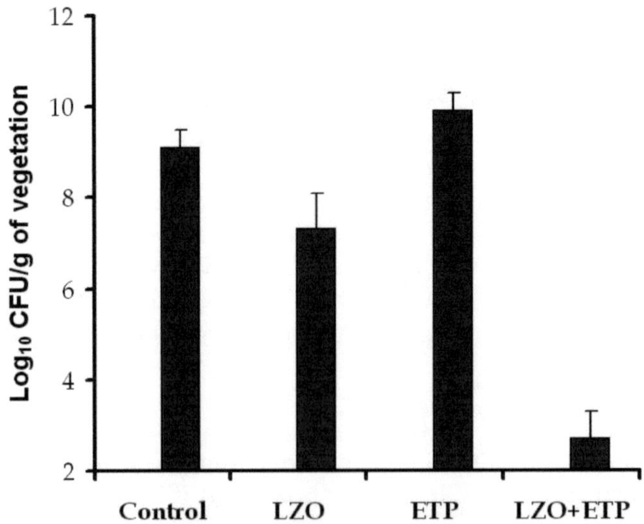

Fig. 6. In vivo synergy between linezolid (LZO) and ertapenem (ETP) against an MRSA strain in the endocarditis model. Error bars represent standard deviations (adapted from Jacqueline et al., 2006)

4. Quinupristin-dalfopristin: A therapeutic option for MRSA endocarditis?

Streptogramins inhibit protein synthesis by binding to the ribosomal 50S subunit, and the most frequent mechanism of quinupristin resistance encountered is target modification by methylation of an adenine residue in 23S rRNA (encoded by the *ermA*, *ermB*, or *ermC* gene). Constitutively expressed *erm* genes confer in vitro cross-resistance to macrolides, lincosamides, and streptogramin B. Quinupristin and dalfopristin are water-soluble injectable streptogramin B and streptogramin A antibiotics, respectively, whose combination in a 30:70 (wt/wt) ratio acts synergistically on Gram-positive bacteria (Bouanchaud, 1992). Despite in vitro susceptibility to quinupristin-dalfopristin, mutations in the L22 ribosomal protein are correlated with resistance to quinupristin in *S. aureus* (Bruni et al., 2000). The experimental model of infective endocarditis was used to address the efficacy of quinupristin-dalfopristin against susceptible and resistant *S. aureus* strains to quinupristin (but not quinupristin-dalfopristin). If quinupristin-dalfopristin remained active against quinupristin-susceptible MRSA after 4 days of treatment, a significant decrease of the activity was observed against a quinupristin-resistant strain. Nevertheless, the impact of the resistance on the activity of the combination can differ between studies (Batard et al., 2002; Pavie et al., 2002).

Combination with vancomycin improved the in vivo activity for susceptible and resistant strains (Pavie et al., 2002), but the benefit was less important against the resistant MRSA. Despite clinical interest in adding gentamicin (aminoglycosides) to quinupristin-dalfopristin, the combination showed no additive benefit against two MRSA strains (Batard et al., 2002). Although the lack of benefit may be due to the high efficacy of the monotherapies, these data did not argue for its use in clinical practice.

5. Daptomycin: Experimental evaluation of an old new drug

Daptomycin, previously called LY 146032, was first discovered in the 1980s by researchers at Eli Lilly, but an increase in creatine phosphokinase levels in serum in early clinical trials (probably related to skeletal muscle toxicity) led to initial abandonment of this promising compound (Tally & DeBruin, 2000).

Daptomycin is a novel lipopeptide antibiotic active against Gram-positive bacteria, including MRSA strains. It disrupts the bacterial cell membrane by forming transmembrane channels, and causes a calcium-dependent depolarization of the cellular membrane and inhibition of macromolecular synthesis leading to cell death (Silverman et al., 2003).

Daptomycin is a potential alternative to vancomycin for the treatment of severe MRSA infections, with benefits such as once-daily dosing, the lack of need for monitoring serum concentrations, and FDA approval for the treatment of right-sided endocarditis (Cubist, 2003). In vitro, the lipopeptide exerts its bactericidal action in a rapid (60 min) and concentration dependent way exhibiting more powerful activity than glycopeptides.

5.1 *In vivo* antibacterial activity of daptomycin: More bactericidal than glycopeptides?

The endocarditis model was used to assess the activity of daptomycin against MRSA and to confirm the highly bactericidal activity observed in vitro, especially in comparison with the reference drug, vancomycin. Effectiveness against three MRSA strains, including one GISA strain (MU50), was tested using computer-controlled simulation to mimic the human dose of 6 mg/kg once daily (Jacqueline et al., 2011). After 4 days of treatment, daptomycin performed well against MSSA, MRSA, and GISA strains (daptomycin MIC= 0.5 mg/L) with a decrease of 5 log_{10} CFU/g (Figure 7).

More than 20 years ago, Kennedy & Chambers evaluated the potent in vivo activity of daptomycin, known at that time as a vancomycin-like lipopeptide, against *S. aureus* (Kennedy & Chambers, 1989). Vancomycin (25 mg/kg twice daily) was as effective as daptomycin (once-daily dose of 10 mg/kg) against both MSSA and MRSA strains in the endocarditis model. The next year Kaatz et al compared daptomycin (8 mg/kg q8hr) with the glycopeptides, vancomycin and teicoplanin (Kaatz et al., 1990). The conclusion of the study was interesting:

"We have established that, in the rabbit model and against the *S. aureus* test strains we used, daptomycin and teicoplanin-HD are as efficacious as vancomycin, but for certain strains of *S. aureus*, diminished susceptibility to both can develop during therapy" (Kaatz et al., 1990). Also at that time, the authors highlighted an important characteristic of daptomycin, its rapid propensity to select resistant variants during therapy. Despite high in vivo bactericidal activity, experimental models were not able to demonstrate that the rapid bactericidal activity of daptomycin observed in vitro was correlated with a better outcome in vivo than glycopeptides, vancomycin, or teicoplanin.

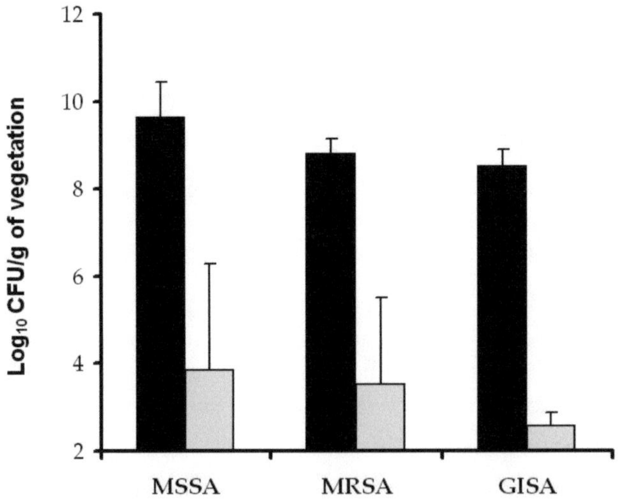

Fig. 7. In vivo activity of daptomycin (human-equivalent (HE) at 6 mg/kg/24 h) against MSSA, MRSA, and GISA strains after a 4-day treatment. Control animals (black); daptomycin-treated animals (grey). Error bars represent standard deviations (adapted from Jacqueline et al., 2011)

5.2 Emergence of daptomycin-resistance during therapy

The experimental endocarditis model is not considered an appropriate model for detection of the emergence of resistant variants. Nevertheless, emergence of daptomycin-resistant variants was observed after only 4 days of therapy in a model using human-equivalent dosage (Jacqueline et al., 2011), as previously shown by Kaatz et al (Kaatz et al., 1990). This strongly suggests that combination therapy may be useful for daptomycin treatment of *S. aureus* infections. In the study by Jacqueline et al, the 6 mg/kg dosage regimen did not prevent the emergence of resistance in two animals (one in the MSSA group (8 animals) and one in the MRSA group (7 animals)) (Figure 8). Moreover, detection of resistant variants was correlated with a failure of daptomycin treatment in those animals. These data support the use of daptomycin dosages exceeding 6 mg/kg to increase bacterial killing and limit the risk of emergence of resistant variants during daptomycin therapy. Case reports have described safe and well tolerated daptomycin treatment at doses up to 12 mg/kg (Benvenuto et al., 2006; Cunha et al., 2006), but adequate dosing of daptomycin remains unresolved. A recent review about clinical utility of daptomycin in infective endocarditis specifies that adequate dosing of daptomycin for the treatment of left-sided or prosthetic valve S. aureus endocarditis should be ≥ 10 mg/kg/day (Cervera et al., 2011).

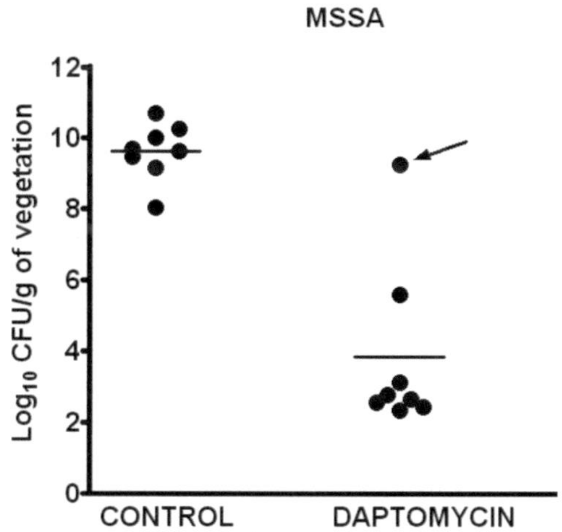

Fig. 8. Bacterial titers in vegetations infected by methicillin-susceptible *S. aureus* after 4 days of treatment with daptomycin (human-equivalent of 6 mg/kg once-daily). Arrows indicate animals with isolates exhibiting increased MICs to daptomycin (adapted from Jacqueline et al., 2011)

5.3 What partner drugs to use with daptomycin? An unresolved question

Faced with rapid emergence of daptomycin-resistant variants during therapy, clinicians should use a combination to limit the risk of resistance development. Rifampicin and gentamicin are often used in combination with antibacterial agents such as glycopeptides, beta-lactams, or linezolid. Two studies investigated the in vivo activity of daptomycin alone and in combination with rifampicin or gentamicin against different MRSA strains (LaPlante & Woodmansee, 2009; Miró et al., 2009). In experiments simulating human PK for all studied drugs, Miro et al demonstrated that daptomycin plus gentamicin was as effective as daptomycin alone (P=0.83). In addition, both were more active than daptomycin plus rifampicin (P<0.05) (Miró et al., 2009). Using an in vitro pharmacodynamic infection model with simulated endocardial vegetations, LaPlante & Woodmansee showed that daptomycin monotherapy displayed better activity than daptomycin in combination with rifampicin or gentamicin (LaPlante & Woodmansee, 2009). These experimental data strongly show that the addition of gentamicin or rifampicin does not aid the in vivo activity of daptomycin. In vitro, Miro et al (Miro et al., 2009) showed a synergistic interaction between daptomycin and fosfomycin against MSSA and MRSA. Further in vivo and clinical studies are strongly needed to determine effective combinations for avoiding the emergence of resistance to daptomycin.

6. Tigecycline

Tigecycline is the first clinically-available member of a new class of broad-spectrum antibacterials, the glycylcyclines, which were specifically developed to overcome the two major mechanisms of tetracycline resistance (Zhanel et al., 2004). By binding to the 30S ribosomal subunit, tigecycline blocks the entry of aminoacyl-tRNA into the A site of the ribosome during translation (Slover et al., 2007). Like other protein synthesis inhibitors, the drug is bacteriostatic. Tigecycline is an obvious choice to treat MRSA endocarditis, however its potent in vitro activity against MRSA suggests that it should be used as a last resort.

Few studies have valuated the activity of tigecycline in experimental model of MRSA endocarditis. A study using a rat model of endocarditis showed a dose-effect relationship, with a >2-$\log_{10}$ decrease in bacterial counts with doses greater than 10 mg/kg/day for the course of treatment (Murphy et al., 2000). Using a computer-controlled simulation mimicking the human dose of 100 mg initially, followed by 50 mg twice daily, tigecycline demonstrated a significant and homogeneous activity against MSSA, MRSA, and GISA strains (Jacqueline et al., 2011). Nevertheless, the drug failed to exhibit a bactericidal effect versus the effect of the control treatment, despite 4 days of treatment (reduction, 2-$\log_{10}$ CFU/g compared with the controls) (Figure 9). This moderate activity could be improved

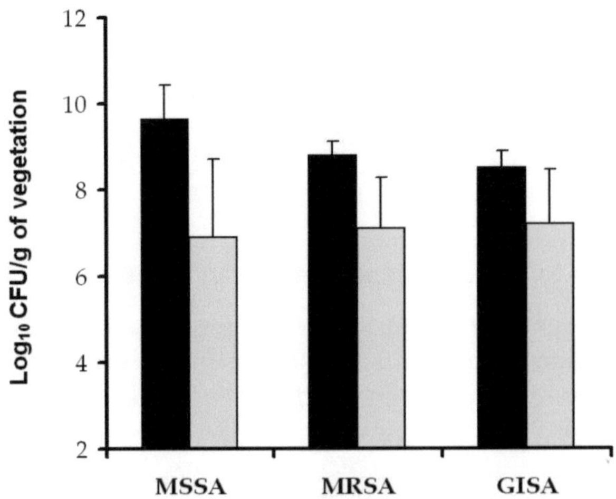

Fig. 9. In vivo outcome after a 4-day treatment of tigecycline (human-equivalent of 100 mg initially, followed by 50 mg twice daily) against MSSA, MRSA, and GISA strains. Control animals (black); tigecycline-treated animals (grey). Error bars represent standard deviations (adapted from Jacqueline et al., 2011)

by the use of a partner drug in combination with tigecycline. The addition of gentamicin significantly improved the killing activity of tigecycline in biofilm-forming *S. aureus* using an in vitro pharmacodynamic model (McConeghy KW & LaPlante, 2010). Finally, studies conducted in both animals and humans have demonstrated that tigecycline distributes widely into various tissues and body fluids (Rello, 2005), and peak serum concentrations do not exceed 1 mg/L, which may limit its utility in the treatment of bacteraemia and endocarditis (Paterson, 2006). The recommended dosage of tigecycline may be too low for the treatment of severe infections and assessment of higher doses in severe experimental animal models is needed.

7. Anti-MRSA cephalosporins exhibiting high affinity for PBP2A: A revolution?

PBPs catalyze transpeptidase or transglycosidase reactions, and are essential for the final stages of peptidoglycan synthesis (Spratt, 1977). β-lactam antibiotics, including penicillins and cephalosporins, inhibit PBPs. β-lactams are widely used because of their broad-spectrum activity and favorable safety profiles (Darville & Yamauchi, 1994). MRSA strains are not susceptible to the action of β-lactams because of the low affinity of β-lactams for PBP2a, an additional PBP encoded by the *mecA* gene and conferring methicillin resistance (Lim & Strynadka, 2002). Because β-lactam antibiotics are usually considered the most effective therapeutic option against *S. aureus* infections, researchers have sought to increase the affinity of β-lactams for the modified PBP2a. This is illustrated by the development of two cephalosporins, namely ceftobiprole and ceftaroline, which have potent antimicrobial activities against both Gram-positive (including MRSA) and Gram-negative bacteria. Ceftaroline binds to the four natural PBPs in *S. aureus*, but has maximum affinity for PBP2a (Villegas-Estrada et al., 2008). Because the marketing authorization for ceftobiprole was withdrawn in the United States and the European Union due to unfavorable assessments of the applications, ceftaroline is better studied.

7.1 Ceftaroline, a broad-spectrum cephalosporin active against MRSA

Ceftaroline is a novel broad-spectrum cephalosporin with potent activity against MRSA strains due to its strong affinity for *S. aureus* PBPs, including PBP2a, encoded by the methicillin resistance gene *mecA* (Lim & Strynadka, 2002). Ceftaroline acetate (PPI-0903) is an N-phosphono-water-soluble prodrug rapidly metabolized in vivo into the bioactive metabolite ceftaroline (PPI-0903 M). In vitro, bactericidal activity (≥3 $\log_{10}$ CFU/mL reductions) and time-dependent killing was observed for the cephalosporin from 4 times the MIC against an MRSA strain (Figure 10). Ceftaroline in vivo activity was assessed against two MRSA strains isolated from blood cultures (Jacqueline et al, 2007). The MRSA strain exhibited heterogeneous high-level methicillin resistance (methicillin MIC =128 mg/L), and the heterogeneous glycopeptide- intermediate *S. aureus* strain (hGISA) exhibited homogeneous resistance to methicillin (methicillin MIC >1,024 mg/L) and heterogeneous resistance to glycopeptides. Ceftaroline MICs/MBCs were 1/1 and 2/2 mg/L for the MRSA and hGISA strain, respectively. A human-like simulation was intended to provide apparent values of pharmacokinetic parameters close to those observed in healthy volunteers after a 1-h infusion of a 600-mg dose (approximately 10 mg/kg) of ceftaroline acetate: mean half-life

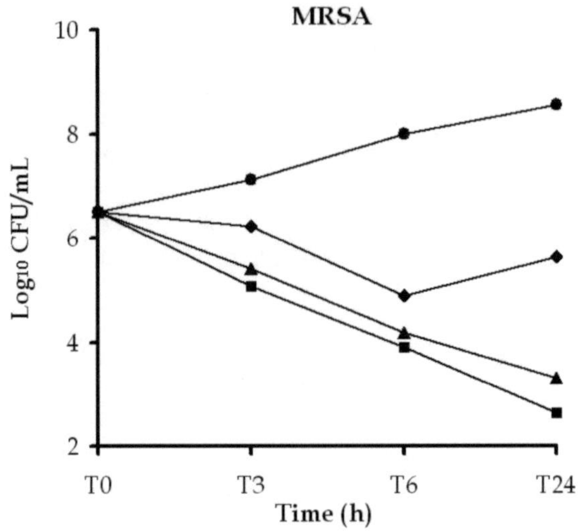

Fig. 10. In vitro activity of ceftaroline against methicillin-resistant *S. aureus*. Control (circles); ceftaroline at 1×MIC (diamonds); ceftaroline at 4×MIC (triangles), ceftaroline at 8×MIC (squares) (Author's unpublished data)

(*t*1/2), 1.57 to 2.63 h; peak concentration (Cmax), 18.96 to 21.02 mg/L; and area under the curve (AUC), 56.08 mg.h/L (Cerexa, Inc., unpublished data). After simulation into the rabbit, the corresponding Cmax, AUC, and *t*1/2 values were 21.9±3.0 mg/L, 71.2 mg.h/L, and 2.4 h, respectively (Figure 11). Ceftaroline in vivo activity was assessed against two MRSA strains isolated from blood cultures (Jacqueline et al, 2007). The MRSA strain was a strain with heterogeneous high-level methicillin resistance (methicillin MIC =128 mg/liter), and

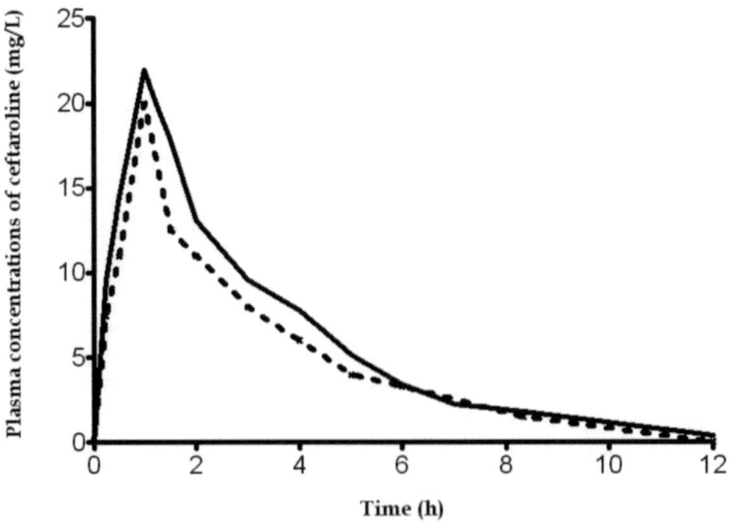

Fig. 11. Pharmacokinetics of ceftaroline in plasma after administration of a dose simulating a 600-mg dose in humans (dashed lines) and the corresponding human pharmacokinetics in animals (solid line) (adapted from Jacqueline et al., 2007)

the heterogeneous glycopeptide- intermediate *S. aureus* strain (hGISA) exhibited homogeneous resistance to methicillin (methicillin MIC >1,024 mg/liter) and heterogeneous resistance to glycopeptides.

Ceftaroline MICs/MBCs were 1/1 and 2/2 mg/L for the MRSA and hGISA strain, respectively. A human-like simulation was intended to provide apparent values of pharmacokinetic parameters close to those observed in healthy volunteers after a 1-h infusion of a 600-mg dose (ca. 10 mg/kg) of ceftaroline acetate: mean half-life ($t1/2$), 1.57 to 2.63 h; peak concentration (Cmax), 18.96 to 21.02 mg/liter; and area under the curve (AUC), 56.08 mg.h/liter (Cerexa, Inc., unpublished data). After simulation into the rabbit, the corresponding Cmax, AUC, and $t1/2$ values were 21.9±3.0 mg/liter, 71.2 mg.h/liter, and 2.4 h, respectively (Figure 11).

In this study, Jacqueline et al evaluated the in vivo activity of ceftaroline in comparison with vancomycin and linezolid, the two main therapeutic options available for the treatment of severe MRSA infections. In vivo outcome after a 4-day treatment is shown in Figure 12. Ceftaroline demonstrated excellent bactericidal and homogeneous activity against MRSA in the endocarditis model with at least a 6-$\log_{10}$ CFU/g decrease as compared to the control animals. In comparison, linezolid displayed moderate activity with a 2-$\log_{10}$ decrease. Vancomycin was as effective as ceftaroline against the MRSA strain (vancomycin MIC = 1 mg/L), but showed only bacteriostatic activity against the hGISA strain (vancomycin MIC = 4 mg/L). In addition, ceftaroline was able to sterilize 90% and 60% of the vegetations produced by the MRSA or hGISA strain, respectively, whereas vancomycin achieved sterilization of 67% and 0% of the vegetations, respectively.

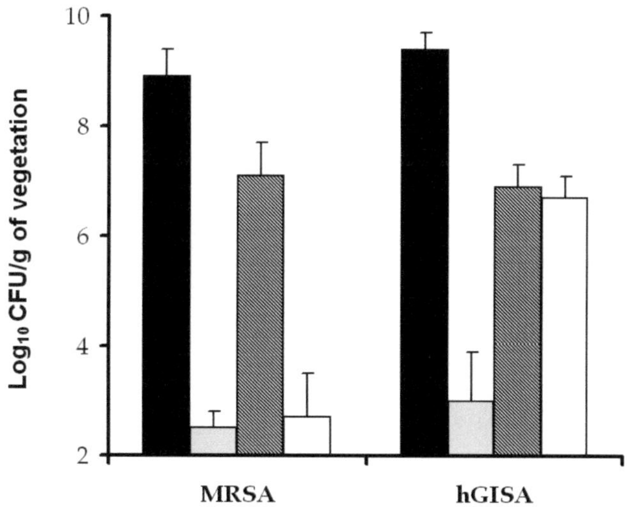

Fig. 12. Bacterial titers in vegetations infected by MRSA or hGISA strains after 4 days of treatment with ceftaroline (human-equivalent of 600 mg twice daily), linezolid (human-equivalent of 600 mg twice daily), and vancomycin (continuous infusion targeting a serum-steady state concentration of 25 mg/L). Control animals (black); ceftaroline-treated animals (grey), linezolid-treated animals (dashed lines), vancomycin-treated animals (white). Error bars represent standard deviations (adapted from Jacqueline et al., 2007)

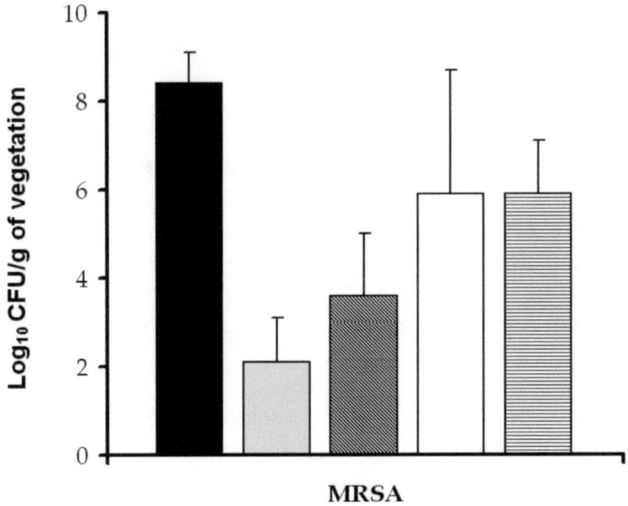

Fig. 13. Bacterial titers in vegetations infected by MRSA after 4 days of treatment with ceftobiprole medocaril (formerly BAL9141) (19 mg/kg of active drug [ceftobiprole] administered intramuscularly thrice daily), daptomycin (intravenous 18 mg/kg once daily), vancomycin (intravenous 30 mg/kg twice daily), and linezolid (75 mg/kg administered subcutaneously three times daily). Control animals (black); ceftaroline-treated animals (grey), linezolid-treated animals (dashed lines), vancomycin-treated animals (white). Error bars represent standard deviations (adapted from Tattevin et al., 2010)

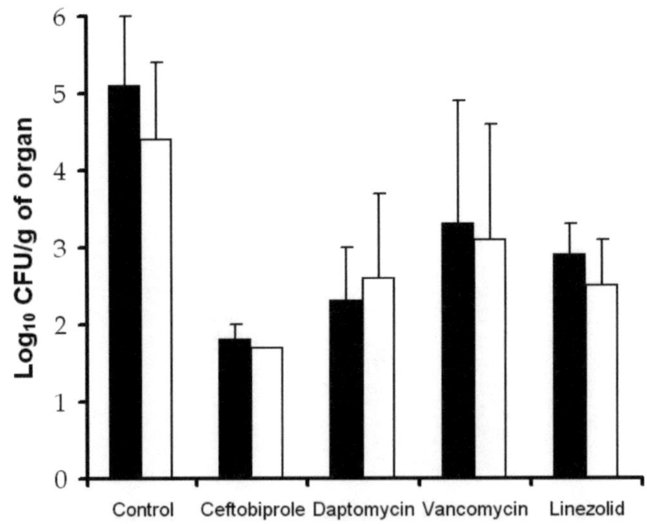

Fig. 14. Bacterial titers in spleens and kidneys after 4 days of treatment with ceftobiprole medocaril (formerly BAL9141) (19 mg/kg of active drug [ceftobiprole] administered intramuscularly thrice daily), daptomycin (intravenous 18 mg/kg once daily), vancomycin (intravenous 30 mg/kg twice daily), and linezolid (75 mg/kg administered subcutaneously three times daily). Spleen bacterial counts (black); Kidney bacterial counts (white). Error bars represent standard deviations (adapted from Tattevin et al., 2010)

Endocarditis studies evaluating the activity of ceftaroline are very limited. However, Tattevin et al have assessed the activity of ceftobiprole (formerly BAL9141), the other anti-MRSA cephalosporin with high affinity for PBP2a, against MRSA in comparison with vancomycin, linezolid, and daptomycin (Tattevin et al, 2010). Using experimental conditions similar to the conditions used by Jacqueline et al, they showed that the burdens of organisms in vegetations were significantly lower in ceftobiprole-treated rabbits than in rabbits treated with vancomycin, linezolid, or daptomycin (4-day treatment) (Figure 13). Moreover, the bacterial titers in spleens and in kidneys were significantly lower in ceftobiprole treated animals than in animals treated by linezolid or vancomycin (Figure 14). A study comparing ceftaroline and daptomycin, and using human-projected doses, demonstrated that both antimicrobial agents displayed highly bactericidal activity against *S. aureus* strains but ceftaroline achieved 100% sterilization of the vegetations infected by the MSSA, MRSA or GISA strains, whereas daptomycin sterilized 62%, 57% and 100% of the vegetations, respectively (Jacqueline et al., 2011).

7.2 Assessment of intramuscular administration of ceftaroline

Pathogens such as MRSA are becoming more virulent and are no longer confined to acute-care settings. There is a clinical need for new antibiotics that can be administered by intramuscular (IM) injection, facilitating outpatient antibiotic therapy for MRSA. The goals of the following experiments were to compare the pharmacokinetic parameters of ceftaroline after intravenous and IM administration and evaluate the in vivo activity of 3 different doses of ceftaroline against MRSA compared with teicoplanin as a positive control after IM administration by using an aortic valve endocarditis rabbit model (Jacqueline et al., 2010).

Six animals were divided into 2 groups, and a 20-mg/kg dose of the prodrug ceftaroline acetate was administered by IM injection into the right thigh or by a short intravenous infusion. Blood samples were obtained from the animals over 8 h (5, 10, 15, 30, and 45 min, and 1, 2, 4, and 8 h post-dose). Results suggest that ceftaroline has an excellent pharmacokinetic profile after IM administration. Bioavailability of IM administration exceeded 90% of intravenous infusion as calculated by AUC (Table 2). C_{max} was decreased with IM administration compared with intravenous infusion as ceftaroline was slowly released from the IM injection site. After IM administration of 5-, 20-, and 40-mg/kg doses, the C_{max} increased approximately in proportion to dose (5.18, 15.75, and 37.85 mg/L, respectively) and plasma half-life increased from 0.74 to 1.14 h (Figure 15). Compared with a short intravenous infusion, IM administration of ceftaroline resulted in longer plasma half-life and percentage of time that the concentration of ceftaroline remained above the MIC (%T>MIC), which is the most critical pharmacokinetic-pharmacodynamic parameter for efficacy (Table 2) (Andes & Craig, 2006).

Using the well-established rabbit endocarditis model, experimental endocarditis was induced with an inoculum of 10^8 CFU of a MRSA strain (ceftaroline MIC = 1 mg/L) with heterogeneous high-level methicillin resistance (methicillin MIC = 128 mg/L). Treatment was started 24 h after inoculation and antibiotics (ceftaroline and teicoplanin) were administered twice daily using the IM route for 4 days. Animals were randomly assigned to no treatment (controls), ceftaroline 40 mg/kg IM twice daily, ceftaroline 20 mg/kg IM twice daily, ceftaroline 5 mg/kg IM twice daily, or teicoplanin 20 mg/kg IM twice daily.

Pharmacokinetic parameter	Ceftaroline 20 mg/kg IM administration	IV administration
C_{max} (mg/L)	16.1 ± 0.7	84.0 ± 7. 5
T_{max} (minutes)	30	5
$t_{1/2}$ (hours)	0.9 ± 0.3	0.2 ± 0.00
$AUC_{0\text{-}8h}$ (mg•h/L)	26.5 ± 2.9	29.2 ± 3. 9
%T>MIC[a] (8-h period)	46.3 ± 2.0	22.5 ± 1.9
%T>MIC[a] (12-h period)	30.9 ± 1.3	15.0 ± 1.3

[a]Methicillin-resistant *Staphylococcus aureus* (MRSA) strain with ceftaroline MIC = 1 mg/L.
AUC = area under the concentration-time curve; C_{max} = peak concentration; T_{max} = time to peak concentration; $t_{1/2}$ = half-life; %T>MIC = time that drug levels in the serum remained above the MIC (Author's unpublished data).

Table 2. Pharmacokinetic parameters following single-dose intramuscular (IM) administration or short intravenous (IV) infusion of ceftaroline (mean ± SD)

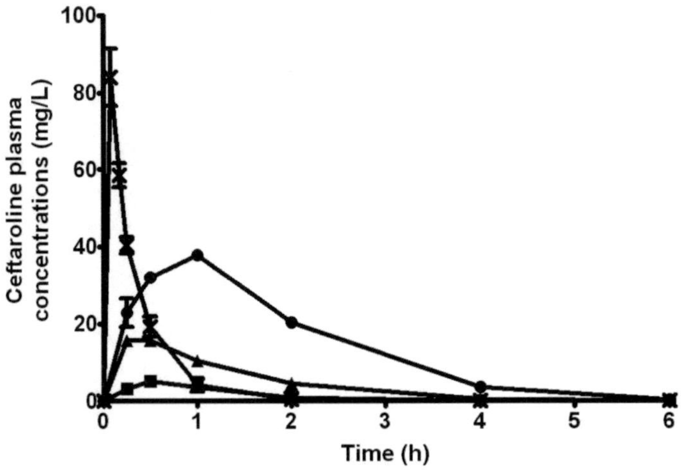

Fig. 15. Ceftaroline concentrations after intramuscular (IM) and intravenous (IV) administration in the rabbit (mean ± SD). ■ = 5-mg/kg IM dose; ▲= 20-mg/kg IM dose; • = 40-mg/kg IM dose; × = 20-mg/kg intravenous dose (Author's unpublished data)

The in vivo outcome after a 4-day treatment regimen and the rate of sterilization of the vegetations produced by the MRSA strain are shown in Table 3 (Jacqueline et al., 2010). A dose-dependent response was observed with sterilization rates for ceftaroline of 100%, 80%, and 33% for the 40-mg/kg, 20-mg/kg, and 5-mg/kg doses of ceftaroline, respectively. The difference between 20-mg/kg and 40-mg/kg doses was not statistically significant (P>0.05). In vivo bactericidal activity was consistent across all animals tested at the 40-mg/kg dose and for 9 of 10 animals at the 20-mg/kg dose of ceftaroline.

The %T>MICs attained with IM administration in this model were associated with bactericidal activity against MRSA (Tables 2 and 3). The efficacy of IM ceftaroline was similar to that achieved previously with intravenous ceftaroline administered in a regimen simulating the human dose (i.e., 600 mg twice daily) (Jacqueline et al., 2007). As expected, the positive control teicoplanin at 20 mg/kg IM displayed activity against the MRSA strain, with a sterilization rate of 60%, and bacterial titers similar to those observed with vancomycin against the same MRSA strain (Jacqueline et al., 2007). Currently, teicoplanin is the only anti-MRSA drug approved as an IM injection; however, it is not available in the United States. Ceftaroline may be a valuable option for the IM treatment of MRSA infections. These findings are consistent with a favorable IM pharmacokinetic profile and strongly support the development of IM ceftaroline as a promising and effective therapeutic option for the treatment of severe MRSA infections.

Regimen	Mean ± SD $\log_{10}$ CFU/g of vegetation (no. of sterile veg./total no. of veg.) (%)
Controls	8.99 ± 0.47 (0/10) (0)
IM ceftaroline 40 mg/kg	2.45 ± 0.14 (10/10) (100)[a,b,c]
IM ceftaroline 20 mg/kg	3.14 ± 1.38 (8/10) (80)[a,d]
IM ceftaroline 5 mg/kg	5.26 ± 2.73 (3/9) (33)[a]
IM teicoplanin 20 mg/kg	3.07 ± 0.66 (6/10) (60)[a,d]

[a] *P*<0.001 vs controls; [b] *P*<0.001 vs IM ceftaroline 5-mg/kg regimen; Bonferroni's test after analysis of variance. [c] The titers for vegetations from all animals in the group were below the limit of detection. [d] *P*<0.05 vs IM ceftaroline 5-mg/kg regimen. IM = intramuscular.

Table 3. Bacterial titers in vegetations after 4 days of treatment with IM ceftaroline (5, 20, and 40 mg/kg) and IM teicoplanin (20 mg/kg) (adapted from Jacqueline et al., 2010)

8. Conclusions

Antimicrobial therapy is the cornerstone of the treatment of infective endocarditis. Although vancomycin still remains the standard treatment for severe MRSA infections, new therapeutic options are now available for the treatment of MRSA infective endocarditis. Introduction of linezolid, the first member of the oxazolidinone class, in the early 2000s, opened a new field of investigation that demonstrated that vancomycin was not the only solution against MRSA infections. Although linezolid was not the most effective option for endocarditis treatment, studies with the oxazolidinone demonstrated that experimental animal models are essential to (i) develop better understanding of the in vivo activity of a new drug, (ii) obtain important information not present in clinical trials.

Among the new recently available antimicrobial agents, experimental data strongly support daptomycin as an effective option in the treatment of MRSA endocarditis. The lipopeptide demonstrated homogeneous in vivo bactericidal activity against *S. aureus*, including methicillin-susceptible, methicillin-resistant, and glycopeptide-intermediate strains. Taking advantage of favourable drug pharmacokinetics (once-daily administration), daptomycin should be considered as a valuable alternative to vancomycin. Nevertheless, clinical use of daptomycin merit further investigation due to unresolved questions, such as adequate dosing, emergence of resistance during treatment, and appropriate combination therapy.

Ceftaroline fosamil (prodrug of the active metabolite) is a new, broad-spectrum cephalosporin recently approved in the USA for the treatment of acute bacterial skin and skin structure infections and community-acquired bacterial pneumonia. Data from both clinical trials (Corey et al., 2010; Wilcox et al., 2010; Rank et al., 2011) and animal studies confirmed ceftaroline as a very promising new cephalosporin for the treatment of serious MRSA infections. Given its safety profile, bactericidal activity, and excellent activity against *S. aureus*, ceftaroline should play an important role in the treatment of MRSA infective endocarditis in the coming years.

9. References

Adembri, C., Fallani, S., Cassetta, M.I., Arrigucci, S., Ottaviano, A., Pecile, P., Mazzei, T., De Gaudio, R. & Novelli, A. (2008). Linezolid pharmacokinetic/pharmacodynamic profile in critically ill septic patients: intermittent versus continuous infusion. *International Journal of Antimicrobial Agents*, Vol.31, No.2, pp. 122-129.

Andes, D. & Craig, W.A. (2006). Pharmacodynamics of a new cephalosporin, PPI-0903 (TAK-599), active against methicillin-resistant *Staphylococcus aureus* in murine thigh and lung infection models: identification of an *in vivo* pharmacokinetic-pharmacodynamic target. *Antimicrobial Agents and Chemotherapy*, Vol.50, No.4, pp. 1376–1383.

Aoki, H., Ke, L., Poppe, S.M., Poel, T.J., Weaver, E.A., Gadwood, R.C., Thomas, R.C., Shinabarger, D.L. & Ganoza, M.C. (2002). Oxazolidinone antibiotics target the P site on *Escherichia coli* ribosomes. *Antimicrobial Agents and Chemotherapy*, Vol.46, No.4, pp. 1080–1085.

Batard, E., Jacqueline, C., Boutoille, D., Hamel, A., Drugeon, H.B., Asseray, N., Leclercq, R., Caillon, J., Potel, G. & Bugnon, D. (2002). Combination of quinupristin-dalfopristin and gentamicin against methicillin-resistant *Staphylococcus aureus*: Experimental rabbit endocarditis study. *Antimicrobial Agents and Chemotherapy*, Vol.46, No.7, pp. 2174-2178.

Benquan, W., Yingchun, T., Kouxing, Z., Tiantuo, Z., Jiaxing, Z. & Shuqing, T. (2002). *Staphylococcus* heterogeneously resistant to vancomycin in China and antimicrobial activities of imipenem and vancomycin in combination against it. *Journal of Clinical Microbiology*, Vol.40, No.3, pp. 1109-1112.

Benvenuto, M., Benziger, D.P., Yankelev, S. & Vigliani, G. (2006). Pharmacokinetics and tolerability of daptomycin at doses up to 12 milligrams per kilogram of body weight once daily in healthy volunteers. *Antimicrobial Agents and Chemotherapy*, Vol.50, No.10, pp. 3245-3249.

Bouanchaud, D.H. (1992). *In-vitro* and *in-vivo* synergic activity and fractional inhibitory concentration (FIC) of the components of a semisynthetic streptogramin, RP 59500. *Journal of Antimicrobial Chemotherapy*, Vol.30 (Suppl. A), pp. 95–99.

Bugnon, D., Potel, G., Caillon, J., Baron, D., Drugeon, H.B., Feigel, P., Kergueris, M.F. (1998). *In vivo* simulation of human pharmacokinetics in the rabbit. *Bulletin of Mathematical Biology*, Vol.60, No.3, pp. 545-567.

Boucher, H.W., Talbot, G.H., Bradley, J.S., Edwards, J.E., Gilbert, D., Rice, L.B., Scheld, M., Spellberg, B. & Bartlett, J. (2009). Bad bugs, no drugs: no ESKAPE! An update from the Infectious Diseases Society of America. *Clinical Infectious Diseases*, Vol.48, No.1, pp. 1-12.

Carbon, C. (1990). Impact of the antibiotic schedule on efficacy in experimental endocarditis. *Scandinavian Journal of Infectious Diseases*, Suppl. 74, pp. 163–172.

Cappelletty, D.M., Kang, S.L., Palmer, S.M. & Rybak, M.J. (1995). Pharmacodynamics of ceftazidime administered as continuous infusion or intermittent bolus alone and in combination with single daily-dose amikacin against *Pseudomonas aeruginosa* in an *in vitro* infection model. *Antimicrobial Agents and Chemotherapy*, Vol.39, No.8, pp. 1797–1801.

Cervera, C., Castañeda, X., Pericas, J.M., Del Río, A., de la Maria, C.G., Mestres, C., Falces, C., Marco, F., Moreno, A. & Miró, J.M. (2011). Clinical utility of daptomycin in infective endocarditis caused by Gram-positive cocci. *International Journal of Antimicrobial Agents*, [Epub ahead of print].

Chiang, F.Y. & Climo, M. (2003). Efficacy of linezolid alone or in combination with vancomycin for treatment of experimental endocarditis due to methicillin-resistant *Staphylococcus aureus*. *Antimicrobial Agents and Chemotherapy*, Vol.47, No.9, pp. 3002-3004.

Corey, G.R., Wilcox, M.H., Talbot, G.H, Thye, D., Friedland, D., Baculik, T. & CANVAS 1 investigators. (2010). CANVAS 1: the first Phase III, randomized, double-blind study evaluating ceftaroline fosamil for the treatment of patients with complicated skin and skin structure infections. *Journal of Antimicrobial Chemotherapy*, 65 Suppl 4, pp. 41-51.

Cubist Pharmaceuticals. (2003). Cubicin (daptomycin for injection). *Cubist Pharmaceuticals*, Lexington, MA, USA.

Cunha, B.A., Eisenstein, L.E. & Hamid, N.S. (2006). Pacemaker-induced *Staphylococcus aureus* mitral valve acute bacterial endocarditis complicated by persistent bacteremia from a coronary stent: Cure with prolonged/high-dose daptomycin without toxicity. *Heart Lung*, Vol.35, No.3, pp. 207-211.

Dailey, C.F., Dileto-Fang, C.L., Buchanan, L.V., Oramas-Shirey, M.P., Batts, D.H., Ford, C.W. & Gibson, J.K. (2001). Efficacy of linezolid in treatment of experimental endocarditis caused by methicillin-resistant *Staphylococcus aureus*. *Antimicrobial Agents and Chemotherapy*, Vol.45, No.8, pp. 2304-2308.

Dailey, C.F., Pagano, P.J., Buchanan, L.V., Paquette, J.A., Haas, J.V. & Gibson, J.K. (2003). Efficacy of linezolid plus rifampin in an experimental model of methicillin-susceptible *Staphylococcus aureus* endocarditis. *Antimicrobial Agents and Chemotherapy*, Vol.47, No.8, pp. 2655-2658.

Darville, T. & Yamauchi, T. (1994). The cephalosporin antibiotics. *Pediatrics in Review*, Vol.15, No.2, pp. 54-62.

Durack, D.T. & Beeson, P.B. (1972). Experimental bacterial endocarditis. I. Colonization of a sterile vegetation. *British Journal of Experimental Pathology*, Vol.53, No.1, pp. 44-49.

Durack, D.T. & Beeson, P.B. (1972). Experimental bacterial endocarditis. II. Survival of a bacterium in endocardial vegetations. *British Journal of Experimental Pathology*, Vol.53, No.1, pp. 50-53.

Entenza, J.M., Que, Y.A., Vouillamoz, J., Glauser, M.P. & Moreillon P. (2001). Efficacies of moxifloxacin, ciprofloxacin, and vancomycin against experimental endocarditis due to methicillin-resistant *Staphylococcus aureus* expressing various degrees of ciprofloxacin resistance. *Antimicrobial Agents and Chemotherapy*, Vol.45, No.11, pp. 3076-3083.

Fowler, V.G. Jr., Scheld, W.M. & Bayer, A.S. (2005). Endocarditis and intravascular infections, In: *Mandell, Douglas, and Bennett's Principles and Practice of Infectious Diseases, Sixth Edition*, pp. 975–1022, Philadelphia: Elsevier Churchill Livingstone.

Garrison, P.K. & Freedman, L.R. (1970). Experimental endocarditis I. Staphylococcal endocarditis in rabbits resulting from placement of a polyethylene catheter in the right side of the heart. *Yale Journal of Biology and Medicine*, Vol.42, No.6, pp. 394-410.

Gonzalez, L.S. 3rd. & Spencer, J.P. (1998). Aminoglycosides: a practical review. *American Family Physician*, Vol.58, No.8, pp. 1811-1820.

Grohs, P., Kitzis, M.D. & Gutmann, L. (2003). *In vitro* bactericidal activities of linezolid in combination with vancomycin, gentamicin, ciprofloxacin, fusidic acid, and rifampin against *Staphylococcus aureus*. *Antimicrobial Agents and Chemotherapy*, Vol.47, No.1, pp. 418-420.

Heep, M., Rieger, U., Beck, D. & Lehn, N. (2000). Mutations in the beginning of the rpoB gene can induce resistance to rifamycins in both *Helicobacter pylori* and *Mycobacterium tuberculosis*. *Antimicrobial Agents and Chemotherapy*, Vol.44, No.4, pp. 1075-1077.

Hiramatsu, K., Hanaki, H., Ino, T., Yabuta, K., Oguri, T. & Tenover, F. C. (1997). Methicillin-resistant *Staphylococcus aureus* clinical strain with reduced vancomycin susceptibility. *Journal of Antimicrobial Chemotherapy*, Vol.40, No.1, pp. 135–136.

Jacqueline, C., Batard, E., Perez, L., Boutoille, D., Hamel, A., Caillon, J., Kergueris, M.F., Potel, G. & Bugnon, D. (2002). *In vivo* efficacy of continuous infusion versus intermittent dosing of linezolid compared to vancomycin in a methicillin resistant *Staphylococcus aureus* rabbit endocarditis model. *Antimicrobial Agents and Chemotherapy*, Vol.46, No.12, pp. 3706-3712.

Jacqueline, C., Caillon, J., Le Mabecque, V., Miegeville, A.F., Donnio, P.Y., Bugnon, D. & Potel, G. (2003). *In vitro* activity of linezolid alone and in combination with gentamicin, vancomycin or rifampicin against methicillin-resistant *Staphylococcus aureus* by time-kill curve methods. *Journal of Antimicrobial Chemotherapy*, Vol.51, No.4, pp. 857-864.

Jacqueline, C., Asseray, N., Batard, E., Le Mabecque, V., Kergueris, M.F., Dube, L., Bugnon, D., Potel, G. & Caillon, J. (2004). *In vivo* efficacy of linezolid in combination with gentamicin for the treatment of experimental endocarditis due to methicillin-resistant *Staphylococcus aureus*. *International Journal of Antimicrobial Agents*, Vol.24, No.4, pp. 393-396.

Jacqueline, C., Navas, D., Batard, E., Miegeville, A.F., Le Mabecque, V., Kergueris, M.F., Bugnon, D., Potel, G. & Caillon, J. (2005). *In vitro* and *in vivo* synergistic activities of linezolid combined with subinhibitory concentrations of imipenem against methicillin-resistant *Staphylococcus aureus*. *Antimicrobial Agents and Chemotherapy*, Vol.49, No.1, pp. 45-51.

Jacqueline, C., Caillon, J., Grossi, O., Le Mabecque, V., Miegeville, A.F., Bugnon, D., Batard, E. & Potel, G. (2006). *In vitro* and *in vivo* assessment of linezolid combined with ertapenem: a highly synergistic combination against methicillin-resistant *Staphylococcus aureus*. *Antimicrobial Agents and Chemotherapy*, Vol.50, No.7, pp. 2547-2549.

Jacqueline, C., Caillon, J., Le Mabecque, V., Miègeville, A.F., Hamel, A., Bugnon, D., Ge, J.Y. & Potel G. (2007). *In vivo* efficacy of ceftaroline (PPI-0903), a new broad-spectrum cephalosporin, compared with linezolid and vancomycin against methicillin-resistant and vancomycin-intermediate *Staphylococcus aureus* in a rabbit endocarditis model. *Antimicrobial Agents and Chemotherapy*, Vol.51, No.9, pp. 3397-3400.

Jacqueline, C., Caillon, J., Batard, E., Le Mabecque, V., Amador, G., Ge, Y., Biek, D. & Potel, G. (2010). Evaluation of the in vivo efficacy of intramuscularly administered ceftaroline fosamil, a novel cephalosporin, against a methicillin-resistant *Staphylococcus aureus* strain in a rabbit endocarditis model. *Journal of Antimicrobial Chemotherapy*, Vol.65, No.10, pp. 2264-2265.

Jacqueline, C., Amador, G., Batard, E., Le Mabecque, V., Miègeville, A.F., Biek, D., Caillon, J. & Potel G. (2011). Comparison of ceftaroline fosamil, daptomycin and tigecycline in an experimental rabbit endocarditis model caused by methicillin-susceptible, methicillin-resistant and glycopeptide-intermediate *Staphylococcus aureus*. *Journal of Antimicrobial Chemotherapy*, Vol.66, No.4, pp. 863-866.

Kaatz, G.W., Seo, S.M., Reddy, V.N., Bailey, E.M. & Rybak, M.J. (1990). Daptomycin compared with teicoplanin and vancomycin for therapy of experimental *Staphylococcus aureus* endocarditis. *Antimicrobial Agents and Chemotherapy*, Vol.34, No.11, pp. 2081-2085.

Kaatz, G.W. & Seo, S.M. (1996). *In vitro* activities of oxazolidinone compounds U100592 and U100766 against *Staphylococcus aureus* and *Staphylococcus epidermidis*. *Antimicrobial Agents and Chemotherapy*, vol.40, No.3, pp. 799–801.

Kennedy, S. & Chambers, H.F. (1989). Daptomycin (LY146032) for prevention and treatment of experimental aortic valve endocarditis in rabbits. *Antimicrobial Agents and Chemotherapy*, Vol.33, No.9, pp. 1522-1525.

LaPlante, K.L. & Woodmansee, S. (2009). Activities of daptomycin and vancomycin alone and in combination with rifampin and gentamicin against biofilm-forming methicillin-resistant *Staphylococcus aureus* isolates in an experimental model of endocarditis. *Antimicrobial Agents and Chemotherapy*, Vol.53, no.9, pp. 3880-3886.

Lefort, A., & Fantin, B. (1999). Rabbit model of bacterial endocarditis, In: *Handbook of animal models of infection*, O. Zak & M.A. Sande, (Ed.), 611-617, ISBN 0-12-775390-7.

Lim, D. & Strynadka, N.C. (2002). Structural basis for the beta lactam resistance of PBP2a from methicillin-resistant *Staphylococcus aureus*. *Nature Structural Biology*, Vol.9, No.11, pp. 870-876.

McConeghy, K.W. & LaPlante, K.L. (2010). *In vitro* activity of tigecycline in combination with gentamicin against biofilm-forming *Staphylococcus aureus*. *Diagnostic Microbiology and Infectious Disease*, Vol.68, No.1, pp. 1–6.

Malbruny, B.; Canu, A., Bozdogan, B., Zarrouk, V., Fantin, B. & Leclercq, R. (2000). Quinupristin/Dalfopristin resistance Mutation Reveals the Involvement of L22 Ribosomal Protein in Synergy Between Quinupristin and Dalfopristin, *Proceedings of 40th Interscience Conference Antimicrobial Agents and Chemotherapy*, p. 118, Abstr. No. 1928, Toronto, Ontario, Canada, September 17-20, 2000.

Maltezou, H.C. (2009). Metallo-beta-lactamases in Gram-negative bacteria: introducing the era of pan-resistance? *International Journal of Antimicrobial Agents*, Vol.33, No.5, pp. 405-407.

Miró, J.M., García-de-la-Mària, C., Armero, Y., Soy, D., Moreno, A., del Río, A., Almela, M., Sarasa, M., Mestres, C.A., Gatell, J.M., Jiménez de Anta, M.T., Marco, F. & Hospital

Clinic Experimental Endocarditis Study Group. (2009). Addition of gentamicin or rifampin does not enhance the effectiveness of daptomycin in treatment of experimental endocarditis due to methicillin-resistant *Staphylococcus aureus*. *Antimicrobial Agents and Chemotherapy*, Vol.53, No.10, pp. 4172-4177.

Miró, J.M., Entenza, J.M., del Río, A., García-de-la-Mària, C., Giddey, M., Armero, Y., Cervera, C., Mestres, C.A., Almela, M., Falces, C., Marco, F., Moreillon, P. & Moreno, A. (2009). Daptomycin (DAP) plus Fosfomycin (FOM) is Synergistic against Methicillin-Susceptible (MSSA) and Methicillin-Resistant *Staphylococcus aureus* (MRSA) Strains: From Bench to Bedside. *Proceedings of 49th Interscience Conference Antimicrobial Agents and Chemotherapy*, Abstr. No. E-1449, San Francisco, CA, USA, September 12-15, 2009.

Murphy, T.M., Deitz, J.M., Petersen, P.J., Mikels, S.M. & Weiss, W.J. (2000). Therapeutic efficacy of GAR-936, a novel glycylcycline, in a rat model of experimental endocarditis. *Antimicrobial Agents and Chemotherapy*, Vol.44, No.11, pp. 3022-3027.

Nakazawa, H., Kikuchi, Y., Honda, T., Isago, T. & Nozaki, M. (2003). Enhancement of antimicrobial effects of various antibiotics against methicillin-resistant *Staphylococcus aureus* (MRSA) by combination with fosfomycin. *Journal of Infection and Chemotherapy*, Vol.9, No.4, pp. 304-309.

Paterson, D.L. (2006). Clinical experience with recently approved antibiotics. *Current Opinion in Pharmacology*, Vol.6, No.5, pp. 486–490.

Pavie, J., Lefort, A., Zarrouk, V., Chau, F., Garry, L., Leclercq, R. & Fantin, B. (2002). Efficacies of quinupristin-dalfopristin combined with vancomycin *in vitro* and in experimental endocarditis due to methicillin-resistant *Staphylococcus aureus* in relation to cross-resistance to macrolides, lincosamides, and streptogramin B- type antibiotics. *Antimicrobial Agents and Chemotherapy*, Vol.46, No.9, pp. 3061-3064.

Rank, D.R., Friedland, H.D. & Laudano, J.B. (2011). Integrated safety summary of FOCUS 1 and FOCUS 2 trials: Phase III randomized, double-blind studies evaluating ceftaroline fosamil for the treatment of patients with community-acquired pneumonia. *Journal of Antimicrobial Chemother*, 66 Suppl 3, pp. 53-59.

Rello, J. (2005). Pharmacokinetics, pharmacodynamics, safety, and tolerability of tigecycline. *Journal of Chemotherapy*, Vol.17 (Suppl 1), pp. 12–22.

Rochon-Edouard, S., Pestel-Caron, M., Lemeland, J.F. & Caron, F. (2000). *In vitro* synergistic effects of double and triple combinations of beta-lactams, vancomycin, and netilmicin against methicillin-resistant *Staphylococcus aureus* strains. *Antimicrobial Agents and Chemotherapy*, Vol.44, No.11, pp. 3055-3060.

Sahuquillo Arce, J.M., Colombo Gainza, E., Gil Brusola, A., Ortiz Estévez, R., Cantón, E. & Gobernado, M. (2006). *In vitro* activity of linezolid in combination with doxycycline, fosfomycin, levofloxacin, rifampicin and vancomycin against methicillin-susceptible *Staphylococcus aureus*. *Revista Espanola de Quimioterapia*, Vol.19, No.3, pp. 252-257.

Sakoulas, G., Eliopoulos, G.M., Alder, J. & Eliopoulos, C.T. (2003). Efficacy of daptomycin in experimental endocarditis due to methicillin-resistant *Staphylococcus aureus*. *Antimicrobial Agents and Chemotherapy*, Vol.47, No.5, pp. 1714-1718.

Silverman, J.A., Perlmutter, N.G. & Shapiro, H.M. (2003). Correlation of daptomycin bactericidal activity and membrane depolarization in *Staphylococcus aureus*. *Antimicrobial Agents and Chemotherapy*, Vol.47, No.8, pp. 2538-2544.

Singh, S.R., Bacon, A.E. 3rd., Young, D.C. & Couch, K.A. (2009). *In vitro* 24-hour time-kill studies of vancomycin and linezolid in combination versus methicillin-resistant *Staphylococcus aureus. Antimicrobial Agents and Chemotherapy*, Vol.53, No.10, pp. 4495-4497.

Slover, C.M., Rodvold, K.A. & Danziger, L.H. (2007). Tigecycline: a novel broad-spectrum antimicrobial. *Annals of Pharmacotherapy*, Vol.41, No.6, pp. 965-972.

Soriano, A., Jurado, A., Marco, F., Almela, M., Ortega, M. & Mensa, J. (2005). *In vitro* activity of linezolid, moxifloxacin, levofloxacin, clindamycin and rifampin, alone and in combination, against *Staphylococcus aureus* and *Staphylococcus epidermidis. Revista Espanola de Quimioterapia*, Vol.18, No.2, pp. 168-172.

Spratt, B.G. (1977). Properties of the penicillin binding proteins of *Escherichia coli* K12. *European Journal of Biochemistry*, Vol.72, No.2, pp. 342-352.

Tally, F.P. & DeBruin, M.F. (2000). Development of daptomycin for Gram-positive infections. *Journal of Antimicrobial Chemotherapy*, Vol.46, No.4, pp. 523–526.

Tattevin, P., Basuino, L., Bauer, D., Diep, B.A. & Chambers, H.F. (2010). Ceftobiprole is superior to vancomycin, daptomycin, and linezolid for treatment of experimental endocarditis in rabbits caused by methicillin-resistant *Staphylococcus aureus. Antimicrobial Agents and Chemotherapy*, Vol.54, No.2, pp. 610-613.

The 10 x '20 Initiative: pursuing a global commitment to develop 10 new antibacterial drugs by 2020. (2010). Infectious Diseases Society of America. *Clinical Infectious Diseases*, Vol.50, No.8, pp. 1081-1083.

Totsuka, K., Shiseki, M., Kikuchi, K. & Matsui, Y. (1999). Combined effects of vancomycin and imipenem against methicillin-resistant *Staphylococcus aureus* (MRSA) *in vitro* and *in vivo. Journal of Antimicrobial Chemotherapy*, Vol.44, No.4, pp. 455-460.

Tsaganos, T., Skiadas, I., Koutoukas, P., Adamis, T., Baxevanos, N., Tzepi, I., Pelekanou, A., Giamarellos-Bourboulis, E.J., Giamarellou, H. & Kanellakopoulou, K. (2008). Efficacy and pharmacodynamics of linezolid, alone and in combination with rifampicin, in an experimental model of methicillin-resistant *Staphylococcus aureus* endocarditis. *Journal of Antimicrobial Chemotherapy*, Vol.62, No.2, pp. 381-383.

The bacterial challenge: time to react, In: European Centre for Disease Prevention and Control, European Medicines Agency Joint Technical report, September 2009, Available from
http://www.emea.europa.eu/pdfs/human/antimicrobial resistance.

Uete, T. & Matsuo, K. (1995). Synergistic enhancement of *in vitro* antimicrobial activity of imipenem and cefazolin, cephalothin, cefotiam, cefamandole or cefoperazone in combination against methicillin-sensitive and -resistant *Staphylococcus aureus. Japanese Journal of Antibiotics*, Vol.48, No.3, pp. 402-408.

Villegas-Estrada, A., Lee, M., Hesek, D., Vakulenko, S.B. & Mobashery, S. (2008). Co-opting the cell wall in fighting methicillin-resistant *Staphylococcus aureus*: potent inhibition of PBP 2a by two anti-MRSA beta-lactam antibiotics. *Journal of the American Chemical Society*, Vol.130, No.29, pp. 9212-9213.

Wilcox, M.H., Corey, G.R., Talbot, G.H., Thye, D., Friedland, D., Baculik, T. & CANVAS 2 investigators. (2010). CANVAS 2: the second Phase III, randomized, double-blind study evaluating ceftaroline fosamil for the treatment of patients with complicated skin and skin structure infections. *Journal of Antimicrobial Chemotherapy*, 65 Suppl 4, pp. 53-65.

Zak, O., Sande, M., & O'Reilly, T. (1999). Introduction: the role of animal models in the evaluation of new antibiotics, In: *Handbook of animal models of infection*, O. Zak & M.A. Sande, (Ed.), 611-617, ISBN 0-12-775390-7.

Zhanel, G.G., Homenuik, K., Nichol, K., Noreddin, A., Vercaigne, L., Embil, J., Gin, A., Karlowsky, J.A. & Hoban, D.J. (2004). The glycylcyclines: a comparative review with the tetracyclines. *Drugs*, Vol.64, No.1, pp. 63-88.

Zhanel, G.G., Johanson, C., Embil, J.M., Noreddin, A., Gin, A., Vercaigne, L. & Hoban, D.J. (2005). Ertapenem: review of a new carbapenem. *Expert Review of Anti-Infective Therapy*, Vol.3, No.1, pp. 23-39.

Zyvox [package insert]. (2000). *Pharmacia & Upjohn Company*, Kalamazoo, MI, USA.

7

Ocular Complications of Endocarditis

Ozlem Sahin
Middle East Technical University Health Sciences Department of Ophthalmology, Ankara Turkey

1. Introduction

Cardiac complications are the most common complications in patients with infective endocarditis, and they can be related to significant mortality and morbidity. (1) Extra-cardiac manifestations along with their historical descriptions such as splinter hemorrhages, emboli, Osler's nodes, Janeway and Bowman lesions of the eye, Roth's spots, patechiae and clubbing generally result from thromboemboli or septic emboli. (2) Inflammatory complications may occur as a result of septic emboli, and these include endogenous (metastatic) endophthalmitis, focal abscess, and vasculitis. (3) In this chapter we mainly focus on the endogenous endophthalmitis arising as a complication of infective endocarditis.

Endogenous (metastatic) endophthalmitis is an inflammatory condition of the intraocular structures including the aqueous, iris, lens, ciliary body, vitreous, choroid and retina. (4-6) It results from the hematogenous spread of organisms from a distant source of infection, most commonly infective endocarditis, gastrointestinal tract and urinary tract infections and wound infections. (7-9) Other sources of infection have included pharyngitis, pneumonia, septic arthritis and meningitis. (10,11) Compared with endophthalmitis following trauma or surgery, endogenous endophthalmitis is relatively rare, accounting 2-8% of all reported endophthalmitis cases. (5) However, endogenous endophthalmitis carries with it the danger of bilateral infection in 15-25% of cases. (6,12)

2. Epidemiology

Endogenous endophthalmitis has been reported to occur at any age and no sexual predilection. (13) However, in the recent years the mean age of endogenous endophthalmitis has shifted to 65 years possibly because of the reduction in the incidence of rheumatic heart disease. (14)

The mean incidence of endogenous endophthalmitis was reported as1.8 cases/year, and 48.1% of patients presented were seen as outpatients. (15) Endogenous bacterial endophthalmitis is recognized as a major cause of visual loss with an associated high mortality rate. (16,17) It is considered a diagnostic challenge in the early stages of the disease, with 16% to 63% of cases being initially misdiagnosed (18). In unilateral cases, the right eye is twice as likely to become infected as the left eye, probably because of the more proximal location and direct blood flow to the right carotid artery. (19)

3. Classification of endogenous endophthalmitis

A classification system introduced by Greenwald et al. takes into consideration the affected areas of the globe and the associated visual prognosis. (20) It is divided as focal anterior or posterior, diffuse anterior or posterior and panophthalmitis. (20) Anterior focal endophthalmitis manifests as localized inflammatory nodules or plaques in the iris and /or ciliary body associated with iridocyclitis and minimal hypopyon. (5,21) (Fig. 1) Intraocular pressure varies from normal to high. (5,21) The anterior vitreous has no or minimal inflammation. (5,21) The retina is normal. (5,21) The prognosis in these cases is good. (21) Anterior diffuse endophthalmitis is characterized by a more severe anterior segment inflammation associated with conjunctival chemosis, marked anterior chamber reaction with fibrin clots and significant hypopyon that hampers the view of retina. (5,21) (Fig. 2)

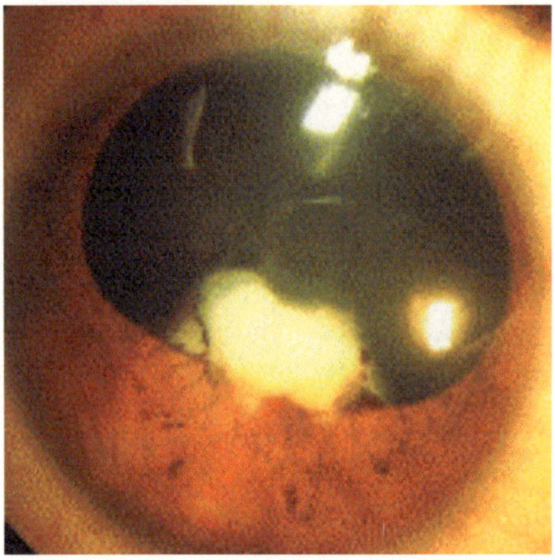

Fig. 1. Anterior focal endophthalmitis presented with an inflammatory nodule in the iris extending from the ciliary body

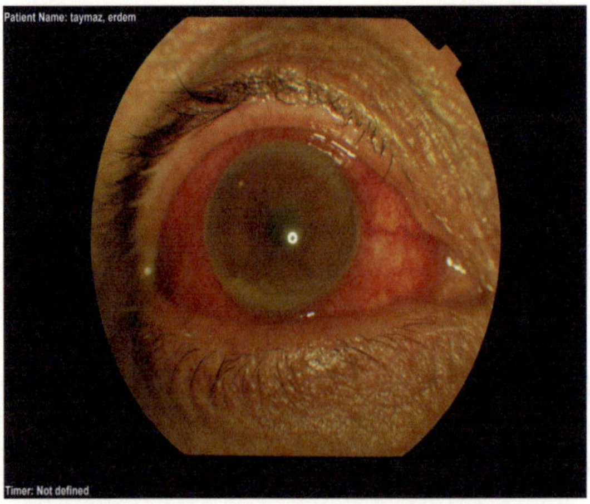

Fig. 2. Anterior diffuse endophthalmitis with a more severe anterior segment inflammation associated with conjunctival chemosis, marked anterior chamber reaction with fibrin clots and significant hypopyon

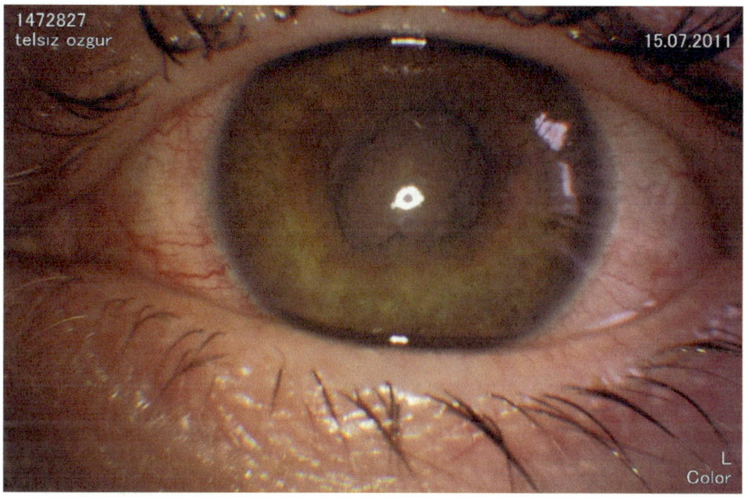

Fig. 3. Anterior diffuse endophthalmitis with posterior synechia and corneal haze

Intraocular pressure is typically elevated. (22) Corneal opacification may occur. (22) (Fig. 3) It is an ocular emergency and if not promptly and adequately treated the infection can spread to the entire eye. (22) The visual prognosis is excellent with aggressive and appropriate treatment. Blindness usually results from delay in treatment. (22) Posterior focal endophthalmitis manifests as white-yellowish retinal or choroidal lesions associated with retinal hemorrhages and vitreous cells and/or debris. (23) (Fig. 4) Infections caused by Gram-positive organisms may show multifocal lesions. (23) However, Gram-negative infections usually cause a single large choroidal abscess involving the posterior pole. (24,25) (Fig. 5) The anterior chamber reaction is usually mild with or without keratic precipitates. (23) (Fig. 6) The intraocular pressure varies from low to normal. (23) Posterior diffuse endophthalmitis may present as multiple whitish lesions located inside the vessels or in the

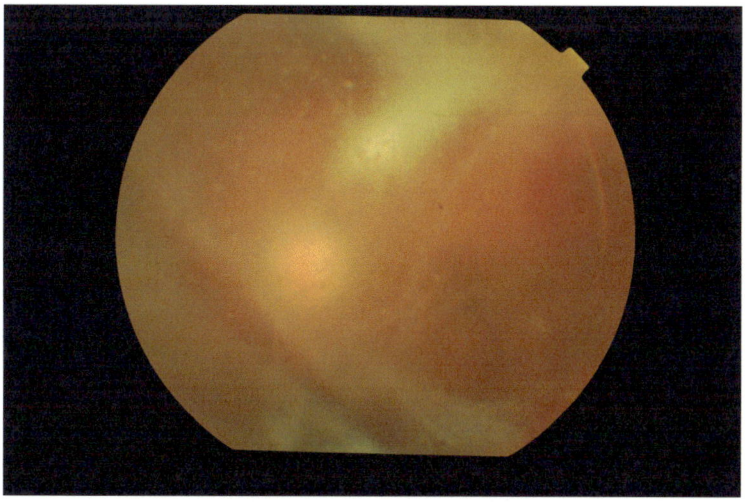

Fig. 4. Posterior focal endophthalmitis manifested as white-yellowish retinal or choroidal lesions associated with vitreous cells and/or debris

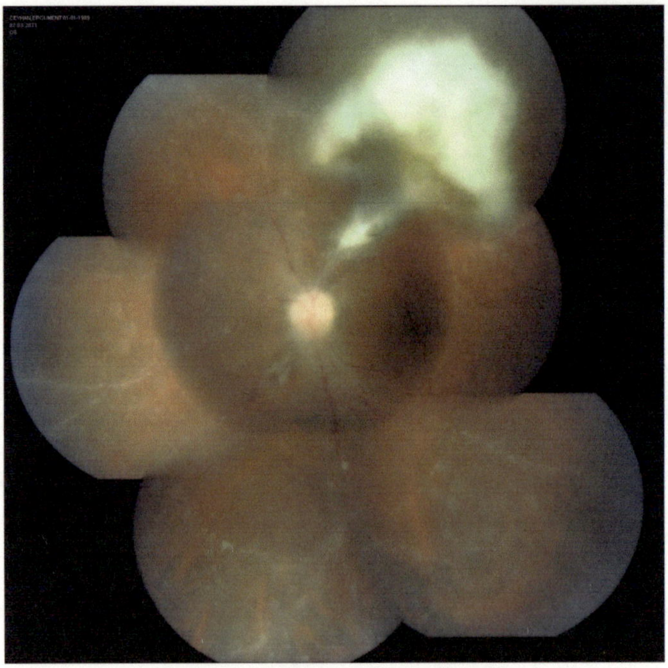

Fig. 5. A single large choroidal abscess involving the posterior pole

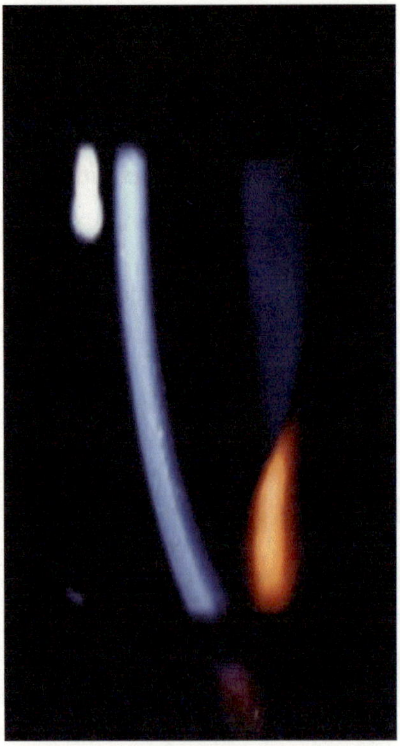

Fig. 6. Mild anterior chamber reaction with keratic precipitates

retina with perivascular hemorrhages in the early stages of the disease. (26) As the infection progresses, the retina becomes necrotic, and vitreous abscess frequently occur. (26) (Fig. 7) The anterior segment is also involved with forward spread of the infection and hypopyon is formed as the disease progresses. (26) (Fig. 8) The intraocular pressure is low. (26) The poor visual prognosis is most likely due to retinal ischemia as a result of occlusion of central retinal artery by a septic embolus. (26) Panophthalmitis is inflammation of all coats of the eye including intraocular structures. (27-29) It presents with marked lid edema, proptosis and limitation of ocular movements. (28) (Fig. 9) All details of anterior as well as posterior chamber are lost because of the prominent hypopyon. (29) (Fig. 10) Typically the intraocular pressure is high. (29)It is a disastrous and rapidly developing infection that destroys the globe and invades the orbit, resulting in blindness, phthisis or enucleation. (28,29) Depending of the virulence of pathogen, progression of panophthalmitis may be life threatening. (28)

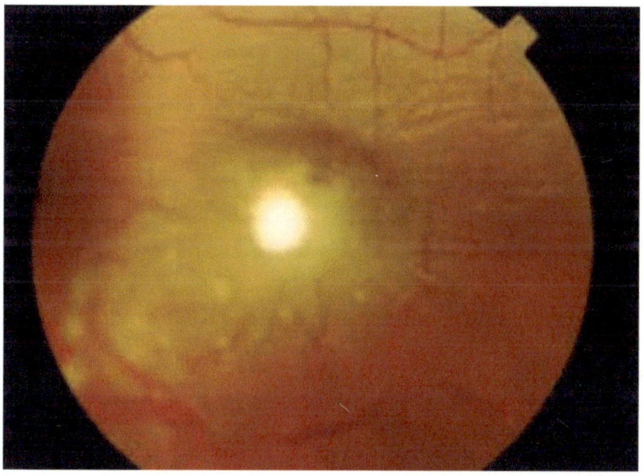

Fig. 7. Necrotic / hemorrhagic retina with vitreous abscess

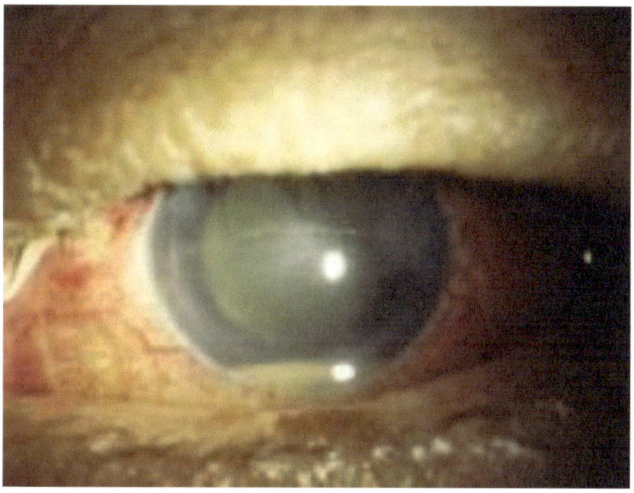

Fig. 8. Forward spread of infection with hypopyon formation

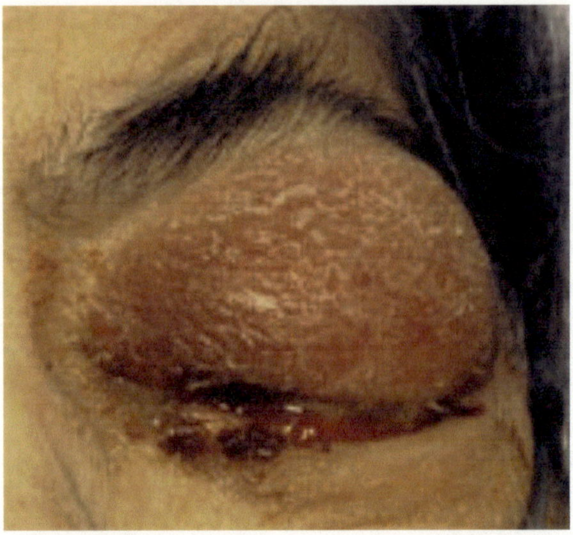

Fig. 9. Panophthalmitis with marked lid edema and proptosis

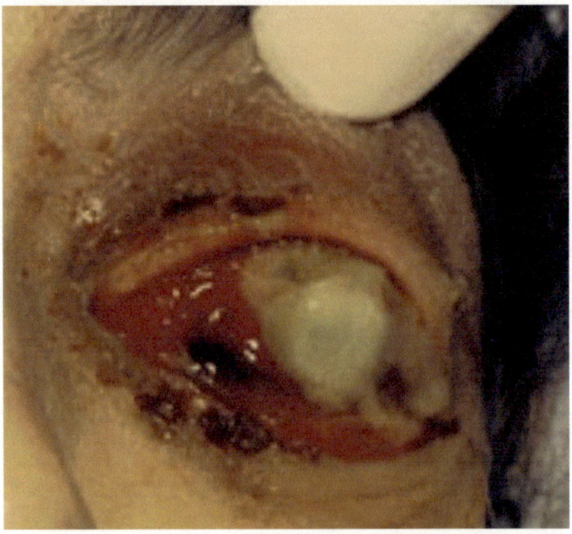

Fig. 10. Severe panophthalmitis with loss of the details of anterior and posterior segments of the eye

4. Pathogenesis

In endogenous endophthalmitis the microorganisms enter into the uveal tract or retinal circulation as scattered organisms or in a bolus, and lodge in small capillaries. (30,31) To invade ocular tissues and produce infection the organisms must cross the blood-ocular barrier either by direct invasion (septic emboli) or by changes in vascular endothelium caused by substrates released during infection. (30) They establish a septic focus that can develop in the retina prior to breaking into the vitreous. (30) The infectious embolus is usually in proximity to the retinal vessels. (30) If a large septic embolus pass through the central retinal artery and disseminates throughout the retina, retinal necrosis and ischemia may occur. (30) This allows the microorganisms to quickly invade the vitreous and further the anterior segment, causing inflammation of intraocular tissues (panuveitis) that may be mixed-up a non-infectious inflammatory disease. (31) Similarly, in cases of fungal endophthalmitis a localized inflammatory reaction surrounding a small nidus of fungi forms in the inner choroid, breaks through Bruch's membrane into the retina forming a microabscess and spreads into the vitreous cavity. (31) It is a destructive process that has a poor visual prognosis that the visual loss rate reaches up to 37.5%. (30) The final visual outcome in patients with endogenous bacterial endophthalmitis in the recent 12 years has not differed significantly from five decades ago. (31) Under normal circumstances, the blood-ocular barrier provides a natural resistance against invading organisms. (30) Destruction of intraocular tissues may be due to direct invasion of the organism and/or from inflammatory mediators of the immune system. (30,31) In any type of endophthalmitis, bacteria are introduced into the intraocular environment, encountering a site of immunological inactivity. (30) The intraocular environment is termed an "immune privileged site", devoid of inflammatory mediators and cells present that would otherwise fight infection. (32) The blood-ocular barrier facilitates maintenance of a sterile environment in the interior of the eye contributing to the immune privileged site. (32) In this environment initial immune responses that would typically handle infection are delayed or absent, providing an optimum growth medium for the organisms that reach the area. (32) Eventually, organisms are recognized and inflammation initiates in an effort to handle the infection. (30) The extent of inflammation in the eye is during endophthalmitis has been shown to be organism dependent. (30,31) The course of endophthalmitis, treatment effectiveness and visual outcome can be unpredictable. (33) Clinical presentation of the disease depends, in part, on the relative virulence of the infecting pathogen, the mechanism of introduction into the eye and how quickly treatment is initiated. (33) Other factors that affect the outcome of infection include the patients' age, how vulnerable the infecting agent is to antibiotic therapy and the anatomic condition of the eye during infection. (33) Clinical studies have reported that increased time between infection and treatment is associated with a worse visual outcome. (19,34) Endophthalmitis may be as subtle as white nodules on the lens capsule, iris, retina, or choroid. (35) It can also be as ubiquitous as inflammation of all the ocular tissues, leading to a globe full of purulent exudate. (36) In addition, inflammation can spread to involve the orbital soft tissue. (37)

5. Mortality/morbidity

Decreased vision and permanent loss of vision are common complications of endophthalmitis. (33,34) Patients may require enucleation to eradicate a blind and painful eye. (38) Mortality is related to the patient's comorbidities and the underlying medical problem, especially when considering the etiology of hematogenous spread in endogenous infections. (39,40)

6. Clinical presentations

Bacterial endophthalmitis usually presents acutely with pain, redness, lid swelling, and decreased visual acuity. (11,16,22) Specific signs have been described which may suggest a specific infecting organism. For example, Bacillus infections characteristically demonstrate chocolate brown anterior chamber exudates with a ring-shaped white corneal infiltrate. (41) Serratia infections may be associated with a pink or dark hypopyon. (42,43) An eye with Klebsiella or Group B Streptoccoccus endogenous endophthalmitis often has a pupillary hypopyon. (44,45) The hypopyon associated with Group B Streptococcus often does not organize and shifts to occupy the most dependent portion of the anterior chamber. This has been termed a "sliding hypopyon". (46) Fungal endophthalmitis may present with an indolent course over days to weeks. (47) Symptoms are often blurred vision, pain and decreased visual acuity. (47) Individuals with candidal infection may present with high fever, followed several days later by ocular symptoms. (48) Persistent fever of unknown origin may be associated with an occult retinochoroidal fungal infiltrate. (48) A characteristic sign of endogenous Candida endophthalmitis is a creamy, white, well-circumscribed lesion, involving the retina and choroid in the posterior pole. (48) Aspergillus endogenous endophthalmitis, although less common, is frequently a more fulminant disease. (40) Nearly all patients have anterior chamber cells and keratic precipitates. (40) The inflammation may result in hypopyon, pupillary membrane, rubeosis iridis, and an anterior chamber inflammatory mass. (40) Posteriorly, chorioretinitis may appear as fluffy yellow-white elevated chorioretinal opacities. (49) Gravitational layering of the inflammatory cells may produce a subhyaloid or subretinal "hypopyon" especially since subretinal and subretinal pigment epithelial infection tends to occur with Aspergillus. (49) Retinal detachment mat complicate the infection. (40) Retinal haemorrhages and perivasculitis may be present. (40) Ultimately full thickness retinal necrosis may occur. (40) The earlier signs of endogenous endophthalmitis include Roth's spot (round, white retinal spots surrounded by hemorrhage) (Fig. 11), hemorrhagic spots in the conjunctiva, superficial or profound retinal hemorrhage, and retinal periphlebitis. (20-22) The occlusion of small arterioles may produce cotton-wool spots, or if the larger vessels are involved, branch retinal or central retinal artery obstruction. (20-22) Slit-lamp examination reveales ciliary injection, keratic precipitates (KP), mild to moderate cells and flare in the anterior chamber or severe iritis with hypopyon formation and fibrin precipitates. (21,22) Ophthalmoscopy shows infiltrations of the retina and vitreous, retinal vasculitis and retinal hemorrhage or dense vitreous opacities progressing to white mass obstructing fundus view. (26,27) If the fundus

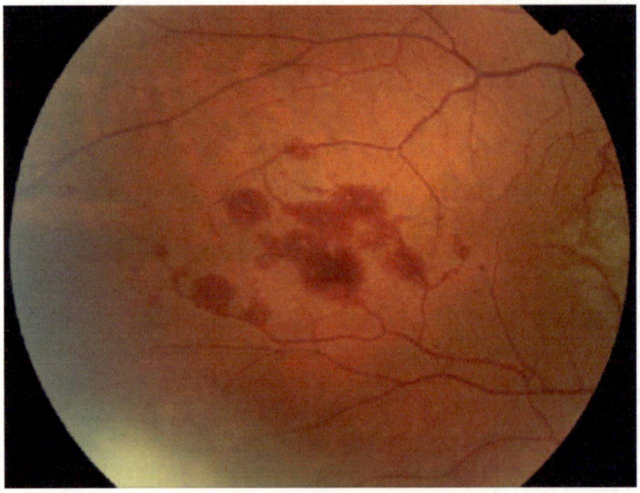

Fig. 11. Roth Spots characterized by round, white retinal spots surrounded by hemorrhage

view is obscured, imaging with optical coherence tomography, ocular ultrasonography, electroretinogram tests are useful in displaying the extent of vitreous involvement, choroidal abscesses, retinal detachment and scleral thickening. (16,18,22) Computed tomography scans allow high resolution orbital imaging in cases of suspected panophthalmitis to detect abscess formation or confirm the presence of contiguous orbital involvement. (37)

7. Causes

Individuals at risk for developing endogenous endophthalmitis usually have comorbidities that predispose them to infection. These include conditions like diabetes mellitus, chronic renal failure, cardiac valvular disorders, prosthetic heart valves, systemic lupus erythematosus, AIDS, leukemia, gastrointestinal malignancies, neutropenia, lymphoma, alcoholic hepatitis, intravenous drug abuse, and bone marrow transplantation. (50,51) Sources of endophthalmitis include most commonly endocarditis followed by urinary tract infection, wound infection and meningitis. (4) Additionally, pharyngitis, pulmonary infection, septic arthritis, pyelonephritis and intraabdominal abscess have also been implicated as sources of infection. (10) About 25% of the cases are bilateral and usually caused by Meningococcus, E.coli and Klebsiella species. (52,53) The most common cause in two-thirds of the infections is Gram-positive bacteria. (31,33) Although the most common agent was S.aureus (25% of patients), the most common group was streptococcus (32%). (31,33) Endogenous endophthalmitis in adults caused by group B Streptococcus has been reported rarely and is almost exclusively related to infective endocarditis. (7,54) Gram-negative organisms cause 32-37% of all endogenous endophthalmitis cases and typically have poor visual outcomes because these infections are difficult to treat. (5,55,56) The low prevalence of Gram-negative bacteria amongst the causative organisms of both infective endocarditis and endogenous endophthalmitis might be related to the absence of an outer capsule, which makes them sensitive to complement mediated lysis and other humoral innate immune defenses, and the lack of surface proteins that specifically bind host matrix molecules and prosthetic material. (57) Moreover, a much higher inoculums of Gram-negative than Gram-positive organisms is required to induce infective endocarditis in laboratory animals. (57) Although aggressive therapy was given, the visual prognosis for all these patients was poor. (56,57) E. coli emphysematous endophthalmitis is a very rare and severe variety of E. coli endophthalmitis. (58,59) The mechanism of emphysematous endophthalmitis has been postulated that a high concentration of glucose in the eye tissue may provide a substrate that bacteria can ferment to produce carbondioxide and hydrogen. (58) A computerized tomography scan of the orbits demonstrate gas bubble in the eye globe indicating emphysematous endophthalmitis. (59) Extra-intestinal pathogenic E.coli (ExPEC) are able to colonize tissue outside the gastrointestinal tract and contain a variety of virulence factors that may enable the pathogens to invade and induce infections in the cardiac endothelia. (57,60) These cases are further complicated by spondylodiscitis and bilateral endophthalmitis. (60) Endogenous endophthalmitis is usually associated with Gram-negative bacteria, most commonly Klebsiella pneumonia (77.4%) among the East Asian population. (6,61,62) The patients at highest risk are diabetic patients with hepatobiliary infections. (6,61) Klebsiella pneumonia endogenous endophthalmitis is a severe but potentially subclinical disease. (62) Early diagnosis requires a high index of suspicion and recognition of risk factors including Asian ancestry and other sources of systemic infection including most commonly liver abscess. (6,61) In contrast, in the Caucasian population, Gram-positive cocci including Staphylococcus aureus, Streptococcus pneumonia and other streptococcal species are the most common causes of bacterial endogenous endophthalmitis. (31,33) Septic metastasis to the iris is a rare manifestation of endogenous endophthalmitis presented with acute painful red eye, hypopyon and iris abscess that might be caused by S.aureus. (63) Subacute bacterial endocarditis caused by viridians streptococci is characterized by a lingering start of the disease with high temperature of unknown origin and an unspecific feeling of illness. (64,65) The ophthalmological findings can manifest itself before the diagnosis of the underlying disease is made. (65) Complications such as blindness after fulminant endophthalmitis and death can be avoided through quick diagnosis and treatment. (64,65) Group B Streptococcus endogenous endophthalmitis is a devastating condition with poor visual prognosis despite therapy. (66,67) It is a rare condition that 17 cases have been reported since 1985. (7) Group B Streptococcus endogenous endophthalmitis was found to arise from hematogenous spread from endocarditis at a rate of 33.3%. (7) Increasing incidence of invasive Group B Streptococcus infection with its varying manifestations including metastatic endophthalmitis has been reported recently in adults with predisposing illnesses. (54,68) Streptococcus anginosus is a member of Streptococcus milleri group and is a commensal found in the mouth, nasopharnyx, throat and sinuses. (69) It is associated with infective endocarditis with a longer than average duration of evolution before diagnosis. (70) S. anginosus should also be considered in the differential diagnosis of a slowly progressive endogenous endophthalmitis when fungal infection is considered likely. (70) Bartonella henselae and Tropheryma whipplei are rare pathogens in humans and were recently recognized as important causative agents of culture-negative endocarditis that the bacteria are indentified by polymerase chain reaction analysis. (71,72) Exposure to cats is an important risk factor for B.henselae which is the causative agent of cat scratch disease characterized by persistent regional lymhadenopathy. (73) B. henselae is responsible for endocarditis in patients with valvular diseases, and may induce retinitis. (73) Whipple's disease is characterized by wide range of clinical manifestations involving diarrhea, weight loss, night sweats, arthritis, vitritis retinitis and papillitis. (74)

Fungal organisms can occur in up to 50% of all cases of endogenous endophthalmitis. (57) Candida albicans is by far the most frequent cause (75-80% of fungal cases). (57) Since 1980, candidal infections reported in intravenous drug users have increased. (57) The number of people at risk may be increasing because of the spread of AIDS, more frequent use of immunosuppressive agents, and more invasive procedures. (57,75) The classic finding of Candida endophthalmitis is white chorioretinal infiltrates with fluffy white vitreous opacities described as "string of pearls" appearance. (76,77) The chorioretinitis may progress and satellite lesions may develop adjacent to the primary lesions. (77) Occasionally anterior uveitis, scleritis and panophthalmitis may also occur. (77) Aspergillus endogenous endophthalmitis, although less common, is frequently a more fulminent disease. (76) It has a predilection for the postequatorial fundus. (78) A confluent yellowish infiltrate is usually seen in the macula beginning in the choroid or subretinal space. (78) Histologically, the retinal and choroidal lesions are angiocentric. (76) Unlike candida endophthalmitis, in which the vitreous is the primary focus of infection, aspergillus endophthalmitis is marked by retinal and choroidal vessel invasion and subretinal pigment epithelial and subretinal infection. (76) The lesions can progress to retinal vascular occlusion and full-thickness retinal necrosis. (78) Intraretinal hemorrhages usually occur. (78) Eventually the infection spreads into the vitreous, producing dense vitritis, and into the anterior segment, producing varying degrees of cell/flare and hypopyon in the anterior chamber. (76,78) The macular lesions heal to form a central atrophic scar. (78) Endogenous cryptococcal endophthalmitis has nonspecific ocular inflammatory signs including intraretinal hemorrhage, vascular sheathing, yellow-white chorioretinal mass or scarlike lesion. (79,80) Retinal detachment may complicate the infection. (79) The infection is usually misdiagnosed as sterile uveitis. (79) Suspicion of infection should be greater in the presence of a yellow or white chorioretinal abscess. (79,80) Coccidioidal endophthalmitis is an uncommon presentation in patients with disseminated disease. (81) Usually a severe granulomatous iridocyclitis characterized by mutton- fat keratic precipitates is present. (81) Multifocal choroiditis, typified by several, scattered, discrete yellow-white lesions measuring less than the disc diameter in size, is observed. (81) Occasionally, vascular sheathing, vitreous haze, serous retinal detachment and retinal hemorrhage may also be seen. (81) Less commonly, Histoplasma capsulatum and other dimorphic fungi have been implicated in endogenous endophthalmitis. (57) Endogenous histoplasmic endophthalmitis has been reported in several patients with disseminated systemic histoplasmosis. (82) The ocular infection may result in a granulomatous anterior uveitis. (82) Vitritis may be mild to severe. (82) The classic fundus lesion is a cream-colored or gray-white chorioretinal infiltrate, often surrounded by hemorrhage. (82) There may be associated retinal pigment epithelial alteration, indicating partial spontaneous healing. (82) The lesions may be solitary or multiple can range from less than a disc diameter to several disc diameters. (83) Histoplasmic optic neuritis has also been reported in association with the chorioretinitis. (83) The ocular findings are not specific for histoplasmic endophthalmitis, and the diagnosis should be suspected in any immunosuppressed patient living in an area endemic for histoplasmosis. (83) Rare causes of endogenous fungal endophthalmitis include Fusarium species, Mucormycosis, Paecilomyces species, Pencillium species, Bipolaris hawaiiensis, and Trichosporon beigelii. (84,85) Endophthalmitis due to systemic fungaemia is less commonly reported in East Asian countries. (57)

8. Diagnosis

The high incidence of misdiagnosis of endogenous endophthalmitis ranging from conjunctivitis, acute glaucoma or other ocular conditions should alert the ophthalmologist to make a correct diagnosis of this insidious entity. The possibility of endogenous endophthalmitis should be considered in any patient who manifests a pronounced anterior reaction that is refractory to steroid treatment. The appropriate diagnosis is necessary to start the appropriate treatment and influence dramatically the visual outcome as well as reduce the incidence of systemic complications, sometime fatal. Therefore the crucial point is diagnostic suspicion. The diagnostic algorithm should include accurate ocular and systemic history, investigation of risk factors, search source of infection, fluorescein angiography, (Fig. 12) B/A scan ocular ultrasonography, (Fig. 13) and computerized tomography of the orbit (Fig. 14) to exclude posterior involvement, and during the follow-up to monitor the adequacy of treatment, anterior aqueous tap, vitreous tap or vitrectomy, gram stain and culture of ocular and non-ocular fluids including blood, urine, cerebrospinal fluid. Organisms are cultured from ocular fluid in 36-73% of cases. (50) In many cases, prior treatment for systemic infection with intravenous antibiotics had already been instituted and this would reduce the culture positive rate from ocular fluids. A second factor resulting

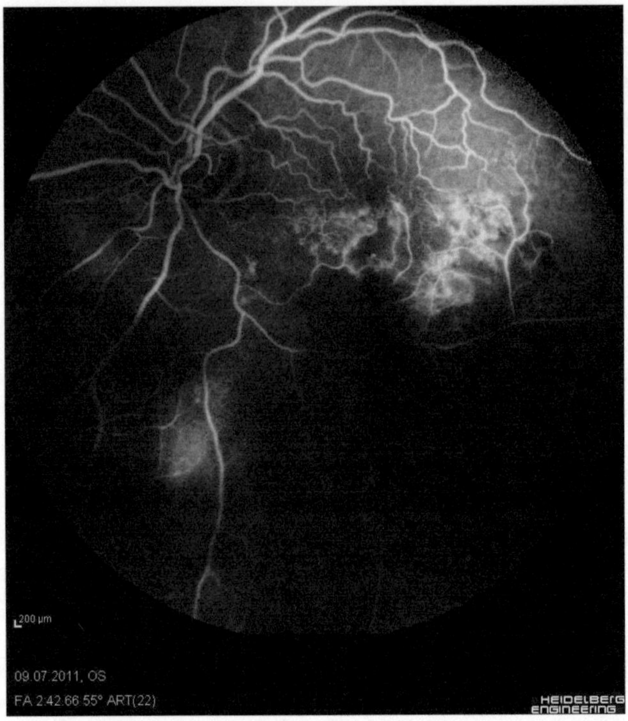

Fig. 12. Fluorescein angiography showing the areas of vascular leakage (hyperfluorescent) and the areas of retinal hemorrhage (hypofluorescent)

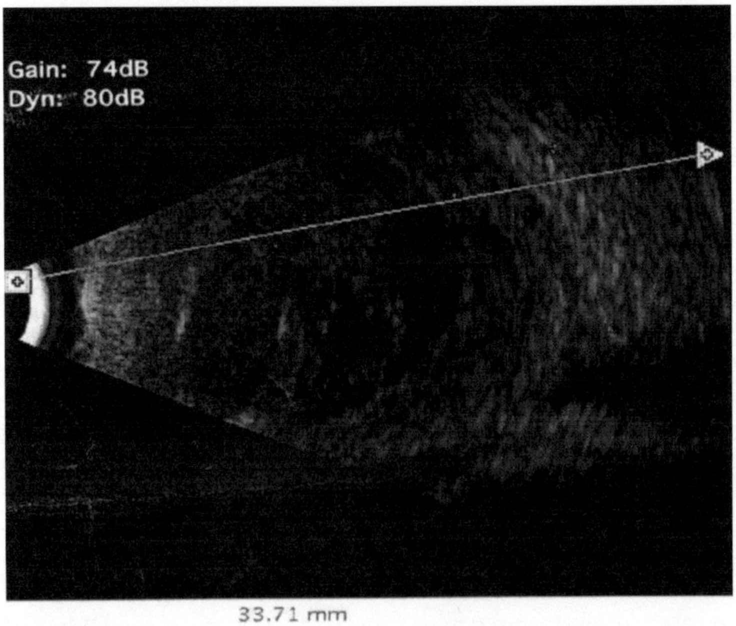

Fig. 13. B-Scan ultrasonography of the eye showing scleral thickening and dense vitreous inflammatory opacifications

in a negative culture is sampling from an inappropriate compartment within the eye. Both aqueous and vitreous cultures should be obtained unless the organism has been identified from a non-ocular source. Beyond an initial diagnostic aqueous and vitreous tap, a pars plana vitrectomy can provide additional material for culture. It should be inoculated in blood agar, chocolate agar, brain-heart infusion broth/agar, thioglycollate broth and Sabouraud agar. (50) A specimen sent for Gram stain may allow provisional categorization of the organism. Polymerase chain reaction (PCR) may allow rapid identification of organism with high sensitivity, but specificity may be a problem and facilitates for this test are not widely available. (50) In comparison with bacterial endogenous endophthalmitis, those case caused by fungi rarely have a positive blood culture. (86) Systemic fungaemia is either transient or not recognized prior to eye infection. (47) On the other hand, screening of several series of patients with candidaemia has not revealed any cases of endophthalmitis. (47) The benefit of screening lucid, asymptomatic patients thus remains doubtful at this point of time. (47,50) However, vitreous cultures will often reveal the offending organisms in these cases. (86) Vitrectomy samples are more sensitive for fungal cultures than vitreous needle biopsies. (86) The cultures must be kept at the laboratory for at least 4-6 weeks to ensure that slow-growing or fastidious fungal organisms are not missed. (86) PCR is also used as a diagnostic tool for fungal endophthalmitis. (87,88) The main advantage of PCR over conventional fungal cultures are the higher sensitivity and the rapid results. (87,88) Although PCR does not replace conventional mycologic methods, it helps to make an early differentiation between bacterial endophthalmitis and fungal endophthalmitis. (88) Candida species grow well on Sabouraud media without cycloheximide. (89) The colonies are white and pasty. (89) Aspergilli species are observed best with Grocott Methenamine Silver (GMS) or Periodic acid-Schiff (PAS) stains. (90) Aspergilli cultures are initially flat, white and filamentous. (90) Within 48 hours, conidia are produced with a concomitant change in

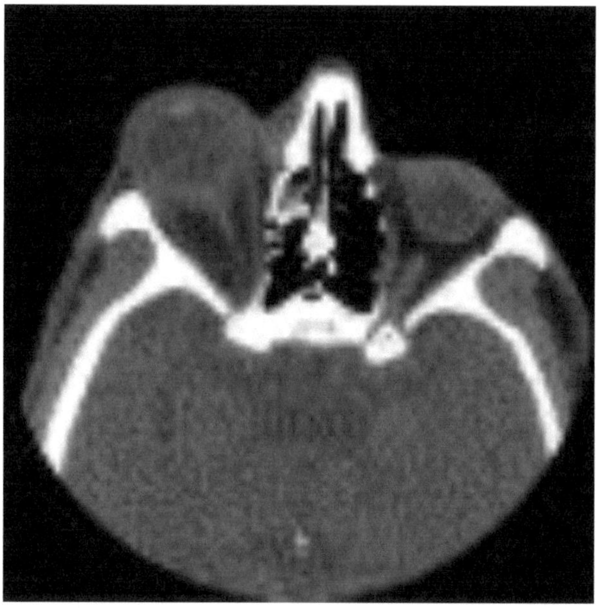

Fig. 14. Orbital tomography showing proptosis, extraocular muscle enlargement, soft tissue swelling and retrobulbar fat stranding of the left eye

pigmentation. (90) Cryptococci also grow well in Sabouraud agar. (91) It may be identified by India ink. (91) Coccidioidomycosis can be diagnosed using a 10% KOH mount and identifying endospores that contain spherules. (92)

Apart from microbiological investigation, other tests may be required according to the clinical picture. These would include complete blood cell count with differential, erythrocyte sedimentation rate, blood urea nitrogen and creatinine.

8.1 Differential diagnosis

Endogenous endophthalmitis should always be considered early in the differential diagnosis of anterior uveitis. (87) The common causes of anterior uveitis must be excluded by the usual serological tests. (87) Glaucoma, CMV retinitis, toxoplasma chorioretinitis, primary intraocular lymphoma, syphilitic chorioretinitis, autoimmune causes, malignancies, masquerade, metastatic tumors, and other infectious diseases should also be ruled out. (93) Rarely, cavernous sinus thrombosis, corneal abrasion, corneal laceration, corneal ulceration and ulcerative keratitis, globe rupture, herpes zoster ophthalmicus and vitreous hemorrhage are included in the differential diagnosis. (78,94)

9. Medical treatment

9.1 Systemic therapy

Prompt administration of antibiotic therapy is the key in the acute management of endogenous endophthalmitis. Systemic antibiotics also treat distant foci of infection and prevent continued bacteremia, thereby reducing the chances of invasion of the unaffected eye. Prolonged intravenous therapy is usually required for 2-4 weeks, until it is certain that the systemic infection is eradicated. (33) Empiric broad-spectrum antibiotic therapy with vancomycin and aminoglycoside or a third-generation cephalosporin is recommended at the highest theurapeutic doses. (33,52) Gentamycine has the coverage of gram-negative organisms including Pseudomonas aeruginosa. (25,44) It is the first choice aminoglycoside for systemic gram-negative coverage. (25,44) It has bacteriocidal activity by binding to 30S ribosomal subunit and inhibiting protein synthesis. (44) Ceftazidime is the third-generation cephalosporin with broad gram-negative coverage but decreased efficacy to gram-positive organisms. (95,96) It binds to one or more of the penicillin-binding proteins and prevent cell wall synthesis inhibiting bacterial growth. (95) Ceftriaxone is another third-generation cephalosporin is active against the resistant gram-negative organisms. (12) For Gram-positive cover, intravenous vancomycin is warranted in the view of the potential severity of the disease and consequences. (95,96) Good Gram-negative coverage is provided by third-generation cephalosporins, ciprofloxacin and aminoglycosides. (25,44) Although intravenous antibiotics can reach therapeutic concentrations in affected eyes, the use of systemic antibiotics that have good intraocular penetration and bioavailability is preferred. (97,98) In particular, aminoglycosides do not have good intraocular bioavailability when given intravenously. (44) In specific situations, certain antibiotics should be preferred. For example, bacillus infections mandate the initial use of either vancomycin or clindamycin. (41) In cases of fungal sepsis and endophthalmitis amphotericin B provides good efficacy and broad coverage. (99,100) It is fungostatic or fungocidal depending on concentration attained in body fluids. (101) It is an polyene antibiotic and it changes permeability of fungal cell membrane by binding to sterols, which causes fungal cell death as intracellular components leak out. (101) Treatment duration and total dose of intravenous drug are determined by the clinical response and the degree of systemic or non-ocular involvement. (102) Toxic side effects including renal and hepatic toxicity must be carefully monitored. (102) The penetration of amphotericin B into vitreous cavity is poor. (103) Doses of 5-10 microgram of intravitreal amphotericin is used for treatment. (103) However, retinal toxicities have also been reported in animal models at these doses. (103) The azole antibiotics are less toxic and have better ocular penetration. (104) Fluconazole and flucytosine have good intraocular penetration, but Candida species show high resitance to flucytosine. (104) Flucytosine can be used in combination with amphotericin B in cases of macular involvement and extensive inflammatory response. (100,104) Itraconazole is useful in Aspergillus and Fusarium infections. (99) A new systemic voriconazole, when administered orally or intravenously, it has good intravitreal concentrations. (100) Intravitreal administration of voriconazole is also safe without evidence of retinal toxicity with concentrations up to 25 microgram/ml. (105) The echinocandins (caspofungin, micafungin, and anidulafungin) are newer agents that exert their antifungal activity by binding D-glucan synthase, an enzyme involved in fungal cell wall synthesis. (106,107) Because mammalian cells lack a cell wall, it also represents an ideal and specific target for antifungal therapy. (106) Echinocandins exert antifungal activity against Candida and Aspergillus species. (106,107) However, they have limited penetration into the vitreous cavity so their role in the treatment of fungal endophthalmitis needs to be determined. (107)

9.2 Intravitreal therapy

Although the value of intravitreal antibiotics over and above the use of intravenous antibiotics has not been definitively established, most cases in our experience are of posterior diffuse disease and panophthalmitis which denote severe infection with extension of organisms into the vitreous. These cases should be treated aggressively as possible with both systemic and intravitreal antibiotics. In cases caused by bacteria, intravitreal injection of vancomycin 1mg/0.1ml and ceftazidime 2mg/0.1 ml provides good coverage and avoids the toxicity associated with aminoglycosides. (41,108) Repeated injections may be required since the half-life of these drugs in the vitreous cavity is short. (108) In most cases of fungal endophthalmitis, an intravitreal injection of 5-10 microgram amphotericin B is recommended. (103) Using amphotericin B in this manner avoids its numerous systemic side effects, but its potential for retinal toxicity should be noted. (103) The use of intravitreal, topical and subtenon steroids should be avoided in fungal endophthalmitis. (99) However, the use of intravitreal steroid, dexamethasone in addition to intravitreal antibiotics is recommended for suppression of inflammatory mediators released in the vitreous in bacterial endophthalmitis. (108-111) The histopathological changes of the eyes treated with intravitreal vancomycin with dexamethasone (0.4 mg/ml) had less conjunctival inflammation, mild iridocyclitis, less vitreous cells, less choroidal vasculitis and retinitis compared to antibiotic treatment alone. (109,110)

Topical steroids are also used in patients with anterior focal or diffuse endophthalmitis to reduce the number of inflammatory cells in the anterior chamber, thereby preventing the complications such as formation of synechiae and secondary glaucoma. (112-114)

Topical antibiotics are definitively indicated if keratitis develops and adjunctive therapy includes the use of cycloplegics, ocular hypotensives and topical steroids. (113,114)

9.3 Surgical treatment

The timing of and necessity for vitrectomy remains unclear in endogenous endophthalmitis. (115,116) The benefits of vitreous tap outweigh the benefits of vitrectomy for anterior focal or diffuse and posterior focal cases with endogenous endophthalmitis. (38) In general vitrectomy is indicated in cases of posterior diffuse cases with prominent vitreous involvement, and also for cases showing progressive disease despite intensive medical therapy. (116) In these cases small gauge vitrectomy is effective in clearing the vitreous from the inflammatory debris, cells and mediators. (117) Other advantage includes the possibility to have larger sample to make the diagnosis and also to deliver a therapeutic level of drug in the vitreous. (118,119) In these cases vitrectomy and intravitreal antibiotics may, however, prevent ocular atrophy or the necessity for enucleation. (119)

10. Prognosis

The visual outcome is usually good in the anterior form of endophthalmitis, differently from posterior diffuse and panophthalmitis forms. (19) The outcome of posterior diffuse endophthalmitis or panophthalmitis is frequently blindness, regardless of the treatment measures. (19) In a recent study surveying cases in Singapore over a 4-year period, 17 of 32 affected eyes ended up with no light perception. (4) In only 40% of patients with endogenous endophthalmitis vision is preserved with ability to count fingers or better. (4)

The virulence factor of the organism and age of the patient are important factors predicting outcome. (4,5) Other variables resulting in poorer outcome include severity of underlying systemic illness, misdiagnosis or delay in diagnosis, and inappropriate, inadequate or delayed treatment, low intraocular pressure, initial visual acuity of light perception, severe hypopyon and absent red reflex. (5,6) Ultrasonography negative prognostic factors are vitreous and subhyaloid opacities, choroidal and retinal detachments. (35) In general Gram-positive infections involving microbes such as Staphylococcus and Streptococcus species result in a better outcome. (112,120) However, Bacillus infections are typically rapidly progressive with a poorer prognosis. (120) Gram-negative organisms, including Klebsiella pneumonia, E. coli, P aeruginosa, often result in severe infection and a very poor prognosis. (6,12) Exceptions include Haemophilus and Neisseria, but these are uncommon causes of endogenous endophthalmitis. (121,122) Fungal endogenous endophthalmitis usually result in very poor outcomes, but those caused by Candida species can often be treated effectively if early and appropriate antifungals are used. (98,99)

11. Conclusion

Endogenous endophthalmitis continues to occur among the patients with infective endocarditis despite the continuing development of effective antibiotics. Although it is devastating, vision can sometimes be salvaged, especially if diagnosis is made early and prompt systemic therapy instituted. The role of intravitreal antibiotics and vitrectomy is not well defined but they have a definite role in cases which progress despite medical therapy and also where fungi are implicated. Future challenge ahead include the aging population and the development of new microbial antibiotic resistance. A coordinated multidisciplinary effort will be required to keep abreast of this difficult condition.

12. References

[1] Lopez J, Revilla A, Vilacosta I, et al. Multiple-valve infective endocarditis: Clinical, microbiologic, echocardiographic and prognostic profile. Medicine (Baltimore) 2011 Jun 18 (Epub ahead of print)
[2] Silverman ME, Upshaw CB Jr. Extra-cardiac manifestations of infective endocarditis and their historical descriptions. Am J Cardiol 2007;100:1802-7.
[3] Walpot J, Klazen C, blok W, et al. Embolic events in infective endocarditis: a review and report of 4 cases. Acta Clin Belg 2005;60:139-45.
[4] Ming PY, Phaik CS. Endogenous endophthalmitis SGH Proceedings 2004;13:113-20.
[5] Okada AA, Johnson RP, Liles WC, et al. Endogenous bacterial endophthalmitis: report of a ten-year prospective study. Ophthalmology 1994;101:832-8.
[6] Wong JS, Chan TK, Lee HM, et al. Endogenous bacterial endophthalmitis: an East Asian experience and a reappraisal of a severe ocular affliction. Ophthalmology 2000;107:1483-91.
[7] Lee SY, Chee SP. Group B Streptococcus endogenous endophthalmitis. Case reports and review of the literature. Ophthalmology 2002;109:1879-86.
[8] Chee SP, Ang CL. Endogenous Klebsiella endophthalmitis- a case series. Ann Acad Med Singapore 1995;24:473-8.
[9] Jain ML, Garg AK. Metastatic endophthalmitis in a patient with major burns: a rare complication. Burns 1995;21:72-3.
[10] Banerjee SN, Emori TG, Culver DH, et al. Secular trends in nosocomial primary bloodstream infections in the United States, 1980-1989. National Nosocomial Infections Surveillance System. Am J Med 1991;91:86S-89S.
[11] Chee SP, Jap A. Endogenous endophthalmitis. Current Opinion in Ophthalmology 2001;12:464-70.
[12] Yang CS, Tsai HY, Sung CS, et al. Endogenous Klebsielle endophthalmitis associated with pyogenic liver abscess. Ophthalmology 2007;114:876-80.
[13] Kiwan YA, Hayat N, Vijayaraghavan DG, et al. Infective endocarditis: A prospective study of 60 consecutive cases. Mater Med Pol 1990;22:173-5.
[14] Al-Tawfiq JA, Sufi I. Infective endocarditis at a hospital in Saudi Arabia: epidemiology, bacterial pathogens and outcome. Ann Saudi Med 2009; 29:433-6.
[15] Binder MI, Chua J, Kaiser PK, et al. Endogenous endophthalmitis. An 18-year review of culture-positive cases at a tertiary care center. Medicine (Baltimore) 2003;82:97-105.
[16] Durand ML. Bacterial endophthalmitis. Curr Infect Dis Rep 2009;11:283-8.
[17] Schiedler V, Scott IU, Flynn HW Jr, et al. Culture-proven endogenous endophthalmitis: clinical features and visual acuity outcomes. Am J Ophthalmol 2004;137:725-31.
[18] Ness T, Serr A. Diagnostics for endophthalmitis. Klin Monbl Augenheilkd 2008;225:44-9.
[19] Liang L, Lin X, Yu A, et al. The clinical analysis of endogenous endophtahlmitis. Yan Ke Xue Bao 2004,20:144-8.
[20] Greenwald MJ, Wohl LG, Sell H. Metastatic bacterial endophthalmitis: a contemporary reappraisal. Surv Ophthalmol 1986;31:81-101.

[21] Puliafito CA, Baker AS, Foster CS. Infectious endophthalmitis. Ophthalmology 1982;89:921-9.
[22] Pflugfelder CS, Flynn HW Jr. Infectious endophthalmitis. Infect Dis Clin North Am 1992;6:859-73.
[23] Davis JL, Nussenblat RB, Bachman DM, et al. Endogenous bacterial retinitis in AIDS. Am J Ophthalmol 1989;107:613-23.
[24] Margo CE, Mames RN, Guy JR. Endogenous Klebsiella endophthalmitis. Report of two cases and review of the literature. Ophthalmology 1994;101:1298-301.
[25] Tseng CY, Liu PY, Shi ZY, et al. Endogenous endophthalmitis due to Escherichia coli:case report and review. Clin Infect Dis 1996;22:1107-8.
[26] Jeng BH, Kaiser BK, Lowder CY. Retinal vasculitis and posterior pole "hypopyons" as early signs of acute bacterial endophthalmitis. Am J Ophthalmol 2001;131:800-2.
[27] Magadur-Joly G, Raffi F, Bouchut P, et al. Hematogenic bacterial endophthalmitis. A rare infection with very poor functional prognosis. Ann Med Interne (Paris) 1996;147:212-7.
[28] Molina DN, Colon M, Bermudez RH, et al. Unusual presentation of Pseudomonas aeruginosa infections: a review. Bol Asoc Med P R 1991;83:160-3.
[29] Treister G, Rothoff L, Yalon M, et al. Bilateral blindeness fron panophthalmitis in a case of bacterial endocarditis. Ann Ophthalmol 1982;14:663-4.
[30] Khan A, Okhravi N, Lightman S. The eye in systemic sepsis. Clin Med 2002;2.444-8.
[31] Ness T, Pelz K, Hansen LL. Endogenous endophtahlmitis: microorganisms, disposition and prognosis. Acta Ophthalmol Scand 2007;85:852-6.
[32] Hori J, Vega JL, Masli S. Review of ocular immune privilege in the year 2010: modifying the immune privilege of the eye. Ocul Immunol Inflamm 2010;18:325-33.
[33] Novosad BD, Callegan MC. Severe bacterial endophthalmitis: towards improving clinical outcomes. Expert Rev Ophthalmol 2010;5:689-98.
[34] Bartz-Schmidt KU, Bermig J, Kirchoff B, et al. Prognostic factors associated with the visual outcome after vitrectomy for endophthalmitis. Graefes Arch Clin Exp Ophthalmol 1996;234:S51-8.
[35] Uchio E, Ohno S. Ocular manifestations of systemic infections. Curr Opin Ophtahlmol 1999;10:452-7.
[36] Riss JM, Righini-Chossegros M, Paulo F, et al. Endogenous bacterial endophthalmitis. Report of three cases. J Fr Ophthalmol 1990;13:327-31.
[37] Hutnik CM, Nicolle DA, Munoz DG. Orbital aspergillosis. A fatal masquerader. J Neuroophthalmol 1997;17:257-61.
[38] Ho V, Ho LY, Ranchod TM, et al. Endogenous methicillin-resistant Staphylococcus aureus endophthalmitis. Retina 2011;31:596-601.
[39] Saffra NA, Desai RU, Seidmann CJ, et al. Endogenous fungal endophthalmitis after cardiac surgery. Ophthalmic Surg Lasers Imaging 2010;28:e1-3.
[40] Willermain F, Bradstreet C, Kampauridis S, et al. different presentations of ophthalmic aspergillosis. Eur J Ophthalmol 2008;18:827-30.
[41] Miller JJ, Scott IU, Flynn HW Jr, et al. Endophthalmitis caused by Bacillus species. Am J Ophthalmol 2008;145:883-8.
[42] al Hazzaa SA, Tabbara KF, Gammon JA. Pink hypopyon: a sign of Serratia marcescens endophthalmitis. Br J Ophthalmol 1992;76:764-5.
[43] Equi RA, Green WR. Endogenous Serratia marcescens endophthalmitis with dark hypopyon: case report and review. Surv Ophthalmol 2001;46:259-68.

[44] Ang LP, Lee HM, Au Eong KG, et al. Endogenous Klebsiella Endophthalmitis. Eye (Lond) 2000;14:855-60.
[45] Hauch A, Elliott D, Rao NA, et al. Dark hypopyon in Streptococcus bovis endogenous endophthalmitis: clinicopathological correlations. J Ophthalmic Inflamm Infect 2010;30:39-41.
[46] Hawkins AS, Deutsch TA. Infectious endophthalmitis. Curr Infect Dis Rep 1999;1:172-77.
[47] Bogadhi B. Fungal endogenous endophthalmitis. J Fr Ophthalmol 2011;34:40-45
[48] Kaburaki T, Takamoto M, Araki F, et al. Endogenous Candida albicans infection causing subretinal abscess. Int Ophthalmol 2010;30:203-6.
[49] Rana M, Fahad B, Abid Q. Embolic aspergillus endophthalmitis in an immunocompetent patient from aortic root aspergillus endocarditis. Mycoses 2008;51:352-3.
[50] Chung KS, Kim YK, Song YG, et al. Clinical review of endogenous endophthalmitis in Korea: a 14-year review of culture positive cases of two large hospitals. Yonsei Med J 2011,1:630-4.
[51] Hueber A, Welsandt G, Grajewski RS, et al. Fulminant endogenous anterior uveitis due to Listeria monocytogenes. Case Report Ophthalmol 2010;27:63-5.
[52] Cornut PL, Chiquet C. Endogenous bacterial endophthalmitis. J Fr Ophthlmol 2011;34:51-7.
[53] Arcieri ES, Jorge EF, de Abrea Ferreira L, et al. Bilateral endogenous endophthalmitis associated with infective endocarditis: case report. Braz J Infect Dis 2001;5:356-9.
[54] Nagelberg HP, Petashnick DE, To KW, et al. Group B streptococcal metastatic endophthalmitis. Am J Ophthalmol 1994;117:498-500.
[55] Wann SR, Liu YC, Yen MY, et al. Endogenous Escherichia coli endophthalmitis. J Formos Med Assoc 1996;95:56-60.
[56] Park SB, Searl SS, Aquavella JV, et al. Endogenous endophthalmitis caused by Escherichia coli. Ann Ophthalmol 1993;25:95-9.
[57] Durante-Mangoni E, Tripodi MF, Albisinni R, et al. Management of Gram-negative and fungal endocarditis. International Journal of Antimicrobial Agents 2010;36:S40-S45.
[58] Faraawi R, Fong IW. Escherichia coli emphysematous endophthalmitis and pyelonephritis. Case report and review of the literature. Am J Med 1988;84:636-9.
[59] Tseng CY, Yuk-Fong Liu P, Shi ZY, et al. Endogenous endophthalmitis due to Escherichia coli: Case report and Review. Clinical ınfectious Diseases 1996;22:1107-8.
[60] Lauridsen TK, Arpi M, Fritz-Hansen T, et al. Infectious endocarditis caused by Escherichia coli. Scand J Infect Dis 2011;43:545-6.
[61] Chen YJ, Kuo HK, Wu PC, et al. A 10-year comparison of endogenous endophthalmitis outcomes: an east Asian experience with Klebsiella pneumniae infection. Retina 2004;24:383-90.
[62] Kashani AH, Eliott D. Bilateral Klebsieela pneumoniae (k1 serotype) endogenous endophthalmitis as the presenting sign of disseminated infection. Ophthalmic Surg Lasers Imaging 2011;10:e12-4.
[63] Ramonas KM, Freilich BD. Irıs abscess as an unusual presentation of endogenous endophthalmitis in a patient with bacterial endocarditis. Am J Ophthalmol 2003;135:228-9.

[64] Seles S, Lang GE. Ocular manifestations of an infectious endocarditis. Klin Monbl Augenheilkd 2007;224:606-8.
[65] McCue JD, Dreher RJ. Bilateral endophthalmitis with Streptococcus viridans endocarditis. J Maine med Assoc. 1979;70:463-5.
[66] Kobayashi K, Fujiseki Y, Takahashi K, et al. Bacterial endophthalmitis caused by B streptococcus endocarditis. Nippon Ganka Gakkai Zasshi 2006;110:199-204.
[67] Chihara S, Siccion E. Group B streptococcus endophthalmitis with endocarditis. Mayo Clin Proc 2005;80:74.
[68] Pokharel D, Doan AP, Lee AG. Group B streptococcus endogenous endophthalmitis presenting as septic arthritis and a homonymous hemianopsia due to embolic stroke. Am J Ophthalmol 2004;138:300-2.
[69] Hui M. Streptococcusanginosus bacteremia: Sutton's law. J Clin Microbiol 2005;43:6217.
[70] Hadid OH, Shah SP, Sherafat H, et al. Streptococcus anginosus-associated endogenous endophthalmitis mimicking fungal endophthalmitis. J Clin Microbiol 2005;43:4275-6.
[71] Dreier J, Vollmer T, Freytag CC, et al. Culture-negative infectious endocarditis caused by Bartonella spp.: 2 case reports and a review of the literature. Diagn Microbiol Infect Dis 2008;61:476-83.
[72] Puechal X. Whipple's disease. Rev Med Interne 2009;30:233-41.
[73] Edouard S, Raoult D. Bartonella henselae, an ubiquitous agent of proteiform zoonotic disease. Med Mal Infect 2010;40:319-30.
[74] Escher R, Roth S, Droz S, et al. Endocarditis due to Tropheryma whipplei: rapid detection, limited genetic diversity, and long-term clinical outcome in a local experience. Clin Microbiol Infect 2010;16:1213-22.
[75] Falcone M, Barzaghi N, Carosi G, et al. Candida infective endocarditis: report of 15 cases from a prospective multicenter study. Medicine (Baltimore) 200988:160-8.
[76] Rao NA, Hidayat A. a comparative clinicopathologic study of endogenous mycotic endophthalmitis: variations in clinical and histological changes in candidiasis compared to aspergillosis. Trans Am Ophthalmol Soc 2000;98:183-93.
[77] Brooks RG. Prospective study of Candida endophthalmitis in hospitalized patients with candidemia. Arch Inter Med 1989;149:226-8.
[78] Weishaar PD, Flynn HW Jr, Murray TG, et al. Endogenous aspergillus endophthalmitis: Clinical features and treatment outcomes. Ophthalmology 1998;105:57-65.
[79] Sheu SJ, Chen YC, Kuo NW, et al. Endogenous cryptococcal endophthalmitis. Ophthalmology 1998;105:377-81.
[80] Crump JR, Elner SG, Elner VM, et al. Cryptococcal endophthalmitis: case report and review. Clin Infect Dis 1992;14:1069-73.
[81] Blumenkranz MS, Stevens DA. Endogenous coccidioidal endophthalmitis. Ophthalmology 1980;87;974-84.
[82] Weingeist TA, Watzke RC. Ocular involvement by histoplasma capsulatum. Int Ophthalmol Clin 1983;23:33-47.
[83] Leung C, Farmer JP, Zoutman DE, et al. Histoplasma capsulatum endophthalmitis in southeastern Ontario. Can J Ophthalmol 2010;45:90-1.
[84] Louie T, el Baba F, Shulman M, et al. Endogenous endophthalmitis due to Fusarium: case report and review. Clin Infect Dis 1994;18:585-8.
[85] McGuire TW, Bullock JD, Bullock JD Jr, et al. Fungal endophthalmitis. An experimental study with a review of 17 human ocular cases. Arch Ophthalmol 1991;109:1289-96.

[86] Kalkancı A, Ozdek S. Ocular fungal Infections. Curr Eye Res 2011;36:179-89.

[87] Vasseneix C, Bodaghi B, Muraine M, et al. Intraocular fluids analysis for etiologic diagnosis of presumed infectious uveitis. J Fr Ophthalmol 2006;29:398-403.

[88] Harper TW, Miller D, Schiffman JC, et al. Polymerase chain reaction analysis of aqueous and vitreous specimens in the diagnosis of posterior segment infectious uveitis. Am J Ophthalmol 2009;147:140-7.

[89] Odds FC, Bernaerts R. Chromagar candida, a new differential isolation medium for presumptive isolation of clinically important candida species. Journal of Clinical Microbiology 1994;32:1923-9.

[90] Piao YS, Liu HG, Liu XJ. Significance of MUC5B antibody in differential diagnosis between Aspergillus species and Mucorales of fungal sinusitis. Zhonghua Bing Li Xue Za Zhi 2008;37:255-8.

[91] Shashikala, Kanungo R, Srinivasan S, et al. Unusual morphological forms of Cryptococcus neoformans in cerebrospinal fluid. Indian J Med Microbiol 2004;22:188-90.

[92] Sarosi GA, Lawrence JP, Smith DK, et al. Rapid diagnostic evaluation of bronchial washings in patients with suspected coccidioidomycosis. Semin Respir Infect 2001;16:238-41.

[93] Turno-Krecicka A, Misiuk-Hojlo M, Grzybowski A, et al. Early vitrectomy and diagnostic testing in severe infectious posterior uveitis and endophthalmitis. Med Sci Monit 2010;16:296-300.

[94] Heidemann DG, Trese M, Murphy SF, et al. Endogenous Listeria monocytogenes endophthalmitis presenting as keratouveitis. Cornea 1990;9:179-80.

[95] Connell PP, O'Neill EC, Fabiyni D, et al. Endogenous endophthalmitis: 10-year experience at a tertiary referral center. Eye (Lond) 2011;25:66-72.

[96] Torii H, Miyata H, Sugisaka E, et al. Bilateral endophthalmitis in a patient with bacterial meningitis caused by Streptococcus pneumonia. Ophthalmologica 2008;222:357-9.

[97] Ang M, Jap A, Chee SP. Prognostic factors and outcomes in endogenous Klebsiella pneumonia endophthalmitis. Am J Ophthalmol 2011;151:338-44.

[98] Connell PP, O'Neill EC, Amirul Islam FM, et al. Endogenous endophthalmitis associated with intravenous drug abuse: seven-year experience at a tertiary referral center. Retina 2010;30:1721-5.

[99] Chakrabarti A, Shivaprakash MR, Singh R, et al. Fungal endophthalmitis: Fourteen years' experience from a center in India. Retina 2008;28:1400-7.

[100] Riddell J 4th, Corner GM, Kaufmann CA. Treatment of endogenous fungal endophthalmitis: focus on new antifungal agents. Clin Infect Dis 2011;52:648-53.

[101] Goldblum D, Rohrer K, Frueh BE, et al. Ocular distribution of intravenously administered lipid formulations of amphotericin B in a rabbit model. Antimic Agents Chemother 2002;46:3719-23.

[102] Narendran N, Balasubramaniam B, Johnson E, et al. Five-year retrospective review of guideline-based management of fungal endophthalmitis. Acta Ophthalmol 2008;86:525-32.

[103] Payne JF, Keenum DG, Sternberg P Jr, et al. Concentrated intravitreal amphotericin B in fungal endophthalmitis. Arch Ophthalmol 2010;128;1546-50.

[104] Annamalai T, Fong KC, Choo MM. Intravenous fluconazole for bilateral endogenous Candida endophthalmitis. J Ocul Phramacol Ther 2011;27:105-7.

[105] Funakoshi Y, Yakushijin K, Matsuoka H, et al. Fungal endophthalmitis successfully treated with intravitreal voriconazole injection. Intern Med 2011;50:941.
[106] Mora-Duarte J, Betts R, Rotstein C, et al. Comparision of capsofungin and amphotericin B for invasive candidiasis. N Eng J Med 2002;347:2020-9.
[107] Gauthier GM, Nork TM, Prince R, et al. Subtheurapeutic ocular penetration of capsofungin and associated treatment failure in candida albicans endophthalmitis. Clin Inf Dis 2005;41:27-8.
[108] Mehta S, Armstrong BK, Kim SJ et al. Long-term potency, sterility and stability of vancomycin, ceftazidime and moxifloxacin for treatment of bacterial endophthalmitis. Retina 2011;Feb 23 (Epub ahead of print)
[109] Albrecht E, Richards JC, Polock T, et al. Adjunctive use of intravitreal dexamethasone in presumed bacterial endophthalmitis: a randomised trial. Br J Ophthalmol 2011;Feb 2 (Epub ahead of print)
[110] Liu F, Kwok AK, Cheung BM. The efficacy of intravitreal vancomycin and dexamethasone in the treatment of experimental bacillus cereus endophtahlmitis. Curr Eye Res 2008;33:761-8.
[111] Ermis SS, Cetinkaya Z, Kıyıcı H, et al. Effects of intravitreal moxifloxacin and dexamethasone in experimental Staphylococcus endophthalmitis. Curr Eye Res 2007;32:337-44.
[112] Nentwich MM, Kampik A, de Kaspar HM. Chronic endogenous endophthalmitis. Klin Monbl Augenheilkd 2008;225:929-33.
[113] Pavesio CE, Decory HH. Treatment of ocular inflammatory conditions with loteprednol etabonate. Br J Ophthalmol 2008;92:455-9.
[114] Smith A, Pennefather PM, Kaye SB, et al. Fluoroquinolones: place in ocular therapy. Drugs 2001;61:747-61.
[115] Laube T, Akgül H, Brockmann C, et al. Endogenous bacterial endophthalmitis: a retrospective study in 22 consecutive cases. Klin Monbl Augenheilkd 2004;221:101-8.
[116] Maguire JL. Postoperative endophthalmitis: optimal management and the role and timing of vitrectomy surgery. Eye (London) 2008;22:1290-300.
[117] Thompson JT. Advantages and limitations of small gauge vitrectomy. Surv Ophthalmol 2011;56:162-72.
[118] Wen X, Zhong K, Wang Z, et al. Vitrectomy combined with intravitreal injection of drugs for the management of advanced suppurative endophthalmitis. Yan Ke Xue Bao 1992;8:164-8.
[119] Yarng SS, Hsieh CC, Chen TL. Vitrectomy for endogenous Klebsiella pneumonia endophthalmitis with massive subretinal abscess. Ophthalmic Surg Lasers 1997;128:147-50.
[120] Vahey JB, Flynn HW Jr. Results in the management of Bacillus endophthalmitis. 1991;22:681-6.
[121] Sullivan P, Clark WL, Kaiser PK. Bilateral endogenous endophthalmitis caused by HACEK microorganism. Am J Ophthalmol 2002;133:144-5.
[122] Balaskas K, Potamitou D. Endogenous endophthalmitis secondary to bacterial meningitis from Neissereia meningitides: a case report and review of the literature. Cases J 2009;2:149.

8

Radiology in Infective Endocarditis

C. Prados, C. Carpio, A. Santiago, I. Silva and R. Álvarez-Sala
Pulmonology Service, La Paz University Hospital, Autónoma University, Madrid
Spain

1. Introduction

In the last 50 years, the incidence of infective endocarditis (IE) has remained between 2 and 6 per 100.000 individuals in the general population per year and its mortality has fluctuated between 10% and 30%, depending on the type of pathogen. Historically, chronic rheumatic heart disease had being the primary risk factor for IE but in the last years, new at-risk groups have emerged like individuals undergoing hemodialysis, patients with catheters and elderly people with degenerative valve lesions. IE is characterized by the infection of the endocardium, most commonly by bacteria. Although the primary focus of the infection is confined to the endocardium, microbial shedding by continuous bacteremia and embolization of vegetation fragments makes IE a true systemic infection. This disease, therefore, is positioned at the crossroads of multiple medical specialties, including cardiology, cardiac surgery, infectious diseases, internal medicine, neurology, and intensive care. Valve vegetations are specific pathologic findings of this disease. They are the result of the combination of thrombus with bacteria and leucocytes. The size and mobility of valvular vegetations are important predictors of whether or not the patient will develop septic emboli. These lesions usually affect valve endocardium, but it also could involve papillary muscles, mural endocardium and the great vessels. IE is fatal if it is not treated early with antibiotics. Negative prognostic factors are fungal etiology, involvement of the aortic valve, and presence of large vegetations. Patients with a left-sided endocarditis have a higher mortality in comparison to patients with right-sided endocarditis

The mean age of patients with IE has increased from 30 years in the 1950s, to 50 years in the 1980s. The higher frequency of IE diagnosis in older individuals probably reflects the clustering of more than one risk factor in the elderly. The results of epidemiological studies vary depending on the population analyzed and the microbial pathogens tend to differ between the various groups.

2. Classification

IE can be classified in four categories:

- Native valve endocarditis
- Intravenous drug abuse endocarditis (IVDA)
- Prosthetic valve endocarditis
- Pacemaker endocarditis and nosocomial endocarditis

Left-sided native valve endocarditis is the most frequent form of endocarditis, representing more than 60% of all cases. In-hospital mortality is approximately 15%. Pre-existing lesions can favor attachment of circulating bacteria and promote IE. Frequently, congenital or acquired valve diseases are present (rheumatic fever, degenerative cardiopathies, mitral valve prolapse). Mitral -valve prolapsed is a relatively common condition and have a 10–100-fold increased risk of IE. Degenerative valve lesions are present in up to 25% of patients with IE and they involve local inflammation, microulcers, and microthrombi of the endothelium. Degenerative valve lesions might increase the risk of IE in up to 50% of patients older than 60 years of age. Alpha-hemolytic streptococci or enterococci typically are the causative agents of this type endocarditis.

IVDA endocarditis usually occurs on healthy right heart valves, and 50% of these infections involve the tricuspid valve. Although highly population-specific, right-sided IE has represented up to 5–10% of cases in general surveys. This form of IE has a better prognosis than left-sided IE and in-hospital mortality is <10%, although mortality of up to 50% has been observed in patients with AIDS, especially in advanced cases. Intravenous-drug users, including those with HIV, are a group that primarily consists of relatively young adults. The risk of IE is approximately four to five times higher in those with < 200 CD4 per mm^3. The tricuspid valve is usually affected in these patients and Staphylococcus aureus is the most common causative organism.

Prosthetic valve endocarditis is the most-severe form of IE, and is associated with high mortality that ranges from 20% to >40%. It occurs in 1–5% of patients with prosthetic valves and accounts for up to 20% of all cases of IE. It is classified as 'early' or 'late' infection on the basis of the time period between surgery and the onset of IE. Early and late prosthetic valve endocarditis are defined, as occurring either within or more than 12 months after surgery, respectively. Early prosthetic valve endocarditis is often caused by surgery-related and drug-resistant microbes such as methicillin-resistant staphylococci and late endocarditis is due to infection with oral streptococci and Gram-negative bacteria of the HACEK group.

Pacemaker endocarditis are produced by infections of these devices within a few months of implantation. The rate of pacemaker endocartditis is estimated at 0.55 cases per 1,000 pacemakers recipients per year. These infections always require ablation of the material in addition to antibiotic therapy. Of pacemaker infections, 75% are produced by staphylococci.

3. Etiology and pathophysiology

The pathogens involved in IE depend on the different categories of endocarditis. The most frequent IE pathogens are Gram-positive bacteria (S. aureus, Streptococcus spp., and enterococci) and they are responsible for more than 80% of all IE cases. These bacteria have great ability to adhere to and colonize damaged valves and are equipped with several surface adhesins that mediate attachment to extracellular host matrix proteins. The clumping factor A and the fibronectin-binding protein A are involved in valve colonization and invasion of S. aureus. Fibrinogen-binding mediates the primary attachment of the bacteria to nonbacterial thrombotic endocarditis, and subsequent binding of fibronectin triggers endothelial cell internalization, followed by local proinflammatory and procoagulant responses.

Skin microorganisms are responsible for the vast majority of infections in IVDA endocarditis but contamination of drugs and material employed by drug abusers, also contribute to the bacteremia. Aortic and mitral valves are affected in 25% of cases of IVDA endocarditis. The pathogenic mechanisms that explain the increased prevalence of right sided IE in injection drug users are not fully elucidated. Damage to the right sided valves from injected particulate matter in the setting of injected bacterial loads is thought to be important, while subtle abnormalities of immune function may also have a role in pathogenesis. Cocaine use is associated with an increased incidence of endocarditis greater than heroin use, but this finding is not fully explained.

Pulmonary valve is only involved in less than 2% of cases. It is also reported that 6% of patients presents both right and left endocarditis at the same time.

With respect to the pathophysiology, there are many mechanisms proposed to the development of this disease. Endothelial damage can be caused by turbulent blood flow associated with congenital heart disease or prosthetic valves, by electrodes or catheters, or, in intravenous-drug users, from repeated intravenous injection of particulate material. Alternatively, endothelial damage can result from inflammation, for example in patients with rheumatic carditis or in elderly individuals with degenerative valve lesions. Other theories, however, defend the so-called "immunological hypothesis" which explains that the valve affection is secondary to immunological mechanisms that cause local inflammation.

4. Clinical manifestations

Symptoms of IE are related to the infectious condition of the process. General manifestations like persistent fever, chills, pleuritic chest pain, cough and hemoptysis have been described. Embolic events occur in approximately one-third of cases, more frequently in patients with intravenous drug use, right-sided endocarditis or positive blood cultures.

The most common extra-cardiac organ system involved in infective endocarditis is the central nervous system and could produce embolic stroke, intracranial hemorrhage, intracranial mycotic aneurysm, brain abscess and meningitis. With respect to the respiratory system, it has been reported septic pulmonary embolism like a clinical presentation of this condition. In right-sided endocarditis, pulmonary embolic manifestations are frequently present. Septic pulmonary emboli are detected in more than 80% of cases, and may be associated with pleuritic chest pain and dyspnea.

5. Radiology

A chest radiograph should be done routinely but the findings are not specified. Fifty percent of patients with IVDA endocarditis have radiologic opacities and 50-60 % of injection drug users with definite IE have multiple pulmonary opacities (figure 1 and figure 2). The typical radiograph pattern of septic emboli is peripheral, poorly marginated bilateral lung nodules that often demonstrate cavitary changes and moderately thick irregular walls. Also cardiomegaly, pleural effusion and radiographic signs of left heart failure (septal thickening, air bronchogram, pleural effusion) are reported.

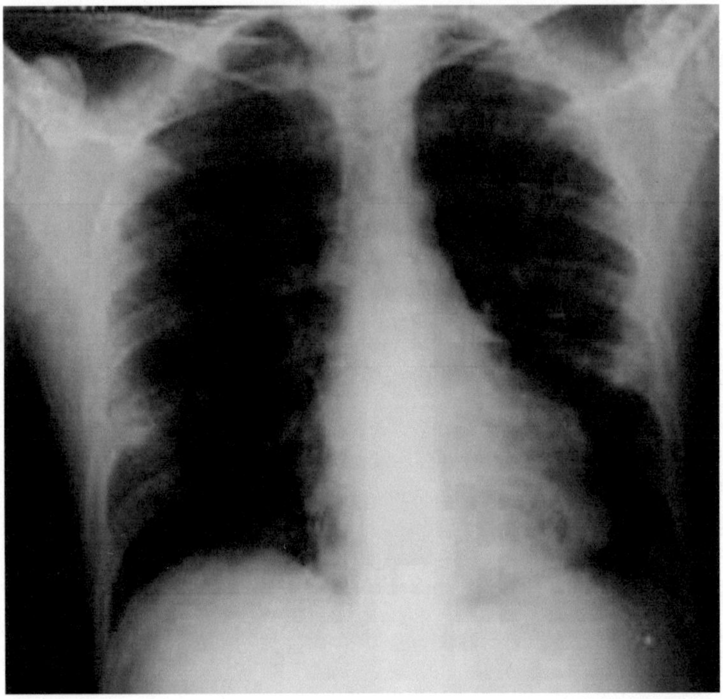

Fig. 1. Chest X-ray showing bilateral opacities and nodules, corresponding to septi emboli

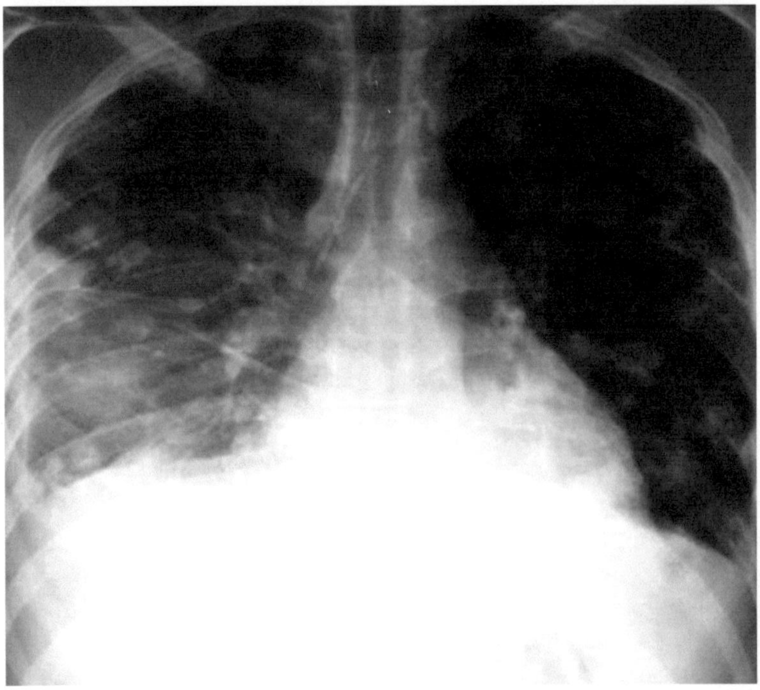

Fig. 2. Chest X-ray showing bilateral opacities. Also it can be observed the presence of pleural fluid

Computed tomography findings include:

- Peripheral triangle opacities, corresponding to regions of pulmonary infarcts produced by septic embolism.
- Peripheral, poorly marginated bilateral lung nodules.
- Cavitary nodules with thick irregular walls. These nodules typically measure 5-35 mm, have a peripheral and basilar predominance, and demonstrate air-bronchograms. The nodule may increase in number and change from day to day (figure 3).
- "Feeding vessel sign" that consists of a distinct vessel leading directly into the center of a nodule.
- Radiologic findings suggestive of empyema like pleural effusion, thickening and enhacement of the visceral and parietal pleurae and inflammation of the extrapleural fat. Also, empyema had been described as a pleural collection that is immnobile on decubitus views. Pleural fluid, pericardic fluid and pneumothorax.
- Unilateral or bilateral interstitial lung infiltrate.

In many instances, these radiological findings precede the clinical manifestations of IE. Also, the follow up of septic emboli could be performed by computed tomography.

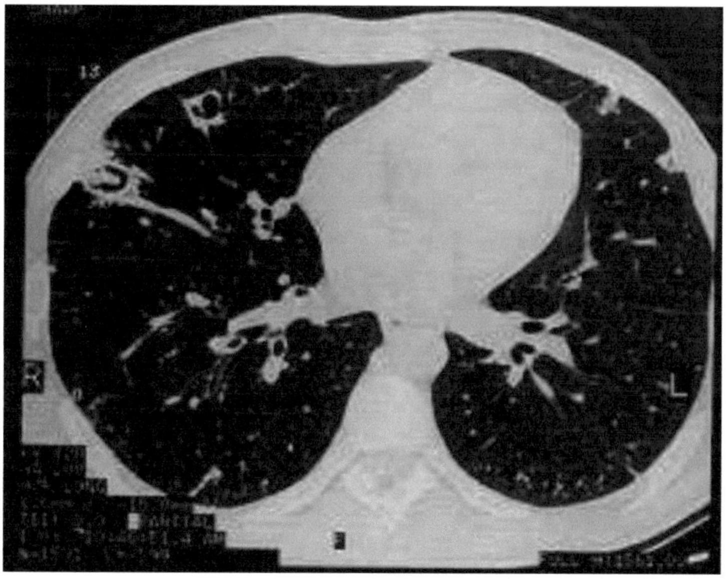

Fig. 3. Computed tomography scan showing peripheral cavitary nodules with thick irregular walls from 1 to 3 cm of size

These radiological findings are more common in IVDA endocarditis but also they can be found, less commonly, in other types of right IE, like endocarditis associated to pacemaker and intravascular devices. It is important to differentiate other radiologic presentation of IVDA, like ground-glass opacities, pulmonary hemorrhage, air trapping and pulmonary hypertension. When IE affects left chambers, radiographic findings are less frequent. Furthermore, they only appear in the context of heart complications: increased cardiothoracic ratio (secondary to pericardial effusion) and signs of left heart failure resulting from chordal rupture or valve failure.

6. Conclusion

Although echocardiography is the gold standard in the diagnosis of IE, the presence of many radiological findings could suggest its diagnosis.

7. References

Bittermann V, Pros SA. Manifestaciones osteoarticulares de endocarditis. *Semin Fund Esp Reumatol.* 2010;11:152-8.

Nandakumar R, Raju G. Isolated tricuspid valve endocarditis in nonaddicted patients: A diagnostic challenge. *Am J Med Sci* 1997;314:207-12.

Lacassin F, Leport C. Infectious endocarditis, risk factors, prevention. Research group for infectious endocarditis and jury of the consensus conference. *Rev Med Interne.* 1993; 14(9):871-6.

Clifford SP, Eykyn SJ, Oakley CM. Sthaphylococcal tricuspid valve endocarditis in patients with structurally normal hearts and no evidence of narcotic abuse. *QJM* 1994;87:755-7.

Naidoo DP. Right-sided endocarditis in the non-drug addict. Postgrad Med J 1993;69:615-20.

Prados C, Galera R, Santiago A. Unilateral interstitial lung pattern as a first sign of a bacterial endocarditis. *Arch Bronconeumol.* 2010;46:206-7.

Nguyen E, Silva I, Souza C, Müller N. Pulmonary complications of illicit drug use differential diagnosis based on CT findings. *J Thorac Imaging* 2007;22:199-206.

TRENDS AND ADVANCES IN VETERINARY GENETICS

Edited by **Muhammad Abubakar**

Trends and Advances in Veterinary Genetics
http://dx.doi.org/10.5772/62718
Edited by Muhammad Abubakar

Contributors

Sven Budik, Aya Mahdy, Fernando Moreira Da Silva, Krishna Pavani, Erica Baron, Edo D' Agaro, Adriana Pires Neves, Eduardo Brun Schwengber, Fabiola Freire Albrecht, Liana de Salles van der Linden, José Victor Vieira Isola, Silvina Elena Gutiérrez, Marcela Alicia Juliarena, Eduardo Néstor Esteban, Claudia María Lützelschwab, Marlene Dinis, Joaquim F. Moreira da Silva, Vijay Kumar

Published by InTech
Janeza Trdine 9, 51000 Rijeka, Croatia

Publishing Process Manager Martina Usljebrka
Technical Editor SPi Global
Cover InTech Design team

First published March, 2017
Printed in Croatia
Legal deposit, Croatia: National and University Library in Zagreb

Additional hard copies can be obtained from orders@intechopen.com

Trends and Advances in Veterinary Genetics, Edited by Muhammad Abubakar
p. cm.
Print ISBN 978-953-51-3041-3
Online ISBN 978-953-51-3042-0

For EU product safety concerns:
IN TECH d.o.o., Prolaz Marije Krucifikse Kozulić 3, 51000 Rijeka, Croatia, info@intechopen.com or visit our website at intechopen.com.

Meet the editor

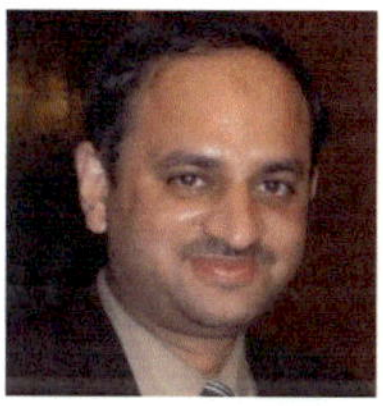

Dr. Muhammad Abubakar, a scientist from the National Veterinary Laboratory, Islamabad, Pakistan, has experience of more than 15 years in various fields of veterinary sciences. He has main expertise on the transboundary animal diseases (TADs) in the country as well as in the region. He has worked with local and international projects for the establishment of diagnostic laboratories for TADs in the country. He has published numerous research papers, review articles, and book chapters on different issues of veterinary medicine especially on TADs. He is the coeditor of the book *The Role of Biotechnology in Improvement of Livestock* by Springer Publisher, Germany. He is currently working as an editor in chief of two journals in the area of veterinary sciences (*Research Journal for Veterinary Practitioners and Veterinary Sciences*; *Research and Reviews*).

Contents

Preface

It is very crucial to understand the recent advances and trends of veterinary genetics to recognize and control diseases and disorders in animals. They are also critical for enhancing animal production and reproduction. Accessible and clearly offered, *Trends and Advances in Veterinary Genetics* provides a concise introduction and details to the aspects of genetics relevant to animal science and production. This is the first edition of the book so it covers the introductory level of topics which are written specifically for veterinary and animal science students. Molecular techniques especially the epigenetics and NGS (next-generation sequencing) that are revolutionizing are covered and discussed in the book, including the areas of basic genetics of lactation, environmental control of inherited disorders, animal breeding, and selection. These topics provide an excellent introduction to molecular techniques and their application to animal disease and production. The book is self-contained, with everything needed for one to understand the latest concepts and trends in the veterinary genetics.

If we observe in detail, the book provides an introductory and up-to-date overview of those aspects of genetics that are relevant to animal disease and animal production. It provides an excellent introduction to anyone interested in acquiring a basic understanding of genetics. Examples are drawn from the field of veterinary science, and a clear account is provided of the importance of molecular biology to genetics. The various concepts are clearly and concisely expressed. The writing is generally clear, realistic, and quite positive on various aspects, so that many students should be tempted to get more involved in genetics.

The book coverage includes the following main areas:

- Biotechnology and Reproductive Genetics
- Advances in Embryonic Genetics
- Conservation and Basic Genetics
- Veterinary Genetics and Future

Each book section comprises two chapters from renowned experts from the area and gives readers a unique opportunity to explore the topic.

I would like to express my gratitude to all the contributors of this book including the authors of the accepted chapters. My special thanks to the Publishing Process Manager, Ms. Martina Usljebrka, and other staff of InTech publishing for their kind support and great efforts in bringing the book to completion. In addition, I am also thankful to my colleagues, friends, and family for all their support in the fulfillment of this project.

Dr. Muhammad Abubakar
National Veterinary Laboratory,
Islamabad, Pakistan

Section 1

Biotechnology and Reproductive Genetics

Chapter 1

Genetic and Breeding Aspects of Lactation

Vijay Kumar

Additional information is available at the end of the chapter

http://dx.doi.org/10.5772/66179

Abstract

Animal breeding is the most important tool to improve milk productivity in dairy animals. Identification of better animals as parent for the next generation is the approach to generate high-producing animals. Genetic disease is the main problem in livestock sector. Complex vertebral malformation (CVM), bovine leukocyte adhesion deficiency (BLAD) syndrome, bovine factor xi deficiency, deficiency of uridine monophosphate synthase (DUMPS), and bovine citrullinemia are some of the main genetic disorders, which should be studied in Holstein and its cross. Recent developments in biotechnology have made it feasible to reveal a large number of genetic polymorphisms at the DNA level. As a result, researchers have been encouraged to use them as markers in order to evaluate genetic basis for the observed phenotypic variability. The selection of genetically superior sires is of utmost importance for any successful breed improvement program as semen of sires is disseminated in various herds under progeny testing program. The investigations on mode of genetic improvement around the world indicated that proper genetic evaluation and selection of bulls bring about more than 75% of the actual genetic improvement.

Keywords: molecular markers, genetic disorder, part-lactation milk yield, test-day milk yield

1. Introduction

Lactation is one of the most important economic characters of dairy animals. Genetic aspect of lactation includes those concepts, which are important for milk production in an individual animal. On the other hand, breeding aspect is important for improvement in milk production in a population of dairy animals. Milk production is largely affected by a combination of factors, namely, genetic makeup, a favorable nutritional environment and improved managerial practices. Consequently, genetic makeup of dairy animals plays a great role in the variation of milk yield and composition. Lactation is, therefore, a factor of genotype-environment interactions. Animals are subjected to constant improvement for this trait, which is based on phenotypic observations of cattle and evaluation of the progeny and kins. These processes are both time-consuming and expensive. With the observed advances in molecular genetics, one may presume, however, that this may dramatically accelerate genetic improvement of dairy cattle, especially due to genotyping of young animals. Identification of various genetic factors involved in regulating the lactation and involution in farm animal would enable to reveal the molecular basis of milk production. This would serve as a platform to direct future research to enhance the productivity of cattle. The identification and characterization of these factors will pave the way to design appropriate approach to ameliorate the problem of lactation. The availability of fully sequenced genomes and further development of DNA sequencing techniques allowed gaining of complex genomic data from a number of animals and promises to overcome traditional problems with understanding of fragmented genomic data provided by other genomic techniques. Association studies using whole genome sequence from animals with different phenotypic performances will permit identification of genomic regions with significant effect on main economic traits. Genetic improvement includes selection of excellent animals from a population to produce higher yields in future generations. Since long back, livestock breeders have used genetic evaluations to identify best animals. Selective use of these livestock improved phenotypic measures for milk production and milk components.

2. Molecular markers and milk production

Recent developments in biotechnology have made it feasible to reveal a large number of genetic polymorphisms at the DNA level. As a result, researchers have been encouraged to use them as markers in order to evaluate genetic basis for the observed phenotypic variability. The distinctive genetic properties as well as methodological advantages of molecular markers make them helpful and amenable, to a greater extent, for genetic research than other genetic markers. Nowadays, molecular markers are being identified on a vast variety of genes of economic importance and are widely accepted. Association between DNA polymorphism and milk production traits has been studied for a number of genes, including prolactin; leptin; diacylglycerol acyltransferase (DGAT1); bovine leukocyte antigen (BoLA)-DRB3, growth hormone receptor gene, ATP-binding cassette, and protease inhibitor gene; proliferator-activated receptor gamma and coactivator (CoA) 1α gene; growth hormone (GH) gene; signal transducer and activator of transcription (STAT)1; thyroglobulin gene; β-lactoglobulin gene; STAT5A; and stearoyl-CoA desaturase. Out of the different marker studies, molecular markers for prolactin, leptin, and DGAT1 show their association with milk traits.

2.1. Pit-1 transcription factor

Pit-1 transcription factor regulates the expression of growth hormone and prolactin in the anterior pituitary gland [1]. The bovine Pit-1 gene is located in centromeric region of chromosome 1 in bovine [2]. Bovine Pit-1 is a 291 amino acid protein. This gene is a candidate for lactation yield because of its role in regulating expression of bovine growth hormone (bGH) and the prolactin genes. Association studies have shown that Pit-1 is associated with milk production in domestic animals. Pit-1 was found to be related to birth weight weaning and average daily gain. Quantitative trait loci (QTL) detection revealed that the region surrounding POU domain, class 1, transcription factor 1 (POU1F1) on cattle, 1q21–q22, had an effect on animal production. POU1F1 gene is also a possible candidate for growth traits. In cattle, Pit-1 was found to be associated with milk production traits. *Hinf*I polymorphism has been reported in exon 6 of the bovine Pit-1 gene by polymerase chain reaction-restriction fragment length polymorphism (PCR-RFLP) technique. This single nucleotide polymorphism (SNP) was found in the coding region of the bovine Pit-1 gene. Moreover, four intronic polymorphisms were also reported: two located in intron 3, one in intron 4, and the last in intron 5.

2.2. Growth hormone receptor (GHR)

The growth hormone plays a critical endocrine role controlling nutrient metabolism in dairy cattle. In the liver, growth hormone receptor (GHR) is dynamically regulated by lactation and energy balance. GH receptor is determined by a single gene with a length of 110 kbp, consisting of ten exons, located on chromosome 20 of cattle [3]. The gene of this receptor (*GHR*) is characterized by the existence of numerous exons whose transcripts undergo alternative splicing. Growth hormone activity depends on the receptor, and consequently its gene may be a potential candidate gene.

2.3. Insulin-like growth factor 1 (IGF-1)

Insulin-like growth factor 1 (IGF-1) is produced in the liver and body tissues. Important role for IGF-1 is to promote cell growth and division. The bovine *IGF*-1 gene is located on the long arm of chromosome 5. It contains seven exons, separated by long introns. As stated, IGF-1 regulates cell growth, development, and division; it can stimulate growth in both normal and cancerous cells. Even small increases in serum levels of IGF-1 are associated with increased risk for several common cancers.

2.4. Diacylglycerol acyltransferase 1 (DGAT1)

DGAT1 is the main enzyme for the synthesis of triacylglycerols, the major fraction of milk fat compounds. Bovine *DGAT1* locus is found on chromosome 14. Milk is the main source of saturated fatty acids, which are a valuable source of nutrients. Recently, a dinucleotide substitution located in the exon 8 of the gene coding for acyl-CoA, diacylglycerol acyltransferase 1 (DGAT1), that modifies the amino acid order from a lysine to an alanine (Lys232Ala) in the mature protein was shown to have an immense effect on milk fat content in some cattle breeds. The frequency of polymorphism in *DGAT1* gene has been found to be very high in dairy cattle. The attention in the bovine *DGAT1* gene has increased during the previous few years. *DGAT1* is also important for the physiological processes involving triacylglycerol metabolism such as intestinal fat absorption, adipose tissue formation, and lactation.

2.5. Leptin (LEP)

Leptin is a 16-kDa protein secreted from white adipocytes, which is involved in regulation of feed intake, milk yield, energy balance, fertility, and immune functions in animals. Leptin is considered as a powerful biomolecule for enhancing productivity in farm animals. Its role in lactogenesis, colostrum secretion, galactopoiesis, and immunity to mastitis has made it an important candidate gene for genetic studies. Since the bovine leptin gene has been recognized on chromosome 4, several SNPs have been in the past identified in introns and exons of leptin among different breeds of cattle. Several investigations have revealed that polymorphisms were associated with lean and fat cattle [4, 5] and with the fat contents and feed intakes [6–8]. Important profitable factors for livestock production may be affected by leptin including feed conversion competence and intramuscular fat, which is considered to improve meat quality [9].

Nutrition is a main determinant of productive potential in cattle and other mammals. Therefore, responses of the productive system to changes in nutrition and metabolic status influence reproductive and economic efficiency of food-producing species in a variety of contexts. As the hormone leptin is involved in regulation of nutritional status and reproductive function, this hormone is an interesting protein to investigate during the periparturient period in dairy cattle. Leptin may help regulate ovarian development and steroidogenesis and serve as either a primary signal initiating puberty or as a permissive regulator of sexual maturation. Leptin is supposed to be necessary by the mammary growth, development, and function, when mammary fat cell leptin expression requires prolactin which then cooperates with leptin to influence mammary activity. The ruminant mammary epithelial cells also synthesize leptin during pregnancy and during established lactation. In dairy cattle, the increase in milk yield has been accompanied by a more negative energy balance during early lactation and a decrease in fertility. The polymorphism in LEP gene was associated with milk performance and increased perinatal mortality in dairy calf birth and weaning weights in beef and dairy and reproductive performance in dairy cattle. Exogenous administration of leptin in ob/ob mice leads to a significant improvement in reproductive and endocrine status as well as reduced food intake and weight loss.

2.6. Prolactin

The bovine prolactin gene (*bPRL*) is regarded as a good candidate gene for marker-assisted selection (MAS) for milk production parameters. Bovine prolactin spans approximately 9.4 kb and consists of five exons and four introns, which encode a mature protein with 199 amino acids first mapped it on the bovine chromosome 23. Prolactin gene disruption experiments proved its important roles in mammary gland development (mammogenesis), lactogenesis, maintenance of milk secretion (galactopoiesis), and expression of milk protein genes [10]. It is also chiefly accountable for synthesis of lactose, lipids, and all other major components of milk [11]. Consequently, the bovine prolactin gene seems to be an outstanding candidate for linkage analysis with quantitative trait loci (QTL) affecting milk production traits. Prolactin is a polypeptide hormone and plays crucial roles in mammary gland development, initiation, and maintenance of lactation, which is synthesized in lactotroph cells of the anterior pituitary gland of vertebrate. Prolactin is a protein hormone primarily, but not solely produced by lactotroph cells of the anterior pituitary. Its role in maintenance of milk secretion is well demonstrated. As a result, the gene encoding prolactin is assumed to be one of the key links in constituting the hereditary component of milk productivity. Therefore, the bovine prolactin gene seems to be an excellent candidate for quantitative trait loci (QTL) affecting milk production traits.

3. Genetic disorders and animal selection

Apart from selection of bulls on the basis of milk production and reproductive abilities, some of the genetic disorders should also be taken care of. Chromosomal abnormalities in domestic animals are one of the very important causes of reproductive impairment. The impairment in reproduction leads to loss of germplasm, and there is every possibility that these chromosomal aberrations are transmitted from one generation to another. Several centric fusions, i.e., *Robertsonian* translocation, have been reported in cattle. The animals carrying this translocation are phenotypically normal but have reproductive problems. In this translocation, two nonhomologous chromosomes break at the extreme end at the short arm. These small segments are lost, and the large segments fuse at their centromeric region and produce a new large metacentric or submetacentric chromosome. The exchange of segment between two nonhomologous chromosomes is a type of structural variation called a reciprocal translocation. In this, the genetic information is neither lost nor gained rather there is a rearrangement of genetic material. The least complex way for this event to occur is for nonhomologous chromosome arms to come close to each other so that an exchange is facilitated. For this type of translocation in which the ends of chromosomes are involved, only two breaks are required. Heterozygous homologues for a reciprocal translocation undergo unorthodox synopsis during meiosis, resulting in a cross-like configuration. By whatever mechanism produced, the translocated region may nevertheless act normally with respect to homologous pairing. Thus, a translocation homozygote forms the same number of homologous pairs as the normal homozygote as long as centromeres are not lost. In several countries, there is restriction on the export and import of semen from bulls without normal karyotype. In the United Kingdom, all the bulls used for artificial insemination are subjected to routine screening for cytogenetic abnormality.

Selection is based on genetic markers and also universally checking up of the breeding bulls for heritable diseases. Many heritable mutations and diseases have been traced to autosomal chromosomes of different cattle breeds; most of these mutations are lethal or bring about deficiencies in the defense mechanism if they occur in the homozygous recessive manner. Moreover, due to coverage of wild-type allele on mutant allele in heterozygotes, carrier animals may not show any phenotypic abnormality but are most likely to transmit the mutant alleles to the next generation. The same problem may assume catastrophic significance if the carrier is a bull intended to be used in artificial breeding programs.

3.1. Complex vertebral malformation

The complex vertebral malformation (CVM) is a recessively inherited congenital disorder leading to frequent abortion of fetuses or vertebral anomalies and prenatal death [12–14]. It is characterized by growth retardation and bilateral flexure of the carpal and metacarpophalangeal joints along with rotation of the digits. In stillborn, aborted, and preterm calves, CVM has been characterized by shortened cervical and thoracic regions of the vertebral column and symmetric arthrogryposis. Multiple hemivertebrae, scoliosis, and synostosis and fused and misshaped vertebral column have also been described. The syndrome was first discovered in the Danish Holstein population in 1999, but, shortly thereafter, its occurrence was reported in the Netherlands, in the United States, in the United Kingdom, and in Japan.

Studies of Danish Holstein showed that the extent of fetal mortality was approximately 77% prior to gestation day 260. This is reflected in a significantly reduced ratio of CVM-affected calves in breeding studies. Through increased fetal mortality, the status of the fetus has a significant effect on calving interval and involuntary culling of cows. The symptoms of the defect have not been observed in carriers of CVM. No productive and reproductive differences between carrier and noncarrier animals have been reported. The only difference which is very important was increase in the rate of intrauterine mortality. The risk of return to service was higher in carrier animals.

When studying the postpartum recommencement of ovulation—the carry-over of ovarian cycles after the birth of one calf—the researchers recognized that there was no major difference in the rate at which resumption occurs in carriers as compared to Holstein cows that were not carriers for CVM. However, CVM carrier cows were recognized to have drastically lower conception rates than control cows, with the gap between calves observed at 463 days in carriers than 399 days for control cows, telling the possibility of heightened death of embryos in CVM carrier cows.

3.2. Bovine leukocyte adhesion deficiency syndrome

Bovine leukocyte adhesion deficiency (BLAD) syndrome is an autosomal recessive hereditary disease affecting young Holstein calves characterized by recurrent bacterial infections, progressive periodontitis, ulcers of oral mucosa, and impaired inflammatory responses [15, 16]. These clinical findings are associated with impaired neutrophil functions such as markedly decreased adherence, chemotaxis, and phagocytosis. In 1990, a lack of β_2 integrin molecules expressed on the leukocytes from affected animals was found in a calf with granulocytopathy syndrome, and this disease was termed bovine leukocyte adhesion deficiency, which was considered to be analogous to human leukocyte adhesion deficiency (LAD). BLAD causes immune deficiency in the early days of life. The affected animal is prone to all infectious agents which can cause death. BLAD was first documented in Holstein-Friesian cattle, and no study has reported the incidence of this disorder in other breeds. The affected cattle with BLAD was linked to common ancestral sires that had been documented to be carriers.

3.3. Deficiency of uridine monophosphate synthase

Deficiency of uridine monophosphate synthase (DUMPS) is a genetic disorder which interferes with pyrimidine biosynthesis. Uridine monophosphate synthase (UMPS) has a key role on the pyrimidine nucleotide synthesis, which is essential for normal growth and development for several ruminant and nonruminant species [17]. Inactivation of this enzyme is caused by an autosomal recessive heredity mutation, which takes place in the gene of uridine monophosphate synthase. The mutation (cytosine to thymine) leads to the loss of the restriction site of *Ava*I site at nucleotide position 405 of the gene. This disorder is named as DUMPS in the Holstein cattle and characterized by lowered blood activity of enzyme UMPS [17]. DUMPS leads to embryonic death in the early stage of pregnancy. So some serious reproductive problems take place in dairy herds.

3.4. Factor XI deficiency syndrome

Factor XI (FXI) deficiency is an autosomal recessive disorder, with partial deficiency of FXI coagulant activity in heterozygotes and considerable deficiency in homozygotes [18]. One of the protein factors concerned in blood coagulation is a serine protease—factor XI. It is produced in the liver as a zymogen, and after alteration to a proteolytic enzyme. FXI deficiency has been recognized in humans and cattle. FXI gene is located on chromosome number 4 in human and on chromosome number 27 in cattle. FXI gene encodes coagulation factor XI of the blood coagulation cascade, and it is one of more than a dozen proteins involved in blood clotting.

In cattle, FXI-deficient animals may be asymptomatic or display several symptoms, like prolonged bleeding, anemia, greater prevalence of repeat breeding, or even lower resistance to pneumonia, mastitis, and metritis. *FXI* deficiency has been recognized in a number of species of mammals, including humans, dogs, and cattle. *FXI* deficiency possibly will result in delayed bleeding and anemia. Persistent bleeding from the umbilical cord is occasionally seen in affected calves. Delayed emission of blood following dehorning or castration may also be observed. Affected cows repeatedly have pink-colored colostrum.

3.5. Bovine citrullinemia

Bovine citrullinemia is a genetic disorder, which has been reported in Holstein cattle [19]. It has been established that bovine citrullinemia is a consequence of a deficiency of argininosuccinate synthetase (ASS), one of the enzymes of the urea cycle. A shortage of the urea cycle enzyme consequences in a lethal neurological disease in newly born calves. The urea cycle entails a series of biochemical steps in which waste product of protein metabolism is removed from the blood in the form of urea. The deficiency of ASS occurs when a calf inherits a copy of the mutant gene encoding for ASS from each parent. The gene is located on chromosome number 11 (BTA11). The mutation is caused by a transition of cytosine to thymine at codon 86 within exon 5 in the gene coding for ASS leading to impaired enzyme, which cannot participate in urea cycle. Calves affected with the disorder appear normal immediately after birth. However, by the second day of birth, they become depressed. By the third day, they are seen wandering or standing with their head pressed against a wall. Death usually takes place within 12 hours of start of these clinical signs. The clinical signs of citrullinemia are believed to be as a consequence of accumulation of ammonia in the brain of the affected calves.

4. Factors affecting milk production

The success of dairy industry is much dependent on productivity and efficient reproduction performance of animals. Genetic progress may be done by selection. The nongenetic factors such as management, housing, feed, season, etc. also control production. The genetic improvement of growth of dairy animals is of great importance in the large ruminant industry.

4.1. Dry period

Dry period is an important economic trait which has the direct effect on lifetime milk production. There is a lot of variability observed in the dry period. It is the period from the date of drying to the next calving. Animals should be given proper rest, when they are in pregnancy, before the next calving to compensate for growth of fetus.

4.2. Growth

The genetic improvement of growth is of great importance in the large ruminant industry. The growth rate of a heifer calf until it matures to a cow is also a significant trait since it characterizes the adaptability and economic appropriateness of the animal. It is anticipated that animals growing faster may also begin physiological performance of reproduction and milk production earlier.

4.3. Age at first calving

Age at calving is an important trait because lower age at first calving (AFC) leads to shorter generation interval and hence increases genetic gain. AFC has a considerable influence on the total expenditure of raising dairy replacements. Older calving heifers are being more expensive to raise than younger calving heifers. Moreover, reducing AFC can also increase the profitability by increasing lifetime milk production and milk production per year of herd life. The most important drawback of reducing AFC is that it is commonly associated with a reduction in the first lactation milk yield. Regardless of this decline in the first lactation milk yield, production per year of herd life is characteristically increased by reduced AFC. In addition, while the first lactation may be affected by AFC, future lactations are absolutely not. Furthermore, stayability and health of cows are not affected by reduced AFC as long as the first calf heifers freshen at a sufficient weight.

4.4. Service period

Service period is the duration between date of calving and date of successful conception. The finest service period facilitates the animal to recover from the stress of calving and also for reproductive organs back to its usual shape. Usually for cattle the best service period is 60–90 days.

4.5. Calving interval

The interval between two successive calvings is referred to as calving interval (CI) which consists of two components—service period and gestation period. Among the traits of dairy animals, calving interval is the most important trait as it determines the number of lactations possible in the lifetime of an animal, thereby influencing its production of an animal. It is generally held that shorter calving intervals favor a large yield for the lifetime of the cow. That frequent calving should give maximum lifetime yield seems in harmony with the known facts of the physiology of reproduction and lactation. The natural need of milk develops with birth of the young. The need increases with growth of the young so long as milk is the only food. As other food is taken, the need for milk decreases and finally disappears. In milch animals, where we have adequate information as to the amount of milk produced day by day, it is found that the rate of milk secretion parallels roughly the rising and declining needs of the young. That is, the rate of milk secretion is most rapid in the cow shortly after calving and slows up quite markedly and continuously thereafter. It would seem that frequent calving by giving more high points in the lifetime lactation curve should result in a greater total yield than less frequent calving. Another way of putting the matter is to relate the length of the calving interval to the average yield of milk per day over the calving interval. This relation may be derived in relative terms from the known characteristics of the lactation curve. The indication is that the highest lifetime yield should be obtained from calving intervals of less than a year rather than from calving intervals of more than a year.

4.6. Days to first service or waiting period

Waiting period (WP) or days to first service (DFS) is one of the important reproduction traits. WP or DFS is the initial phase of lactation during which no inseminations occur. The lower the WP or DFS shows, the higher the breeding efficiency in dairy animals. Reducing WP is tempting because of associated reductions in calving interval. Getting cows pregnant is perhaps one of the major challenges faced by the dairy farmers. Cows that do not become pregnant at a rational interval after calving will remain in the herd, reduced overall milk yield, and if they do become pregnant, they likely to develop post-parturient diseases in the subsequent lactation. Conversely, on the other hand, cows that become pregnant too early after calving would be dried off too early in lactation when they are still producing a reasonable amount of milk.

The voluntary waiting period (VWP) is a time during the early lactation in which cows are purposely not inseminated even though they show estrus signs, to allow for optimum uterine involution. The VWP is fairly inconsistent across dairy herds. Decision over the optimal VWP should be made according to individual situations and after careful analysis of probable gains and losses. The suggestion of extending the VWP is based on the reality that during the early lactation cows are recovering from a condition of negative energy balance. Therefore, extending the VWP may allow cows to recover from a metabolic state that is deleterious to reproductive efficiency and display estrus a few times prior to the first insemination, which has been correlated with improved fertility.

4.7. Daughter pregnancy rate

A genetic evaluation tool for reproduction exists in the form of daughter pregnancy rate (DPR). DPR is calculated from days open and is directly related to the proportion of females eligible to become pregnant in a 21-day period that actually become pregnant (i.e., the 21-day pregnancy rate).

DPR forecasts genetic improvement (or deterioration) in pregnancy rate for future daughters of a bull compared to a bull that is expected to produce no change. Better pregnancy rates decrease semen usage and can be an essential part of efforts to reduce service period. Workers also comment that genetics do not control fertility adequately to justify selection. Heritability of DPR is low—only about 4%—so producers should not expect dramatic improvement in fertility from selection. However, genetic control of fertility is real. DPR needs to be included with all the other traits of economic significance in dairy cattle breeding.

5. New breeding approaches to improve dairy animals

The selection of genetically superior sires is of utmost importance for any successful breed improvement program as semen of sires is disseminated in various herds under progeny testing program. The investigations on mode of genetic improvement around the world indicated that proper genetic evaluation and selection of bulls bring about more than 75% of the actual genetic improvement. The accuracy of estimating the breeding value of an animal is the major factor that affects the genetic progress from selection. The success of a breeding program depends on how early and how accurately young bulls can be evaluated at a minimum possible cost.

Animal breeding is the most important tool by which one can think about improving livestock sector in comparatively faster rate. Animal breeding is all about selecting best animals from population which are used as parent for the next generation. Milk yield is the single most important economic trait determining economic returns from the dairy animals. In animal breeding selection of animals is almost considered as selection of bulls since the progeny-producing ability of bull is many folds more than a cow and progeny testing is the most acceptable technique for the selection of bulls.

5.1. Part-lactation milk yield for genetic evaluation

The first important advancement was the use of part-lactation milk yield for genetic evaluation of cattle and buffalo bulls. The genetic and phenotypic correlation between 305-day and part-lactation monthly and cumulative monthly milk yields in cattle reported that the genetic correlation of monthly yields with 300-day yield was high up to the fifth month and thereafter the estimates declined. The phenotypic correlations among these traits were high and statistically highly significant. There is significant correlation between 100-day and 300-day milk yields, and selection on the basis of 100-day production was sufficiently accurate to select the animal for 300-day production in Gir cattle. In Sahiwal cattle selection on the basis of individual third month milk yield and cumulative 90-day milk yield was at least 89 and 79% as effective as on the basis of first lactation 305-day milk yield. Definitely, these findings will be very helpful in reducing duration for evaluating bulls as only 4–5 months milk records are sufficient enough to evaluate bulls. Hence, the application of part-lactation records of daughters will be helpful in ranking the sires at younger age resulting in reduced generation interval

http://dx.doi.org/10.5772/66179

and increased intensity of selection credited to the availability of more numbers of records on daughters even having part-lactation records.

5.2. Test-day milk yield for genetic evaluation

The second important advancement is the use of test-day milk yield for genetic evaluation of cattle and buffalo bulls. The use of test-day record is easier and advance than part-lactation record as in this case only one or two particular day (test day) record is required instead of taking all-day records up to a certain part of lactation. Genetic correlations between observed milk yield and predicted milk yield under various test-day sampling schemes (fortnightly, monthly, and bimonthly) were very high being greater than 0.95 for Karan Swiss cattle and to be nearly united in Karan Fries cattle. There are higher phenotypic correlations among test-day milk yields ranging from 0.55 to 0.93 in Murrah buffaloes. The genetic correlations among test-day milk yields and 305-day milk yield were close to unity and phenotypic correlations among test-day milk yields and 305-day milk yield were quite high and positive (0.60–0.99) in Murrah buffaloes. So this technique was also explored at research level and found that test-day records could also be used for fast progress in livestock improvement.

At the present time, test-day model is thus used instead of 305-day model for the genetic evaluation of dairy cattle. Test-day model is the statistical method that thinks about all genetic and environmental effects straight on a test-day basis. The test-day models have been recommended as the method of choice for the study of milk yield traits in order to maximize the use of all accessible information. This method becomes significant with smaller herd size and without well-established milk recording systems.

6. Conclusion and future perspectives

A variety of molecular markers for improving milk production and their association with disease and productive and reproductive traits have proved to be beneficial to the livestock breeders. They can also be used economically in breeding and management decisions. The application of diverse molecular markers in determining the vulnerability to economically significant diseases proves to be helpful to minimize loss of animals and their productivity. Advancement of technologies to evaluate polymorphisms provides an idea about the development in the field of genetics to improve cattle health and production. The genetic disease causes heavy losses because of poor animal performance; structural unsoundness reduces the production and reproductive potential of the animal. The massive spread of genetic defects like CVM and BLAD in recent years is caused by the extensive use of elite carrier sires. Artificial insemination hastens the spread of detrimental recessives worldwide. The new technologies of molecular genetics facilitate to find the cause at gene level. This makes it possible to identify heterozygous animals and to manage the genetic health of the cattle population. The use of molecular methods into animal research promises quick progress in animal potential. If no cases are found in routine screening even then, extensive screening programs for identification of genetic disorders appear necessary to guarantee the utilization of bulls free from genetic disorders for artificial insemination programs.

Author details

Vijay Kumar

Address all correspondence to: jaisvet@gmail.com

Department of Animal Genetics and Breeding, U.P. Pt. Deen Dayal Upadhyaya Pashu Chikitsa Vigyan Vishwavidyalaya Evam Go Anusandhan Sansthan, Mathura, Uttar Pradesh, India

References

[1] Lin C, Lin SC, Chang CP, Rosenfeld MG. Pit-1-dependent expression of the receptor for growth hormone releasing factor mediates pituitary cell growth. Nature. 1992;**360**:765–768. DOI: 10.1038/360765a0

[2] Moody DE, Pomp D, Barendse W. Restriction fragment length polymorphism in amplification products of the bovine PIT1 gene and assignment of PIT1 to bovine chromosome 1. Animal Genetics. 1995;**26**:45–47. DOI: 10.1111/j.1365-2052.1995.tb02620.x

[3] Moody DE, Pomp D, Barendse W, Womack JE. Assignment of the growth hormone receptor gene to bovine chromosome 20 using linkage analysis and somatic cell mapping. Animal Genetics. 1995;**26**:341–343. DOI: 10.1111/j.1365-2052.1995.tb02671.x

[4] Stone RT, Kappes SM, Beattie CW. The bovine homolog of the obese gene maps to chromosome 4. Mammalian Genome. 1996;**7**:399–400. DOI: 10.1007/s003359900119

[5] Fitzsimmons CJ, Schmutz SM, Bergen RD, McKinnon JJ. A potential association between the BM 1500 microsatellite and fat deposition in beef cattle. Mammalian Genome. 1998;**9**:432–434.

[6] Konfortov BA, Licence VE, Miller JR. Re-sequencing of DNA from a diverse panel of cattle reveals a high level of polymorphism in both intron and exon. Mammalian Genome. 1999;**10**:1142–1145. DOI: 10.1007/s003359901180

[7] Buchanan FC, Fitzsimmons CJ, Van Kessel AG, Thue TD, Winkelman-Sim DC, Schmutz SM. Association of a missense mutation in the bovine leptin gene with carcass fat content and leptin mRNA levels. Genetics Selection Evolution. 2002;**34**:105–116. DOI: 10.1051/gse:2001006

[8] Lagonigro R, Wiener P, Pilla F, Woolliams JA, Williams JL. A new mutation in the coding region of the bovine leptin gene associated with feed intake. Animal Genetics. 2003;**34**:371–374. DOI: 10.1046/j.1365-2052.2003.01028.x

[9] Wheeler TL, Cundiff LV, Koch RM. Effect of marbling degree on beef palatability in *Bos taurus* and *Bos indicus* cattle. Journal of Animal Science. 1994;**72**:3145–3151.

[10] Horseman ND, Zhao W, Montecino-Rodriguez E, Tanaka M, Nakashima K, Engle SJ. Defective mammopoiesis, but normal hematopoiesis, in mice with a targeted disruption of the prolactin gene. EMBO Journal. 1997;**16**:6926–6935. DOI: 10.1093/emboj/16.23.6926

[11] Le Provost E, Leroux C, Martin P, Gafe P, Dijane J. Prolactin gene expression in ovine and caprine mammary gland. Neuroendocrinology. 1994;**60**:305–313.

[12] Agerholm JS, Andersen O, Almskou MB, Bendixen C, Arnbjerg J, Aamand G, Nielsen US, Panitz F, Petersen AH. Evaluation of the inheritance of complex vertebral malformation syndrome by breeding studies. Acta Veterinaria Scandinavica. 2004;**45**(3):133–137. DOI: 10.1186/1751-0147-45-133

[13] Agerholm JS, Bendixen C, Andersen O, Ambjerg J. Complex vertebral malformation in Holstein calves. Journal of Veterinary Diagnostic Investigation. 2001;**13**:283–289. DOI: 10.1177/104063870101300401

[14] Nielsen US, Aamand GP, Andersen O, Bendixen C, Nielsen VH, Agerholm JS. Effects of complex vertebral malformation on fertility traits in Holstein cattle. Livestock Production Science. 2003;**79**(2):233–238. DOI: 10.1016/S0301-6226(02)00170-7

[15] Kehrli ME, Ackermann MR, Shuster DE, Maaten VD, Schmalstieg FC, Anderson DC, Hughes BJ. Bovine leukocyte adhesion deficiency. β_2 integrin deficiency in young Holstein cattle. American Journal of Pathology. 1990;**140**:1489–1492.

[16] Nagahata H, Noda H, Takahashi K, Kurosawa T, Sonoda M. A suspected case of neutrophil dysfunction in a Holstein heifer. Japanese Journal of Veterinary Science. 1987;**49**(6):1165–1167.

[17] Healy MH, Shanks RD. Performance of females heterozygous for deficiency of uridine monophosphate synthase. Journal of Dairy Science. 1987;**70**(5):945–951.

[18] Gentry PA, Ross ML. Coagulation factor XI deficiency in Holstein cattle: expression and distribution of factor XI activity. Canadian Journal of Veterinary Research. 1994;**58**(4):242–247.

[19] Fesus L, Anton I, Zsolnai A. Marker assisted selection in livestock. DUMPS, weaver-diseases and citrullinaemia in cattle population. Allatt-es-Takarm. 1999;**48**(2):193–203.

Chapter 2

Genetics in Domestic Animal Reproduction

Sven Budik

Additional information is available at the end of the chapter

http://dx.doi.org/10.5772/67132

Abstract

Reproduction and early development in domestic animals are biological processes in which complex genetic events like formation of the germ cells, meiosis, syngamy, zygote formation, cleavage, midblastula transition, dose compensation of sex chromosomes, genetic imprinting, and multiple cell differentiation take place. Many of these processes have great impact in veterinary reproductive medicine and are influenced by the assisted reproductive techniques applied. Altered environmental and metabolic conditions caused by intensive livestock farming influence reproductive success by altered gene expression via epigenetic changes.

Keywords: reproductive genetics, developmental genetics, domestic animals

1. Genetics during germ cell production

Genetics during germ cell production: Mammalian oocytes and sperms originate from the primordial germ cells (PGCs) located in the embryonic mesoderm. Their development is initiated by signals from the extra embryonic ectoderm and the visceral endoderm. In mammals the primordial germ cells invade the genital ridge where they proliferate by mitosis and give rise to either oogonia or spermatogonia. Migration, proliferation, and colonization of PGCs to the developing gonads are controlled by many factors and depend as well on the interaction of PGCs and their surrounding somatic cells. Around the period of PGC migration into the genital ridges sex determination starts. Absence of the expression of the Y-linked gene "sex determining region of Y" (SRY, a transcription factor of the high mobility group box family) leads to female differentiation, therefore the gonads develop into ovaries [1]. Presence of SRY gene expression leads to differentiation of the gonads into testes. As soon as PGCs are formed, the initially bi-potential gonad will continue its differentiation mostly under the influence of somatic cell-derived transcription factors. In female animals after colonization of the gonad, PGCs will undergo a phase of mitotic proliferation leading to the formation of germ cell nests. Following this event, around birth, the germ cell nests break down and mitotic divisions stop. Germ cells initiate meiosis, become primary oocytes which are surrounded by somatic cells leading to the formation of primordial follicles which continue the female program of development.

Meiosis can be divided into two divisions: meiotic division I and II. The prophase of meiotic division I is extended and can be divided into the following parts: leptotene, zygotene, pachytene, diplotene, and diakinesis. During leptotene, progressive condensation of the chromosomes takes place and the telomeres become associated with the inner nuclear membrane. In zygotene, the homologous chromosomes pair due to the formation of the synaptonemal complex in a zipper-like way. The pachytene is characterized by further condensation of the chromosomes and by occurrence of cross-over events leading to intrachromosomal recombination. In the course of the diplotene, the chromosomes separate again except small anchoring regions the so-named chiasmata. Oocytes progressed to the diplotene stage enter into a prolonged resting phase called dictyotene. Oocytes remain at the dictyate stage of meiosis I throughout oogenesis, until luteinizing hormone (LH) induces final oocyte maturation to metaphase II [2]. Cell division during oocyte meiosis is asymmetrically leading to one oocyte containing most of the cytoplasm and three polar bodies. Formation of the second polar body is a requisite of oocyte maturity.

Spermatogenesis, the process that gives rise to fertile sperm, occurs in a similar manner in many animal species, including domestic mammals and birds. Male germ cell development starts with emergence of primordial germ cells (PGCs), which migrate and associate with somatic cells that form the testes. Within the gonad, PGCs localize to regions that are competent to serve as stem cell (SC) niches, where they develop into spermatogonial SCs (SSCs). SCs divide to form new SCs and spermatogonial daughter cells. The daughter cells proliferate, undergoing sequential rounds of mitosis and incomplete cytokinesis to form syncytial groups of spermatogonia. Following a series of synchronous mitotic amplification divisions, spermatogonia differentiate into spermatocytes, which then undergo meiosis. As in the earlier mitotic divisions, meiotic cytokinesis is incomplete, resulting in syncytia of interconnected haploid spermatids. Postmeiotic spermatids undergo an extensive period of differentiation, or spermiogenesis, in which they form sperm-specific organelles, including the sperm head, acrosome, basal body, specialized mitochondria, and flagellum. At the end of spermiogenesis, mature sperm are separated from each other by removal of the remnants of incomplete cytokinesis, released from the gonad, and stored prior to delivery by ejaculation.

In both, oogenesis and spermatogenesis meiosis leads to intrachromosomal recombination (cross-over occurring in prophasis of meiosis I) and in interchromosomal recombination (random mixture of maternal and paternal chromosomes during both meiotic divisions), reducing the diploid chromosome complement to a haploid level. As a result of oogenesis, one haploid oocyte and three haploid polar bodies develop. In spermatogenesis four haploid sperm come into being. In female eutherian mammals meiosis is continued by luteal hormone stimulation and finished during fertilization. In male eutherian mammals meiosis takes place all the time.

http://dx.doi.org/10.5772/67132

2. Genetics during fertilization

During their active and passive migration in the femal genital tract, the sperms obtain their fertilization capacity by capacitation and hyper activation two processes which seem to proceed largely independent. The glycoprotein composition changes during capacitation of the cell membrane. In domestic mammalian species fertilization takes place in the ampulla of the oviduct where the metaphase II oocyte surrounded by the acellular zona pellucida and the cellular cumulus (corona radiata) is present. The sperm leading to fertilization has to fulfill its acrosomal reaction. This is mediated by partial fusion of the cell membrane with the outer acrosomal membrane leading to the release of hyaluronidase. This enzyme enables the sperm to cross the corona radiata. At the zona pellucida binding to species specific zona proteins is necessary (species specificity). After detachment of the cell and outer acrosomal membrane the inner acrosomal membrane rises to the top delivering the protease Acrosin which enables the penetration of the zona pellucida. Now the sperm enters to the perivitelline space and the inner acrosomal membrane and the cell membrane of the oocyte fuse. In natural fertilization, only the head of the sperm enters the cytoplasm of the oocyte meaning that no mitochondria from the sperm can participate (maternal inheritance). After entrance of the first sperm, depolarization of the cell membrane, degranulation of the corticalis granula, shrinkage of the ooplasm, and zona hardening takes place in order to avoid multiple fertilizations. Fertilization by more than one sperm would lead to aneuploid ($n = 3, 4, 5\ldots$) chromosome complement. These embryos stop development before reaching the blastocyst stage. After entrance of the sperm the oocyte finishes the second meiotic division. Female and male pronuclei form and fuse to form a diploid nucleus in a process named syngamy leading to the zygote entering now into cleavage.

3. Genetics of eutherian sex determination and dose compensation

Sex determination in eutherian mammals is mediated by the chromosomes X and Y. Absence of the Y chromosome (SRY gene) leads to female development. Male genital development is mediated by production of the anti-Müllerian hormone (AMH) produced by the Sertoli cells of the embryonal testes. This peptide hormone, belonging to the transforming growth factors (TGF) family, leads to the regression of the Müllerian duct from which in the female the oviduct, the uterus, and the vagina are formed.

Aberrant sex chromosome numbers can arrive by false segregation during meiosis leading to multiple X or Y chromosome numbers. If one or more Y chromosomes are present the sex is male, if no Y chromosome is present the sex is female. Additional X chromosomes will be inactivated to a large extend (only a few genes escape from this inactivation) according to the Lyon hypothesis. This inactivation is mediated by the noncoding X inactive-specific transcript (XIST) RNA. The corresponding gene is located at the X Inactivation Center (XIC) at the X chromosome. Coating of the X chromosome to be inactivated by the XIST RNA leads to the deactivation of most of the genes: Only the XIST gene itself and about one quarter of the genes present mainly in the pseudo autosomal regions of the X chromosome escape from this inactivation. Before inactivation starts small quantities of XIST RNA are produced by both X chromosomes. After inactivation XIST is expressed from the inactivated X chromosome, whereas XIST expression from the active X chromosome ceases. Cytologically the inactivated X chromosome can be visualized as Barr body. The XO syndrome named Turner syndrome is sometimes observed in mares which are not fertile. In cats, the coat color gene is located at the X chromosome leading to the absence of tortoiseshell and calico coats in the X0 (Turner syndrome) female cat. In male cats, this coloring is only possible in the rare case of the Klinefelter syndrome [3]. These animals typically have an extra X chromosome (XXY) and their cells undergo an X-inactivation process like that in females. Additional Y chromosomes are described in humans as a result of a nondisjunction in meiosis II. This chromosomal aberration seems to have less influence since only a few genes are transcribed from the Y chromosome. Nevertheless, in humans, a higher testosterone concentration was observed in chromosome pair in their pseudoautosomal region(s) (PAR). In the horse this region was very helpful in mapping of the euchromatic region of the equine Y- chromosome. These investigations were very helpful for the prediction of male fertility in horses and are therefore considered in horse breeding [4, 5].

Rarely as a consequence of a translocation, the SRY region containing the testes determining factor (TDF) to the X chromosome during meiosis a male cytological having two X chromosomes can be created. These XX men are infertile since they lack other genes necessary for the production of mobile spermatozoa [6].

Before fertilization the XIST gene in the ripe oocyte is inactive, meaning that the X chromosome is active. Fertilization by a male (Y) sperm does not change this status. If a femal (X) sperm enters the oocyte one active XIST gene is now present producing XIST RNA which inactivates also the second X chromosome. This status is not stable since for maintenance of inactivation a protein named EED (polycomb protein EED, responsible for maintaining the transcriptional repressive state of genes over successive cell generations) also coded at the X chromosome is necessary [7, 8]. Therefore, both X chromosomes and also the XIST genes become active again at the morula stage leading to random inactivation of either the matenal or paternal X chromosome. That means that female eutherian mammals are mosaics in relation to maternal or paternal X inactivation, a phenomenon which becomes evident in X coded genes like coat color of the domestic cat.

4. Genomic imprinting

Genomic imprinting became evident by nuclear transplantation experiments at the pronuclear stage in mice [9]. Enucleated oocytes reconstructed with either only two femal or two male pronuclei exhibited different developmental potential concerning the embryo proper and the extraembryonic tissue. Further investigations revealed the nature of this phenomenon: In imprinted genes the female and male promotor regions have different methylation status leading to different gene expression in the early embryo. In humans and mice about 80 imprinted genes are known many of which are involved in embryonic and placental growth and development. Sometimes hybrid offspring of two different species may exhibit unusual growth due to the novel combination of imprinted genes. This becomes especially evident in reciprocal Lion-Tiger crosses [10]. The majority of imprinted genes are found in clusters, the so-called imprinted domains, suggesting a high degree of coordinated regulation. Imprinting is a dynamic process: imprints can be generated and removed at different time points of development from one generation to the other. In the germ line the imprints are erased and then reestablished according to the sex of the individual. In the developing sperms (during spermatogenesis), paternal imprints are established, whereas in developing oocytes (during oogenesis) a maternal imprints are established. In mammals genomic imprinting is present in therian mammals (marsupials and placental mammals) [11, 12].

5. Genetics during preimplantative eutherian embryo development

The eutherian oocyte is oligolecithal. After fertilization, the femal and male pronuclei fuse to establish the diploid zygote nucleus. The eutherian zygote undergoes now rotational holoblastic cleavage. These fast cell divisions consist only in synthesis phase and mitosis and subdivide the former ooplasm onto the blastomeres. Zygotic transcription starts dependent on the species at the two-, four-, or eight-cell stage. This process is named midblastula transition (MBT). So far the early embryo translates only maternally inherited mRNAs just present in the oocyte. So far the zygotic chromatin is hypo-acetylated and methylated, which means that most of the genes are repressed in a heterochromatic state. Now embryo starts to transcribe its own DNA and its cells become motile and the cell divisions loose synchrony. At the eight-cell stage most of the blastomeres become polarized and develop tight junctions with the other blastomeres. At the 16-cell state, the embryo is named morula. The outer cells become bound tightly together by the formation of cell junctions (compact morula). This process initiates the differentiation of two distinct cell populations: outside cells characterized by polarity and undifferentiated inside cells. The outer cells develop into trophoblast cells, which are epithelial cells connected by tight junctions in order to seal the extracellular passage. They express Na+/K+ ATPases and aquaporins at the apical and basal membranes in order to exchange sodium in from the outside by cellular potassium. This leads to electrochemical gradient which is equalized by water influx from the outside leading to blastocoel formation. The embryo is now called a blastocyst. At least in the horse expansion of the blastocyst seems to be under hormonal control [13, 14]. After implantation the trophoblast cells will develop into the fetal part of the placenta. The undifferentiated inner cells are displaced by the water influx to one side of the cavity to form the inner cell mass (ICM). It will develop into the embryo proper and some extraembryonic membranes.

So far the blastocyst like all previous embryonic stages are still surrounded by the acellular zona pellucida since the size of the embryos increased only marginally. Now a rapid expansion mainly due to fluid accumulation takes place and therefore the embryo hatches (human, mouse, pig, cow, sheep, goat, camels) or the zona pellucida is replaced by an embryonic capsule participating in enlargement. Hatched embryos show early placenta formation whereas encapsulated embryos exhibit prolonged preimplantative phase. At that time in most species the maternal recognition of pregnancy (MRP) takes place ensuring the maternal changes necessary for further development.

6. Genetics during mammalian placentation and fetal development

Mammalian placentation can be rated according to the implantation depth and surface expansion. Concerning implantation depth the invasiveness of the chorion is the crucial factor: epitheliochorial (pig, horse, ruminants), endotheliochorial (dog, cat), or hemochorial (human) describe implantational depth. Surface expansion is also influenced by placental capacities and number of fetuses: diffuse, cotelydonaria, zonaria, and discoidal. Implantational depth influences the quality of exchange of substances: The human hemochorial placenta enables the transfer of maternal antibodies into the fetal blood which is very important during the first weeks after birth. From the fetal face also a transfer of fetal cells into the maternal blood stream is probable. This microchimerism can persist even for some years and might be responsible for occurrence of autoimmune diseases in women [15]. In carnivoral placentation, such a microchimerism seems to be probable but was not investigated so far. The circumstances concerning the antibodies seem to be similar like in humans: "In carnivora and rodentia the blood of the newborn has roughly the same globin content as the maternal blood, whereas in those animals in which the placental barrier is relatively thick, such as the cow and pig, the fetus receives few if any antibodies before it is born" [16]. In horses despite their epitheliochorial placentation a microchimerism was proven recently by detection of SRY by means of digital PCR [17]. One of the most probable explanations for this microchimerism seems to consist in the migration of the chorionic girdle cells forming the endometrial cups.

Another form of microchimerism often arrives in cattle during twin pregnancies with different fetal sex named Freemartin syndrome: In most bovine twin pregnancies anastomoses form between the fetal circulations leading to exchange of male hormones (anti-Müllerian hormone, testosterone). Depending on the time of anastomose formation during pregnancy the femal fetus becomes masculinized resulting in intersexuality and infertility. In other domestic ruminantia the occurrence of freemartin syndrome is very rare [18].

7. Genetic alterations caused by assisted reproduction techniques

During *in vitro* maturation (IVM) and *in vitro* fertilization (IVF) the gamets respectively the early embryo are exposed to artificial environments which can differ in both directions from the natural conditions. Absence of essential substances often leads to the termination of development, whereas supernutrition can result in epigenetic changes which manifest later in pregnancy and during birth. One of the most frequent abnormities connected with IVF is the large offspring syndrome in cattle and sheep resulting in oversized fetuses [19].

Somatic nuclear transplantation of domestic animals can cause incomplete epigenetic reprogramming of the somatic nucleus leading to incapacity of blastocyst formation. Therefore, blastocyst rates are relatively low around 2–3%. High rates of embryonic loss, abortions due to placental aberrations, and high postnatal mortality were observed in cloned animals. Directed epigenetic changes during somatic cell culture can ameliorate the blastocyst rate obtained (up to 10%) and reduce the problems during pregnancy and birth [20].

http://dx.doi.org/10.5772/67132

During intracytoplasmic sperm injection (ICSI) a mature oocyte is injected with one sperm or a haploid progenitor of the sperm. This leads to omission of the natural selection of sperms in the femal genital tract and sometimes to fertilization with a sperm that under natural conditions never would be able to fertilize an oocyte. Using ICSI no acrosomal reaction and hyperactivation is necessary. Even dead sperms can be used if the nucleus is intact. Different from natural fertilization the whole sperm is injected into the oocyte leading to a mixture of mitochondria. There seems to be a mechanism to favor the mitochondria originally contributed by the oocyte (also in cloned animals). Nevertheless also coexistence and the reverse are possible [21]. In humans oocytes from aged women can be ameliorated by cytoplasma donation from an oocyte of a young women leading to a mixture of different mitochondria similar to the situation after nuclear transplantation.

In all these techniques applied in animal-assisted reproduction, the ability of blastocyst formation is the critical point to rate the success of the method. In human-assisted reproduction, earlier stages are transferred in multiple numbers often leading to twin and multiple pregnancies.

Different other techniques like oocyte transfer (OT) gamete intrafollopian transfer (GIFT), and zygote intrafollopian transfer (ZIFT) have been developed. Depending on the time of incubation of the gametes and the abandonment of embryo culture these techniques have reduced potential for epigenetic alterations.

PCR techniques using genetic material from blastomeres after the puncture of the embryo before transfer can be used for sex determination, preimplantative diagnostic, and marker-assisted selection in animal breeding.

8. Genetics in poultry reproduction

In birds and monotremes the sex is determined genetically but the exact mechanism is still unknown. All species show a ZZ/ZW sex chromosome system. Contrary to therian mammals it is characterized by female (ZW) heterogamety and male homogamety (ZZ). So far different hypothesis exist: Avian sex might be determined by dosage of a Z-coded gene or by a W-coded gene or may be both. A SRY gene or homolog is absent in birds and monotremes [22–24].

High performance chickens are bred by heterosis breed: In grandparent linages different traits (like high laying performance or good eggshell quality) are fixed by linage breed. In the parent generation the most suitable crossing between those linages will be determined. In case of the recurrent selection one father or mother line will be mated to a standard line. In the reciprocal recurrent selection each parent combination will be tested as mother and father line and rated according to the performance of the progeny.

Due to the chicken genome sequencing finished in 2005 many genes affecting vitality and disease resistance are going to be identified and become focused by the breeding organizations. This might lead to a reduction of therapeutic agents in poultry production.

9. Genetics in fish reproduction

Most of the fishes fostered in aquaculture belong to the teleosts. Many of them show hermaphroditism meaning that both sexes are present in one individuum but active at a different time during life. Most of the farmed fishes in aquaculture just release their eggs and sperms at the same time nearby in the water. In farms the eggs and sperms will be delivered artificially by abdominal massage and admixed together. This is the most suitable state for artificial manipulation like chromosome manipulation and gene transfer. Egg size is very important in fish breeding since large fry have to be fed later. Fertilization takes place by entering of the sperm through the micropyle of the fish egg, a narrow channel through the outer egg membrane. It is accomplished by the fish sperm swimming to the egg surface, locating the entry to the micopyle, and swimming down it to make contact with and penetrating the inner egg membranes. The membrane lifts after penetration of the first sperm which seems to be the mechanism for avoidance of polyspermy. Generation of triploid teleosts has become a widely used tool in order to protect wild fishes from hybridization since these animals are sterile. Production of monosex individuals has a similar effect [25]. Genetic engineering will have a great potential for the generation of disease resistance and low oxygen tolerating fish in the future. Interestingly somatic nuclear transplantation in teleosts leads to nucleocytoplasmic hybrids, meaning that the cytoplasm of the oocyte is able to inherit certain features. The molecular basis of this phenomenon is not elucidated so far [25].

10. Further perspectives of genetics in domestic animal reproduction

In many of the domestic animal species genome projects are ongoing or just finalized meaning that genes important for reproduction can be detected easier in order to investigate their specific role and the influences by the environment and metabolic state of the animal. In dairy cows classical selection has shown a negative correlation between daily milk yield and fertility parameters. In this regard, the metabolic state of the animal might be the limiting factor; therefore, the expression of reproductive genes under these conditions should be of high interest [26]. Modulation of gene expression is mediated not only by epigenetics (DNA methylation, histone modulation) but to a large extent also by micro-RNAs affecting mRNA stability. In this context the reproductive performance is influenced by the quality of the allele inherited, their epigenetic status, as well as the metabolic status of the animal.

In assisted reproduction sexing of sperms and embryos will become more important. Improvement of sexing technologies will allow a wider use also in domestic species which so far were excluded due to reproductive necessities (insemination doses, sensitivity of the sperm cells, survival time of the sperm cells). In embryos noninvasive techniques for sexing and preimplantative diagnostic may be possible in the near future. Selection of the sperm used for fertilization in intracytoplasmic sperm injection (ICSI) might change from motility alone to other, more complex criteria. *In vitro* culture conditions will be improved by adaption to natural conditions avoiding aberrant gene expression leading to phenomenon like the large offspring syndrome. In animal cloning the reprogramming of the donor cells will be improved in order to reach blastocyst rates around 20%.

In the social context the techniques applied in assisted reproduction should be rated in the correct light by understanding their way of action and their advantages in comparison to the objective risks.

Author details

Sven Budik (Mag. rer. nat., Dr. rer. nat., Mag. med. vet.)

Address all correspondence to: sven.budik@vetmeduni.ac.at

Platform for Artificial Insemination and Embryo Transfer, University of Veterinary Medicine, Vienna, Austria

References

[1] Sex determination in mammalian germ cells. Spiller CM, Bowles J, Asian Journal of Andrology (2015) 17, 427–432; doi: 10.4103/1008-682X.150037

[2] Molecular control of oogenesis. Sánchez F, Smitz J, Biochimica et Biophysica Acta – Molecular Basis of Disease (2012) 12, 1896–1912.

[3] A tortoiseshell male cat: Chromosome analysis and histologic examination of the testis, Pedersen AS, Berg LC, Almstrup K, Thomsen PD, Cytogenetic and Genome Research (2014) 142, 107–111; doi:10.1159/000356466

[4] The pseudoautosomal region and sex chromosome aneuploidies in domestic species. Raudsepp T, Das PJ, Avila F, Chowdhary BP, Sexual Development (2012) 6, 72–83; DOI:10.1159/000330627

[5] A gene catalogue of the euchromatic male-specific region of the horse Y chromosome: comparison with human and other mammals. Paria N, Raudsepp T, Pearks Wilkerson AJ, O'Brien PC, Ferguson-Smith MA, Love CC, Arnold C, Rakestraw P, Murphy WJ, Chowdhary BP, PLoS One (2011) 6(7), e21374; doi: 10.1371/journal.pone.0021374. Epub 2011 Jul 25.

[6] 46 XX karyotype during male fertility evaluation; case series and literature review. Majzoub A, Arafa M, Starks C, Elbardisi H, Al Said S, Sabanegh E. Asian J Androl [Epub ahead of print] [cited 2016 Dec 30]. Available from: http://www.ajandrology.com/preprintarticle.asp?id=181224

[7] Xist localization and function: new insights from multiple levels. Cerase A, Pintacuda G, Tattermusch A, Avner P, Genome Biology (2015) 16, 166; doi: 10.1186/s13059-015-0733-y

[8] Origin and evolution of X chromosome inactivation. Gribnau J, Grootegoed JA, Current Opinion in Cell Biology (2012) 24(3), 397–404; doi:10.1016/j.ceb.2012.02.004

[9] Role of paternal and maternal genomes in mouse development. Barton SC, Surani MAH, Norris ML, Nature (1984) 311, 374–376; doi:10.1038/311374a0

[10] Ligers and tigons and.....what?....oh my! McKinnell Z, Wessel G, Molecular Reproduction and Development (2012) 79(8), Fm i; doi: 10.1002/mrd.22074.

[11] Mammalian genomic imprinting. Bartolomei MS, Ferguson-Smith AC, Cold Spring Harbor Perspectives in Biology (2011) 3(7).

[12] Genomic imprinting: parental influence on the genome. Reik W, Walter J, Nature Reviews Genetics (2001) 2(1), 21–32; doi:10.1038/35047554.

[13] Significance of aquaporins and sodium potassium ATPase subunits for expansion of the early equine conceptus. Budik S, Walter I, Tschulenk W, Helmreich M, Deichsel K, Pittner F, Aurich C, Reproduction (2008) 135(4), 497–508; doi: 10.1530/REP-07-0298

[14] Increasing expression of oxytocin and vasopressin receptors in the equine concepts between Days 10 and 16 of pregnancy. Budik S, Palm F, Walter I, Helmreich M, Aurich C, Reproduction, Fertility, and Development (2012) 24(5), 641–648; doi: 10.1071/RD11167

[15] Pregnancy-acquired fetal progenitor cells. Seppanena E, Fiska NM, Khosrotehrania K, Journal of Reproductive Immunology (2013) 97(1), 27–35; doi: 10.1016/j.jri.2012.08.004

[16] Vertebrate Reproduction. Blüm V, (1985) Springer, ISBN 978-3-642-71074-2

[17] Equine fetal sex determination using circulating cell-free fetal DNA (ccffDNA). Moura de Leon PM, Campos VF, Dellagostin OA, Deschamps JC, Seixas FK, Collares T, Theriogenology (2012) 77, 694–698; doi: 10.1016/j.theriogenology.2011.09.005

[18] The freemartin syndrome: an update. Padula AM, Animal Reproduction Science (2005) 87, 93–109.

[19] Large offspring syndrome in cattle and sheep. Young LE, Sinclair KD, Wilmut I, Reviews of Reproduction (1998) 3, 155–163.

[20] A New, Dynamic Era for Somatic Cell Nuclear Transfer? Loi P, Iuso D, Czernik M, Ogura A, Trends in Biotechnology (2016) pii, S0167–7799(16)30003-8; doi: 10.1016/j.tibtech.2016.03.008.

[21] Mitochondrial DNA heteroplasmy in ovine fetuses and sheep cloned by somatic cell nuclear transfer. Burgstaller J, Schinogl P, Dinnyes A, Müller M, Steinborn R, BMC Developmental Biology (2007) 7, 141; doi: 10.1186/1471-213X-7-141

[22] Avian sex determination: what, when and where? Smith CA, Roeszler KN, Hudson QJ, Sinclair AH, Cytogenetic and Genome Research (2007) 117, 165–173; doi:10.1159/000103177

[23] Genetics of the Fowl: The Classic Guide to Poultry Breeding and Chicken Genetics. Hutt FB, ISBN: 978-0972177030

[24] Poultry Genetics, Breeding and Biotechnology. Muir WM, Aggrey Stylus Pub Llc, (2003) SE, ISBN 0851996604

[25] A Review of "Aquaculture and Fisheries Biotechnology, Genetic Approaches, Dunham RA, Stylus Cabi Publishing (2010) 2nd Edition," ISBN: 978-1-84-593651-8

[26] Novel approaches to genetic analysis of fertility traits in New Zealand dairy cattle. Bowley FE, Green RE, Amer PR, Meier S, Journal of Dairy Science (2015) 98, 2005–2012; http://dx.doi.org/ 10.3168/jds.2014-8266

Section 2

Advances in Embryonic Genetics

Studies on Gene Expression and Developmental Competence of Bovine Embryos Produced Under Different Conditions of Heat Stress

Aya K. H. Mahdy, Krishna C. Pavani, Erica Baron and Fernando Moreira da Silva

Additional information is available at the end of the chapter

http://dx.doi.org/10.5772/66268

Abstract

Gene expression is required in all steps of embryonic development and therefore heat stress is known to reduce developmental competence after direct exposure of oocytes and embryos to different conditions of heat shock, by decreasing protein synthesis. Moreover, as in somatic cells, the heat stress befuddles the integration of RNA and posttranscriptional modification of RNA, the assumption was that during meiotic maturation heat shock may mutate RNA within oocytes, with the possibility of altering the surrounding cumulus cells, causing, thus, reductions in development. Heat shock proteins (HSP) are among the first proteins produced during embryonic development and are crucial to cell function. The HSP70 (*HSPA14* gene) is an important part of the cell's machinery for folding, unfolding, transport, localization of proteins and differentiation, regulation of the embryonic cell cycle and helping to protect cells from stress. Therefore, *HSPA14* is an apoptotic gene induced by heat shock is associated with embryonic loss, playing an important role of control mechanism of processes involved in growth, cellular differentiation, and embryonic development. In addition the connexin proteins (e.g. *Cx43*), related to gap junctions, are expressed in numerous tissues including gonads, act as a mediator of heat stress effect on cells. In the present review, the effect of heat stress on bovine embryonic development in a physiologic and genetic point of view is fully discussed.

Keywords: heat stress, oocyte, maturation, gene expression, *HSPA14*, *Cx43*, real-time PCR

1. Introduction

Climate changes influence the biogeography and phenology of animals, thus affecting their reproduction, physiological development, and metabolism [1]. The global warming refers to the continued increase of the earth's temperature and ecosystems change, as when the sun heats the earth, the earth radiates only some of the sun's energy into space, while some energy is trapped by atmospheric gases, such as carbon dioxide and water vapor. This energy builds up in the earth's atmosphere, the earth gradually becomes hotter and leads to increase in the temperature, and hence heat stress can happen [2]. Depending on the proportion of CO_2 emission, the global surface temperature is predicted to rise by 1.1–6.4°C. Heat stress is the main factor responsible for lower productive and reproductive performance in cattle during the summer months. The extreme temperature events due to climate change coupled with high rate of relative humidity decrease the ability of reproduction in animals [3]. Heat shock impacts on the ovulatory oocyte, as well as on functions of follicular granulosa and theca cells, therefore delays and alters the efficiency of follicle selection and lengthening of the follicular wave, which adversely affects the quality of oocytes [4]. The first-wave dominant follicle is depressed by heat stress; hence, lactating cows were found to be smaller in diameter. Thus during the first 7 days of the cycle showed that follicular dynamics have been altered, as indicated by the decrease in the number of medium-sized follicles that associated with depressed summer fertility [5, 6]. During hot summer months, high temperature can affect endocrine responses that may increase foetal abortions, shorten the gestation length, lower calf birth weight, and reduce follicle and oocyte maturation associated with the postpartum reproductive cycle. Postpartum heat stress can significantly decrease the pregnancy rates with impacts lingering well into the fall months [7]. The summer period adversely affects endocrine system, follicular phase, metabolism, function of oocytes, and embryos. The towering temperature causes several cellular changes during the maturation period and germinal vesicle stage in the oocytes [8]. Therefore, the heat stress influences and impacts on *in vitro* oocytes maturation, their nuclear maturation, and further embryos development to the stage of blastocysts after *in vitro* fertilization [9]. The low fertility of cattle females has led to an increased interest in *in vitro* embryo production (IVEP) technologies for achieving rapid genetic improvement and providing an excellent source of embryos for carrying out basic research on developmental physiology [10]. Moreover, cytoplasmic and molecular maturation of oocytes are thought to be critically involved in the ability of the oocyte to support fertilization and early development stages. The major activation of the bovine embryonic genome occurs at the 8- to 16-cell stage. Before embryonic genome activation, mRNAs, ribosomes, and proteins synthesized during oocyte growth and maturation contribute to early development [11]. As known, heat stress induces apoptosis or expression of *HSPA14* gene of *in vitro* produced embryos. Stress proteins are assorted into families depending on their molecular weight and provide two main functions: primarily as a molecular chaperone having key roles in folding/unfolding of proteins and secondarily as a stabilizer factor from deteriorating proteins contributing in the protection of cells against stress/apoptosis, granting an opportunity for rehabilitation or degradation in the cells suffering from cellular stress [12]. Some activities of HSP70 include folding, unfolding, transport, and localization of proteins and differentiation and regulation of the embryonic cell cycle [13]. Hence, the piling up of HSPs has long been considered a sign of cellular damage. There is an evident overlap of the signals that induces a protective stress response and those that initiate apoptosis [14]; therefore, heat shock protein HSP70 plays a protective role in the embryos. During the early 2-cell of embryo to the blastocyst stage, the HSP70 is the prevailing gene. The induction of stress proteins (HSP) synthesis during 1- or 2-

http://dx.doi.org/10.5772/66268

cell stage until blastocyst stage is intensely motivated by heat shock [15]. Thus, *HSPA14* gene is produced by embryonic cells, which protect the embryos from environmental stress. During early development, increased temperatures, free radicals, and oxygen stress have deleterious effects on embryonic viability and development. The *HSPA14* confers thermotolerance against variety of stressors. Thus, the preferential maintenance of *HSPA14* gene expression would allow this gene product to help maintain cellular function by acting as molecular chaperones to stabilize or refold proteins damaged by heat, and by blocking apoptosis [16]. There are many ways in which cells communicate with other cells, and gap junctional communication is one of these ways. Ovarian folliculogenesis and the production of fertilizable oocytes depend on gap junction channels which allow inorganic ions, second messengers, and small metabolites to pass from cell to cell, and this permeability is supposedly for underpinning the physiological roles played by gap junctions, for example, connexin 43 (*Cx43*) gene expressed within the oocyte–granulosa cell complex depending on the species [17]. The expression of *Cx43* gene in the ovary is regulated by gonadotropins like follicle-stimulating hormone (FSH) and luteinizing hormone (LH). Increase in the *Cx43* expression in the large antral follicles was observed where FSH was relatively elevated. Moreover, germline and somatic cell during mammalian ovarian follicle have elements for cellular interactions, development, and function. Somatic cell-to-oocyte communication is essential for oocyte growth and the regulation of meiotic maturation via gap junctions [18]. *Cx43* was later detected in the cytoplasm of germ cells. Therefore, tight junction molecules were found and *Cx43* were distributed at the cell–cell contact of the adjacent cells. Such progressive reorganization of germ cells, *Cx43* gene, is probably coupling with conjugation role of other gap junctions and their specific connexins (Cxs), between the different cell types that structure the animal reproductive system [19]. Furthermore, germline and somatic cell during mammalian ovarian follicle have elements for cellular interactions, development, and function, essential for oocyte growth and the regulation of meiotic maturation via gap junctions [23]. On the other hand, during embryonic early development, increased temperatures lead to free radicals and oxygen stress, having also deleterious effects on embryonic viability and development. As far as *in vitro* embryo production is concerned, more and more motives are actually presented in the cattle breeding, such as the faster propagation of superior germplasm because of the low efficiency of superovulation in programs of embryo transfer. Moreover, embryo production is actually also a reproductive method used to improve the number of progeny with high genomic merit from bovines, both *in vivo* and *in vitro*. *In vitro* embryo production (IVEP) also including some of the applications serves to solve infertility problems, genetic recovery, and production of clones or even transgenic animals. In the present review, physiological and genetic factors affecting embryonic development under heat stress conditions are fully discussed.

2. Ovarian physiology: folliculogenesis, oocytes growth, and development: oocytes growth and development

The fertilization of mature oocyte occurs in the oviduct and there are three distinct phases that can be divided during this process. During the first phase (the oocyte growth phase), the developmental competence of the oocyte and cell structure is generated, when oocyte growth accompanies follicular growth from the primordial to the small (2–3 mm) tertiary (antral) follicle. When follicles in a cohort reach a diameter of about 3–5 mm, one dominant follicle is selected during the antral phase. During the third phase, the oocyte undergoes to change (oocyte maturation) almost 24 hours between the peak ovulation and the rise of LH.

2.1. Oogenesis

The mature oocytes are differentiated, released, and established in mammalian ovaries to undergo oogenesis process for fertilization. The ovaries have individual follicles consisting of an innermost oocyte, surrounding granulosa cells, and outer layers of thecal cells, controlled by the endocrine system. Moreover, mammalian ovary produces steroids and peptide growth factors, which allow the development of female secondary sexual characteristics and support pregnancy [20]. The oocytes and surrounding granulosa cells have amiable connections together to support oocyte viability and growth mediated by the gap junctions, which are efficient conduits for low molecular weight substances. The granulosa cells have some metabolized molecules, which play a role in transporting the oocytes. Additionally, the KIT ligands and c-kit receptor are localized to oocytes and granulosa cells, respectively, to promote oocyte growth and follicular development. Moreover, some of the growth factors derived from oocytes, such as GDF-9 and BMP-15, contribute in follicular development by regulating the differentiation of surrounding somatic cells, as these communications are important for oocyte growth and follicular development [21]. The occurrence of events of oogenesis are concomitantly with folliculogenesis, as oogenesis can be explained as the process of formation and maturation of the egg by development and differentiation of the female gamete during the meiotic division, and this is the first phase of progress for the fetus. Thus, female ovaries have fixed number of oocytes, which decreases by time passing with several years, without potential to renew. During the ovarian start to deplete the auxiliary of oocytes, it evolves to a senescence/aging stage born with a fixed number of oocytes, which through several years reduce, without potential to renew. When the ovarian start to deplete the auxiliary of oocytes, it evolves to a senescence stage, leading the female to menopause [22]. During meiosis, mammalian oocytes undergo two consecutive asymmetric cell divisions, which are essential for the formation of a functional female gamete, without an intermediate replicative phase. Each division must ensure accurate segregation of the maternal genome and highly asymmetric partition of the cytoplasm, further that a tiny polar body and a large oocyte are generated. It leads to an asymmetric organization (or polarization) of the egg, which determines the geometry and the success of fertilization. Asymmetric divisions are tightly controlled by microtubule and microfilament cytoskeletons. During the beginning of the first meiotic division, this process allows the separation of the duplicated centrosomes and therefore to the gathering of a bipolar spindle formed by microtubules. Thus, it is referred to as the process that produces gametes with half of the number of chromosomes from the parent cells. For the position of spindle surrounding the oocytes and tossing the first polar body in parallel with separation of chromosome, the microfilaments are carried out in meiosis I. The microtubule spindle is positioned at the surrounding of the oocytes until fertilization, causing the emission of the second polar body during second meiotic division (meiosis II). Additionally, the loss of asymmetry is a mark of low-quality oocytes and a signature of pre- and postovulatory aging [23].

2.2. Folliculogenesis

Meiotic prophase consists of several temporary stages: preleptotene, leptotene, zygotene, pachytene, and the diplotene stage in which the first meiotic division of the ovarian follicles begin to develop as primordial structure that oocyte arrested. Primordial follicle activation is characterized by the possession of complete layer of 11–20 granulosa cells around the oocytes. Secondary follicle stage starts to show features of a second layer of granulosa cells. Zona pellucid is the initial deposition material around the oocyte, and at the same time, cortical granules are formed within the oocyte cytoplasm. It is at this point of development that follicles appear to become responsive to gonadotrophins [24]. The progress of ovarian follicle is a combination of many sides of a compound process that starts with the foundation of limited pool of primordial follicles and attains in either atretic degradation of the follicle or liberation of mature oocytes for fertilization. Through the primary, preantral and antral stages, the primordial follicles must be grown during these stages before reaching to the preovulatory stage where they are eligible to release oocytes for starting the fertilization stage. The corpus luteum structure (CL) is formed from the differentiation of the residual of granulosa and thecal cells after ovulation [25]. Large stock of oocytes is enclosed in primordial follicles in mammalian ovaries, and some of these follicles initiate growth toward a possible ovulation undergoing activity of the ovarian cycle. Additionally, most of these follicles end their growth at any moment and degenerate through atresia. During the growth of follicles, only a subset of oocytes is capable to support meiosis, fertilization, and early embryo development to the blastocyst stage. This proportion of eligible oocytes depends on the size of the follicular cell. Developing lines of evidence propose that the competent oocytes increase the storage of gene production leading to the determinant to support the precocious stages of developmental embryos, before the activation of embryonic genome. Thus, these transcripts may be stored during early folliculogenesis as the oocyte grows and displays high transcription activity [26]. Young and McNeilly [27] classified the system into five types: type I represents the primordial follicles, which are a resting stage before their activity begins. In this stage, follicles have only one layer of granulosa cells and this is the follicle transitioning through the primary stage, when the granulosa cells become cuboidal. The second type of follicles includes one layer of cuboidal granulosa cells. While antral follicles include two to four layers of granulosa cells going to the third type. At this stage, the large preantral follicles consists of four to six layers of granulosa cells, considering this stage as the fourth stage, increasing the number of layers, thus reaching the fifth type. Then, the *antum* arises and the thecal cells start to appear and protrude. Thus, begins the formation of the layer around the granulosa cells of the oocyte. Therefore, most follicles are observed at early stages of development. At the antral stage, follicles become gonadotropin dependent and form large antral follicles, most of which undergo atresia, and few are selected for ovulation. Estrogens produced from the ovary of vertebrates, which have a fundamental endocrine function, leads the females to develop reproductive organs, while the corpus leteum produces progesterone, which is essential for the foundation of pregnancy. Thus, these functions are tightly coordinated during folliculogenesis, in which a dynamic process includes a continuous differentiation of three types of cells, theca of granulosa cells, and the oocytes themselves. The antrum formation from the granulosa cells proliferate, which is directly related to the follicular growth leading to a restricted number of follicles to complete their development to the stage of ovulation, while others undergo atresia. In the stage of antral follicle, theca cells are divided into two layers, internal and external, which can be distinguished by the surrounding selected follicles [28]. After ovulation, which is triggered by a peak of LH, theca cells and mural granulosa cells luteinize to produce progesterone (**Figure 1**). Once an ovarian follicle increase from the pool of resting follicles and initiates growth, it takes approximately around 100 days to arrive to the point where ovulation can execute and the oocyte included within the follicle is released [29].

2.3. Oocytes morphology and classification

In vitro maturation (IVM) is the starting point of a whole lot of biotechnological applications in animals like *in vitro* fertilization (IVF). These techniques combined with marker-assisted selection at embryonic stage will hasten acceleration for improving the production potency of cattle. The selection of oocytes depends only on the good quality cumulus-oocytes complexes (COCs), which were selected based on cumulus cells and ooplasm characteristics. The good oocytes are surrounded with at least three layers of cumulus cells and their ooplasm should be dark and homogeneous. Therefore, the oocytes were classified into four classes: (1) Grade A: oocytes were characterized with more than five

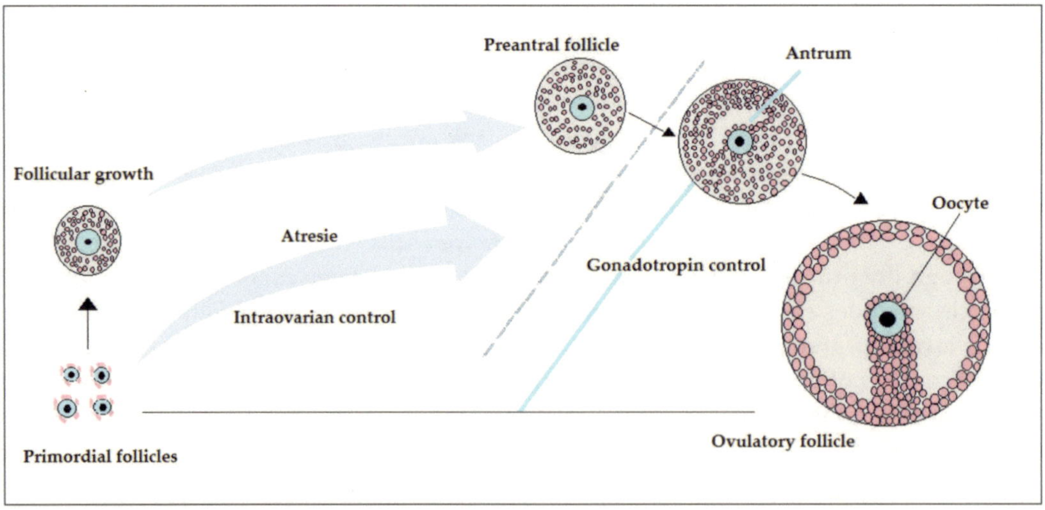

Figure 1. Outline of the main steps of folliculogenesis.

complete layers of cumulus cells, which are uniform granulation of ooplasm and healthy follicle. (2) Grade B: follicles with intact and well-organized granulose cells with three to five complete layers of cumulus cells and uniform granulation of ooplasm. (3) Grade C: follicles with one to two complete layers of cumulus cells and uniform granulation and less regular of ooplasm with some dark area. (4) Grade D: denuded oocytes with uniform granulation of ooplasm [30].

2.4. Oocyte maturation

Immature oocytes begin to develop in the ovaries, with each oocyte possessing a large nucleus that is referred to as the germinal vesicle (GV). Therefore, immature oocytes start to give response and undergo maturation process, which starts the nucleus of oocyte to have disassembly during a sequence called germinal vesicle breakdown (GVBD). After this stage, the immature oocyte turns into mature being eligible for developing until fertilization. Moreover, regardless of the timing of GVBD relative to fertilization and at the end, all oocytes must be matured enough to be able to consequently develop to continue to proceed normally [31]. During dictyate stage of prophase I, the oocytes are arrested, which can be identified by the presence of a germinal vesicle (GV). Additionally, meiosis I is marked by germinal vesicle breakdown (GVBD) following which bivalents are brought to alignment at the spindle equator by metaphase I. Anaphase I then ensues when chromosomes segregate between the secondary oocyte and the polar body. Following first polar body extrusion (PBE), oocytes progress without a hiatus into meiosis II where they are arrested for a second time at metaphase II [32]. During the maturation process, mammalian oocytes accompany a comprehensive, extensive rearrangement of the cytoskeleton and associated proteins. In oocytes, during the MI takes nearby 6-11 hours and the spindle migration toward the egg cortex occurs at this time. When the chromosome-spindle complex moves to the egg cortex, it involves a spindle pole close to the cortex [33]. Spindle movement induces a cortical differentiation performed by the accumulation of actin filaments and a scarcity of microvilli. After polar body extrusion, chromosomes realign progressing to metaphase II.

2.4.1. Nuclear and cytoplasmic maturation

The oocytes for bovine with an inside zona diameter smaller than 95 μm are unable to start meiosis *in vitro*. A high percentage of bovine oocytes are able to start meiosis to the MI stage once the oocyte diameter is at least 100 μm. However, the oocyte must measure 110 μm or more to reach the MII stage. The ability to develop to the blastocyst stage *in vitro* increases with oocyte growth. Cleavage and blastocyst rates increase in parallel with meiotic competence and significantly higher developmental rates have been obtained when the diameter of fertilized oocytes is greater than 120 μm. The developmental potential is apparently similar in oocytes originating from nonatretic and early atretic follicles [34], including spindle transfer, chromosome condensation, germinal vesicle breakdown, the progression to MI, and separation of the homologous chromosomes with polar body extrusion, where the nuclear membrane starts to fold, the nuclear pores disappear, and then the nuclear membrane undergoes fragmentation and rapidly disappears. It appears that nuclear maturation follows the same pattern *in vivo* and *in vitro*. Nuclear maturation involves changes in protein synthesis patterns. Bovine oocytes undergo marked changes in the patterns of protein synthesis after GVBD *in vitro* and *in vivo*, whereas oocytes that remain at GV stage have consistent protein synthesis patterns [35]. Meiotic competence is known as the ability of the oocyte to complete meiosis. Additionally, during follicular growth, the meiotic competence is obtained and is acquired progressively. Oocytes first acquire the capacity to undergo condensation of chromosome, germinal vesicle breakdown, and follicular growth and are desired to acquire the capacity to progress to MI and eventually acquire the capacity to reach MII. The ability to complete the MI to MII transition coincides with the achievement of full size and with the process of nucleolar compaction [36].

The diameter of the follicle increases depending on the number of Golgi apparatus present in the oocyte. The change in location of cortical granules constitutes the most obvious ultrastructure sign of cytoplasmic maturation. According to the oocytes in the GV stage, cortical granules are distributed in clusters throughout the cytoplasm. However, as the oocytes progress to metaphase I stage, the cortical granules translocate to the periphery of the oocyte and become attached to the plasma membrane. At the end of the maturation period, when these oocytes reach the MII stage, the granules are distributed through the inner surface close to the plasma membrane [37]. The mitochondria make a homogeneous distribution throughout the cytoplasmic and are more common at the germinal vesicle (GV) stage, while heterogeneous distribution is more commonly observed in the oocyte of metaphase I or II. During oocyte maturation, the mitochondria disperse distribution throughout the cytoplasm, until reaching metaphase II (MII), when the central position in the cell operates in the mitochondria because high-energy supply around the nucleus is very important during embryonic development. It is also observed that morphologically poor quality embryos are only characterized by the homogenous distribution of the mitochondria [38]. Additionally, the cytoplasmic maturation describes both the ultrastructural changes that take place in the oocyte from the germinal vesicle (GV) to the metaphase II (MII) stage and the possession of developmental competence of the oocyte. Mammalian oocyte's cytoplasmic maturation can be described as the ability of a mature egg to undergo regular fertilization stage, all stages of cleavage, and further development of the blastocyst. Other indirect morphological parameters considered to evaluate cytoplasmic maturation include cumulus cell expansion, polar body expulsion, and increased perivitelline space (PVS) of Ref. [39].

3. RNA synthesis and molecular maturation

The molecular maturation coincides with the maturation and growth of oocyte corresponding with transcription and mRNAs expression by genes of oocytes. In mammalians ovaries, meiosis occurs mainly in two steps: during foetal life (step 1) and through the period of preovulatory life (step 2). The genetic information must be stored in advance because of nuclear instructions, when the chromosomes are the subjects of transformation. Thus, in the form of mRNA, the chromosomes arrive and are silenced at the resumption of meiosis. After DNA synthesis at double helix, the chromosomes are partially condensed and rearranged by the process of crossing over. The chromatin then reaches a special conformation that is an intermediate between chromatin condensation and interphase, the dictyate phase. Additionally, in some species during that special prophase period, the oocyte remains static and the chromosome appearance changes little. When an oocyte begins to grow in the primordial follicle, the uncondensed loops of chromatin in the dictyate state ensure the transcription of required elements. Thus, the mRNA produced is either translated immediately [40]. Through the *in vivo* and *in vitro* maturation, oocytes can have the ability to elucidate the signaling pathways by gene expression. These signaling pathways are involved in the intricate mutual among the oocyte and its somatic compartment through morphogenetic and differentiation processes, and the origin of disturbances in oocyte maturation is theoretically involved in the decrease of the fertility; therefore, molecular maturation of oocytes is characterized by enhanced nucleolar activity and ribosome synthesis, and when the oocyte reaches the meiotic phase, the nucleolus becomes inactivated [41]. During the meiotic phase, for oocyte maturation, large numbers of macromolecules are accumulated. The mRNA and riRNAs produced in these cells are far in excess of those necessary to support protein synthesis. Thus, concomitantly the onset of germinal vesicle breakdown occurs after 6–10 h of IVM. In the course of IVM, *de novo* transcription strongly declines as determined by measuring the incorporation of [3H] uridine into RNA. In contrast to this finding, the incorporation of [3H] adenosine increased and showed a peak during the time interval of 6–10 h of IVM, parallel with the onset of germinal vesicle breakdown (GVBD) and translation. In the further course of maturation, only a moderate decrease of [3H] adenosine incorporation was observed. These findings indicate and betoken that during the time of germinal vesicle breakdown (GVBD) the translation is increased. Additionally, these operations were accompanied by polyadenylation of the mRNA, despite the decline of the transcription and accumulation of polyadenylated mRNA until MII [42]. As known, oocytes' growth normally undergoes cytoplasmic and nuclear maturation, and the bovine embryo has the ability to develop to the blastocyst stage, and it is important to clarify the contribution of the oocyte to the embryo quality. Currently, the most popular hypothesis is that specific mRNA and possibly some proteins are produced and added to the oocyte's stockpile in the last few days before ovulation, it is believed that molecular maturation represents the closest association with the intrinsic capacity of an oocyte to reach the blastocyst stage and probably beyond [43]. Gene expression patterns are responsible for the development of the early embryogenesis. Fertilization and the first zygotic cleavage involve major changes to paternal and maternal genome activation. Additionally, the function of genomes has regulatory mechanisms, including differential promoter activation, alternative RNA splicing, RNA modification, RNA editing, localization, translation and stability of RNA, expression of noncoding RNA, antisense RNA, and microRNAs. All of these mechanisms work together to produce the level of RNA for transcriptome functioning of an organism. Developmental embryonic stage is the first to rely on the stored maternal transcript, which is progressively exhausted untill the production of the embryo on its own transcripts, after shifting to the program for embryonic expression. Moreover, through gene expression patterns and RNA stability, oocytes and early embryos prior to the expression of embryonic activation are dramatically different and it leads to significantly different from what is observed after the main outset of embryonic transcription. The start for transcription of embryonic genes execute at a specific species at a specific time point. In bovine embryos, it occurs at 8- to 16-cell stage [44]. When the immature oocytes are removed from follicle, they spontaneously will convert to mature oocytes. Oocyte maturation can have deficiencies and the incompetence of cellular machinery, frequently causing a failure in embryonic development following fertilization and lower implantation rates. Additionally, the cytoplasmic and molecular maturation of oocyte might fail to promote male pronuclear formation. Hence, it might increase the chromosomal abnormalities after fertilization, and these abnormalities may result in an incompetent embryo in cleavage [45].

4. Production of embryos *in vitro*

There are many reasons for interest in *in vitro* generation embryos that can be produced in the laboratory. Among these reasons is the faster propagation of superior germplasm in cattle because of the low efficiency of superovulation (SO) and embryo transfer (ET) programs. *In vitro* embryo production (IVEP) consists of four steps: (1) aspiration of the ovaries, (2) *in vitro* maturation (IVM) of the recovered oocytes, (3) *in vitro* fertilization (IVF) of the IVM oocytes, and (4) *in vitro* culture of the IVM/IVF zygotes for development to the desired stages [46]. To evaluate the effect of oocyte source (live animals and abattoir ovaries) on subsequent embryo development in cattle, it is essential to perform IVEP from cow ovaries. The beginning of harvest of the oocytes from bovine ovaries and the cumulus-enclosed oocytes (COCs) suitable for IVEP were *in vitro* matured (IVM), fertilized (IVF), and cultured (IVC) to the tight morula (Tm) and blastocyst (Bl) stage. A higher overall IVEP efficiency is mainly related to the higher cleavage rate. Moreover, the production of embryos *in vitro* is a technique largely used as a method for increasing the production of progeny in the bovine with high genetic meritocracy, overcoming several of infertility problems in cattle, genetic recovery, and production of clones and transgenic animals. Despite several studies in this area, the *in vitro* development of cattle embryos to the blastocyst stage rarely surpasses the rate of 40%. Extrinsic and intrinsic oocyte factors can interfere with oocyte fertilization and development to the blastocyst stage. Among the intrinsic factors is the presence of the dominant follicle that, mainly through inhibin and estradiol secretion, has an inhibitory effect on the development of other follicles. Furthermore, they reported that oocytes derived from subordinate follicles have less capacity to become healthy embryos than oocytes derived from growing follicles [47].

In **Figure 2**, it can be observed different stages of embryonic development from day 0 to day 7, monitored by our team. Following fertilization, embryos undergo a series of mitotic cell divisions. Hence, the embryo compacts to form a morula that comprises of cells in a compact cluster including the pellucid zone (i.e., comprising of glycoproteins envelope of mammalian oocytes, which beset the embryo). Then, the blastocyst is formed and finally "hatches" from the zona pellucid. Besides, in humans, all this process takes about 1 week [48], and in cows, it can take up to 10 days.

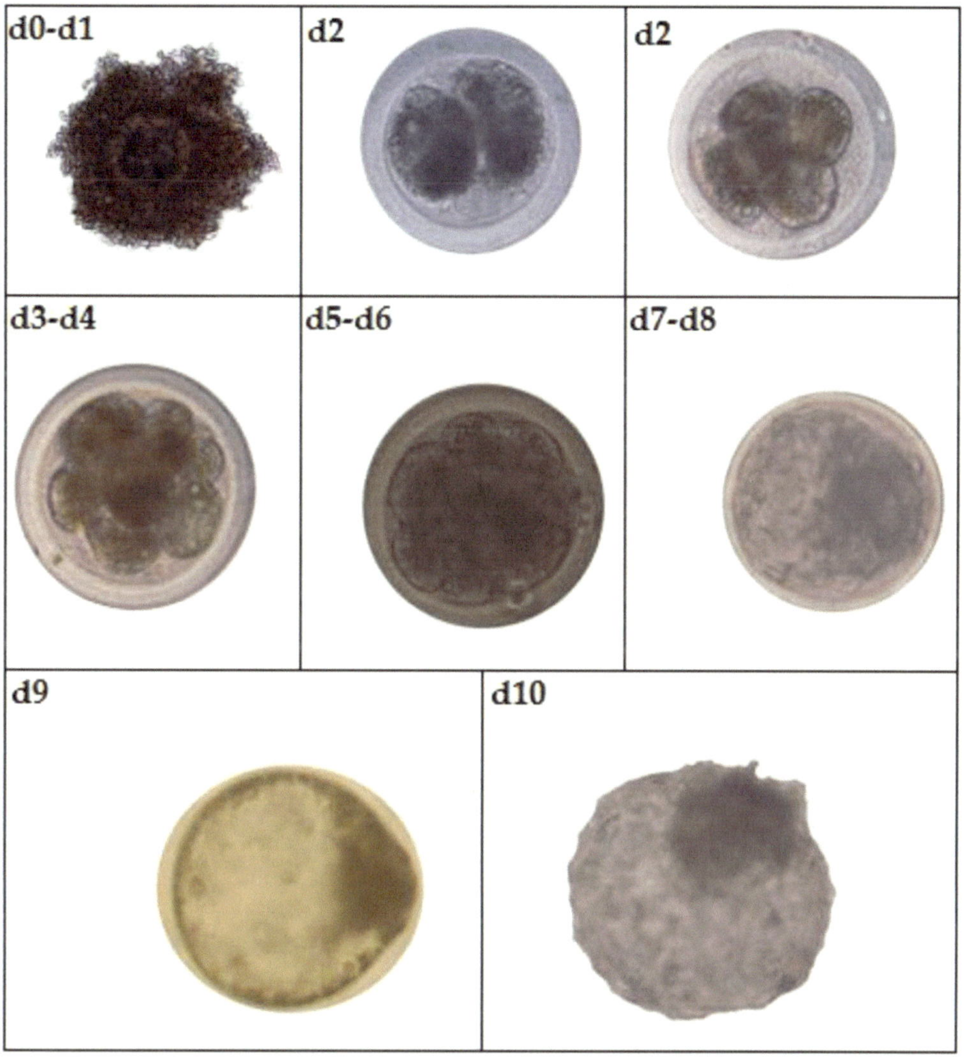

Figure 2. Stages of embryo development (photos made by the authors).

5. Effects of heat stress on animal fertility

During summer, heat shock reduces pregnancy, conception rates, and leads to low fertility in lactating dairy cow. Progesterone secretion by luteal cells is decreased and this is reflected in plasma progesterone concentration, the endometrial function, and alters its secretory activity by high temperature, which leads to the termination of pregnancy. Moreover, heat shock impedes oocytes quality and embryo development and increases the mortality rate of embryos [49]. Therefore, there are different factors that lead to the decrease of fertility in cattle. The most important are the increased humidity and temperature that result in a decreased expression of overt estrus and a reduction in appetite and dry matter intake.

During the postnatal period "puerperium," the exposure to extreme heat stress prolonged, leading to negative energy balance and increase in the calving pregnancy interval. Heat stress influences by decreasing the dominance of the selected follicle and this decreases the steroidogenic ability of its granulose cells and theca cells, which declines the estradiol concentrations in blood. The elevation or reduction of the plasma progesterone levels can be relied on whether it is severe or chronic, and on the cattle metabolism state. The reduction of follicular activity and the alteration of ovulatory pattern execute endocrine changes, leading to the reduction of oocytes and the quality of embryos [50]. Moreover, oocyte's maturation from the meiotic stage of germinal vesicle (GV) to MII is affected by heat stress and it has been shown that high temperatures affect also the cattle cumulus-oocyte complexes (COCs), zona pellucida hardening, fertilization, and further cleavage of putative zygotes after fertilization [51]. In cattle, genes exist for regulation of body temperature and for cellular resistance to elevated temperature. These genes offer possibility for their incorporation into dairy cow through cross breeding or on an individual-gene basis and the physiological and genetic manipulation of the cow to improve embryonic resistance to high environmental temperature, which reduces fertility in lactating dairy cows, and as a result, pregnancy, oocyte, and early embryo are affected by heat stress [52]. Therefore, heat stress reduces gonadotropin secretion and the ovarian pool of oocytes and impairs fertility. Additionally, heat stress has immediate effects on follicle and its enclosed oocyte, follicular function, and follicular growth and disrupts steroidogenesis [53]. Heat stress has an impact on the reproductive function, that is, it reduces the intensity of the behavioral estrus and leads to low fertility in female and compromised sperm output and increased sperm abnormalities in male. The pregnancy rate and the embryos at earlier stages of development during heat stress are affected [54]. Furthermore, oocyte susceptibility to heat shock can be detected during the germinal vesicle (GV) and oocyte maturation periods. The bovine oocytes' exposure to high temperature *in vivo* and *in vitro* affects oocyte maturation, fertilization, and preimplantation of embryonic development. This heat-induced reduction in oocyte function occurs due to a series of cellular alterations that affect nuclear and cytoplasmic compartments of the bovine oocyte. Before ovulation, there are several physiological factors that can disrupt establishment of pregnancy changes by elevated thermal heat. Heat shock effects endometrial prostaglandin secretion, oocytes during maturation period, and decreases low fertility of dairy cows in hot seasons [9]. Moreover, heat stress was suggested to be similar to oxidative stress, because of correspondences in the genes expressed after heat exposure, such as genes encoding heat shock proteins (*HSPA14* gene), demonstrated heat-induced increase of reactive oxygen species (ROS) production, especially the superoxide anion. Additionally, heat stress disturbs protein synthesis, increasing the production of heat shock proteins (HSPs). Due to their chaperone function, HSPs ensure the folding, unfolding, and refolding of nascent or stress-denatured proteins. The HSP70 and HSP90 were correlated with the development of thermotolerance of embryos. Thus, heat stress was shown to increase HSP70 and HSP90 levels and that probably due as a mechanism of cellular defense and/or repair [55]. Dairy cows respond to heat stress in several ways, including reduced feed intake, lower milk yield and quality, and compromised fertility [56]. Thus, fertility traits in dairy animals show a very low heritability value, and this indicates that most of the variations in the fertility are determined by nongenetic factors or environmental effects. Therefore, summer season has been associated with reduced fertility in dairy cattle through its deleterious impact on oocyte maturation and early embryo development. Moreover, the highest pregnancy rate of cow was observed in September–November as 32% while the lowest pregnancy rate of 24% in March–May. The lower pregnancy rate is due to the delay of rebreeding cows in the summer hot months with a high level of heat stress. Additionally, there are some other genes such *ATP1A1* allowing resistance and adaptation to thermal stress in bovine. Whereas *ATP1A1* gene is known as Na+/K+ -ATPase subunit alpha-1, this gene is fully recognized as a nominee to responsd for heat shock because of its assembly to oxidative stress in bovine which have Na+/K+ -ATPase protein complex consisting of α and β subunits. The *ATP1A1* gene encodes the $\alpha 1$ isoform, for α subunit of Na+-K+ ATPase pump is considered as a major isoform. *ATP1A1* gene has been mapped on *Bos taurus* chromosome number 3 and is comprised of 22 introns and 23 exons. *ATP1A1* gene is responsible for the fundamental establishment of the electrochemical gradient of Na+ and K+ across the plasma membrane, which is fundamental for maintaining body fluid and cellular homeostasis. During the elevation of body temperature "hyperthermia," heat stress activates heat shock transcription factor-1 and promotes the expression of HSPs coupled with reduced expression and synthesis of other proteins having a fundamental role to activate the immune and endocrine system. For understanding of genes in the regulation of heat shock response in animals would be helpful to improve their thermal tolerance via gene manipulation. Therefore, the *HSPA14* genes were found highly expressed in summer months in cattle, which enhance their thermotolerance and the ability to adapt to the thermal environment [57]. Genetic adaptation to heat stress for cellular resistance to elevated temperature reduced the levels of gonadotropin receptors, aromatase activity of granulosa cells, the follicular fluid concentrations of oestradiol, and follicular function involving changes at the level of the follicle or the secretion of the pituitary hormones that control development of the follicle. Additionally, oxidative stress is a major cause for thermal damage of spermatogenic cells and leads to apoptosis and DNA strand breaks. Moreover, apoptosis plays a critical role in effects of thermal stress on the maturing of oocyte in cattle. Therefore, the inhibition of apoptosis in bovine embryos with a caspase inhibitor increased the magnitude of the reduction in development caused by the elevated temperature. Thus, apoptosis is limited to the most damaged cells of the embryo. Heat shock caused damage to the oocyte during preovulation, which seems to involve the generation of reactive oxygen species, as both are effects of heat stress *in vivo* and heat shock *in vitro*. Furthermore, there are indications that developmental competence of the resulting embryo can be reduced if fertilization is by a spermatozoon exposed to heat shock. *In vitro* fertilization with sperm recovered from male in which the scrotum was heated to 42°C resulted in embryos with reduced ability to complete development [58]. In cows, heat shock has negative effects on competence of oocytes from antral follicles, granulosa, or theca cells, which are responsible for the production of steroids. Moreover, heat stress applied on bovine oocytes during *in vitro* maturation as well as on embryos during *in vitro* culture reduces both oocyte maturation and embryo development rates. The expression of HSP70 was not affected in the oocyte, but increased in cumulus cells. Therefore, the negative effects in oocytes because of heat shock could be mediated through the surrounding cumulus cells. Interestingly, higher expression of HSP70 in immature bovine oocytes was observed. This mRNA could be translated throughout the IVM and consequently decreases its expression in mature oocytes [59]. Heat stress accelerates cellular metabolism, resulting in the inability of the mitochondria to properly reduce oxygen that remains in its radical state [5, 6]. Thus, the poor developmental competence might be due to the lack of cytoplasmic maturation in oocytes maturing *in vitro*, even though they undergo normal nuclear maturation. In addition to the presence of heat shock proteins, there are several antioxidants, for example glutathione (GSH) that partially imparts the protection against oxidative stress. GSH appears to be the main antioxidant defense system against reactive oxygen species (ROS) in oocytes/embryos [60].

6. Regulation of the cell cycle and oocyte maturation

Several mechanisms are involved in the activation of translationally inactive mRNA. These mechanisms involve the phosphorylation of many factors that initiate translation. Therefore, according to this model, polyadenylation (the addition of adenine) of the 3′ terminal portion of the cytoplasmic mRNA would stimulate the release of repressor molecules linked to the 5′ portion, thus beginning translation. The transport of this mRNA to the cytoplasm occurs through a characteristic splicing of the poly-(A) tail, which, after reaching the cytoplasmic compartment, becomes smaller and heterogeneous in size. The cytoplasmic elongation of the poly-(A) tail has been associated to the translation activation, meaning that during addition of adenine to mRNA in the cytoplasmic of oocyte through maturation leads to deadenylations, leading to the degradation of the particular mRNA. For this reason, protein synthesis starts when the two ribosomal subunits are linked onto the mRNA. This stimulates the degradation of particular mRNA which, when oocytes are acquiring developmental competence, the fundamental transcripts produced encode regulators of the cell cycle such as "maturation promoting factor" (MPF), the protein of the c-mos pro-oncogene (MOS), and mitogen-activated protein kinase (MAPK) [37]. In mitotic cells, S-phase always precedes M-phase in order to maintain euploidy. Additionally, the maturation (M-phase) promoting factor (MPF) plays a pivotal role in oocytes during their maturation. During the mitotic cell cycle, MPF activity shows different stages of vacillation and steadiness, i.e., MPF activity wobbles positively and negatively in time with the beginning and ending of M-phase in succession, while being precisely regulated during the two cell divisions of meiosis. MPF is a heterodimer protein kinase complex consisting of two subunits: the catalytic subunit CDK1 and the regulatory subunit cyclin B1. As phosphorylation is required by CDK1, cyclin B is the main determinant for CDK1 and this is a necessary factor for certain processes during cell cycle as (1) initiating germinal vesicle breakdown (GVBD) through phosphorylation of nucleoporin—a components of nuclear pore complex—among many protein components of nuclear envelope and (2) with a large protein complex termed as condensing that helps in supercoiling the DNA during mitosis. The kinase activity requires more than binding of CDK1 to cyclin B1. MPF, the heterodimer protein, is held in an inactive state termed as PRE-MPF by wee1 kinase that causes inhibitory phosphorylation of CDK1 ($p34^{cdc2}$). However, CDC25 activates CDK1 by dephosphorylation at the same sites. Although binding of CDK1 to cyclin B1 is necessary, it is not sufficient for kinase activity. Switching on MPF in all cells is further governed by the balance in the regulatory activity of Wee1/Myt1 kinases, which cause an inhibitory phosphorylation of CDK1 ($p34^{cdc2}$) (and hold the heterodimer in an inactive state called pre-MPF), and the CDC25 phosphatases, which cause activation of dephosphorylation of CDK1 at the same sites. Thus, the high CDC25 and low Wee1/Myt1 activity are needed for switching on the CDK1 component of MPF. In addition, before entry into mitosis, cyclin B1 (and so MPF) is spatially restricted to the cytoplasm, through a cytoplasmic retention sequence, containing a nuclear export signal. When cells commit to mitosis, cyclin B1 has to become phosphorylated within its cytoplasmic retention sequence, leading to rapid accumulation of cyclin B1 and MPF within the nucleus, and ensuing GVBD [61]. In the mammalian oocytes during the meiotic maturation, two consecutive divisions execute without an intermediate phase of DNA replication where even haploid gametes are produced. In addition, these two divisions are asymmetrical, maintaining and ensuring the maximum number of oocytes possessed for maternal stores. In addition, immature oocyte contains only a small amount of cyclin B, just enough to induce entry into the first meiotic M-phase. Furthermore, MPF activity is regulated by a translation-dependent mechanism that determines the level of cyclin B1 synthesis. Among the different mechanisms that control the expression of maternal mRNAs, polyadenylation has been implicated in cyclin B1 translation in Xenopus and mouse oocytes. The immature oocyte contains only a small amount of cyclin B1, just enough to induce entry into the first meiotic M-phase increases progressively, reaching its maximum at the end of the first meiotic M phase, and the newly synthesized protein becomes associated immediately with the $p34^{cdk1}$ kinase to form an active complex. Cyclin B degradation is required for polar body extrusion. Changes in cyclin B1 levels, through changes in MPF activity, regulate not only the timing of the cell-cycle phases during meiosis but also the orderly events leading to the formation of functional meiotic spindles and asymmetric divisions, MPF activity controls the formation of a functional spindle in the oocyte. The MPF activity required for GVBD (sufficient for entry into M-phase) only allows the formation of a single aster of microtubules around the condensed chromosomes. A first threshold in MPF activity is then required to organize the microtubules into a bipolar structure. In contrast, the further migration of the chromosomes toward the vicinity of the spindle equator does not depend on changes in the MPF level [62]. The meiotic maturation is an essential process for the development of an immature oocyte into fertilization egg. In vertebrates, it is compatible with the transition from the prophase arrest of the first meiotic division to the metaphase arrest of the second meiotic division. Thus, MPF is activated in response to the hormonal signal. Therefore, steroids bring about meiotic maturation through functionally redundant pathways involving synthesis of Mos or of cyclin proteins. The c-mos pro-oncogene (MOS) protein is a Serine/Threonine kinase, which is specifically expressed in germ cells where it functions only during the short period of meiotic maturation from maternal mRNA in vertebrates before being proteolyzed at fertilization. Although it is not necessary for GVBD, Mos remains a powerful inducer of meiotic maturation when microinjected. Two roles could be envisioned for Mos in the process of GVBD induction: (1) The mRNA coding for Mos could, intrinsically or via associated proteins, affect the translation of other mRNA. (2) Synthesized Mos kinase provokes a strong pathway that most certainly participates in the amplification of MPF, as well as being necessary for normal GVBD events (for the repression of DNA synthesis) [63]. Mammalian oocytes reach the prophase diplotene stage of meiosis I before or after birth, and they remain arrested at this stage until resumption of meiosis, characterized by germinal vesicle breakdown (GVBD) that follows preovulatory gonadotropin stimulation after puberty. Thus, family of serine and threonine kinases is activated in the somatic compartment of the follicle. Intra oocyte MAPK cascade activation is more closely related to post-GVBD events such as meiotic spindle organization. Stimulation of meiosis resumption by activation of MAPK can be accomplished by prompting synthesis of downstream meiosis resumption inducing factors. Additionally, the phosphorylation of gap junctional proteins blocks communication between oocyte and around somatic cells, and subsequently prevents the meiosis from inhibiting signals from entering into oocytes from the vicinity of somatic cells. Lutropin causes activation MAPK in follicular somatic cell, which have fundamental role, which in turn phosphorylates connexins, leading to a reduction in gap junction permeability between the somatic cells prior to germinal vesicle breakdown. The suppression of gap junction communication is enough and essential for reinitiating meiosis. Mos kinase is a universal mediator of oocyte meiotic maturation and is produced during oogenesis and destroyed after fertilization. Thus, mos limits the number of meiotic division to just two rounds (meiosis I and II) and to avoid from ingress into meiosis III. Strikingly, the maintaining of Mos/MAPK pathway activities after fertilization close to physiological levels prompts additional rounds of meiosis, and the spindle is positioned symmetrically resulting in further rounds of asymmetric cell division [64]. Additionally, in the mammalian oocytes the meiotic maturation is described by special asymmetric cytokinesis through chromosomes moving from the center toward the cortex zone of an oocyte. After GVBD, a meiotic spindle congregates surrounding centrally positioned metaphase chromosomes and then moves in the vicinity of the cortex in an actin filament relying on the process. Furthermore, cortical reorganization executes an ectopic actin-rich actin cap and a cortical granule-free domain (CGFD) formed in the vicinity of the cortex devoid of microvilli in a MOS-dependent manner. Establishing cortical polarity, including spindle migration, positioning and cortical reorganization is critical for oocyte asymmetric divisions. Then cytokinesis occurs and the polar body extrudes, forming a high-polarized MII oocyte [65]. Additionally, in humans, oocyte growth unfolds over 110–120 days, during which cell mass undergoes an astounding, more than 100-fold, increase and cell diameter shifts from <40 to ~120 mm. At the same time, the macromolecules and organelles are produced and stored in very large amounts. In such a way, the oocyte meets a fundamental for preimplantation embryo developmental growth, storing enough for cytoplasmic mass desired for fertilized egg to accomplish multicellularity without the presence of net growth. Remarkably, the oocyte growth is much more than a quantitative increase in cell mass finalized to the housekeeping needs of the early embryo. For example, maternal effect genes have been characterized as sequences whose transcriptional and translational products are generated during oocyte growth and whose regulatory function is required only after fertilization. In particular, many maternal effect gene products are transcriptional regulators whose loss of function causes major developmental failures, such as arrest at cleavage or blastocyst stages, or inability to activate the zygote genome [66].

7. Regulation of mammalian oocyte gene expression at transcription level

There are six Obox (oocyte-specific homeobox) family transcripts and Obox-1, 2, 3, and 5 mRNA they have been detected in oocytes from growing primary follicles [67], playing then an important role in early embryogenesis [68, 69] by orchestrating gene transcription, either ubiquitously or in a tissue-specific manner. Mice lacking the Obox6 gene grow without morphological abnormalities and with normal fertility, indicating a functional redundancy among the Obox family members [70]. Moreover, several genes play key roles in oogenesis, folliculogenesis, or early embryonic development. In particular, GDF-9 and BMP-15 are necessary for folliculogenesis beyond primary follicles in mouse and sheep, respectively. Gene expression in oocyte is quite different from those in somatic cells. The messenger RNAs produced by these cells are not only required to support germ cell development but, in the case of oocytes, they are also used for maturation, fertilization, and early embryogenesis. It is very important to understand the oocyte mechanisms and transcription factors that play a role in the regulation of the transcriptional activity of the oocyte dictating its ultimate acquisition of developmental competence. The oocyte genome has evolved specialized transcription machinery to ensure proper activation of gene that is required for oocyte growth and early embryonic development [71].

8. Gene expression and the role of the *Cx43* and *HSPA14* genes during the embryonic development

8.1. The *HSPA14* gene

Experiments developed by our team show that exposing cumulus oocyte complexes (COCs) to 41°C did not alter the number of embryos that cleaved but reduced significantly the percentage of development in the blastocyst stage [9]. Additionally, the exposure of bovine embryos to heat shock during oocyte maturation leads to embryos with reduced development and induced alterations in protein synthesis and possibly gene expression as early as the two-cell embryos. In addition, cumulus cells are removed before maturation, which affects and reduces the protein synthesis at 42°C exposure oocytes and COCS. On the other hand, the developed oocytes at 39°C created heat shock protein 70 kDa but oocytes exposure to 42°C did not increase synthesis of any of these proteins, which was shown after examining the methionine- and cysteine-labeled proteins—by two-dimensional SDS-PAGE and fluorography. It has also been noticed that the reduction of protein synthesis caused a prominent decrease in the percentage of protein synthesis in oocytes with intact cumulus compared to those bared oocytes. Therefore, the heat shock increases the steady-state amounts of mRNA for the inducible form of heat shock protein 70 (HSP70) in embryos. The *HSPA14* is the most abundant, highly sensitive to culture environment and it is the major inducible heat shock gene important for protecting embryonic cells from cellular stress in bovine. Thus, HSP70 mRNA in 2- and 4-cell embryos was increased by exposure to 42°C. As findings indicate that the experience for embryos may undergo the transcription of heat shock exposure as early in

2-cell stage, the rates of cleavage and early development are reduced by transcription inhibitors, which show the significance of transcription on the earliest period of fetal life development [72]. The expression of the major heat-inducible protein HSP70 protects cells from a self-destruction known as apoptosis. Cells can also respond to stress by adaptive changes that increase their ability to tolerate normally lethal conditions. The expression of *HSPA14* gene would allow to produce and help maintain cellular function by acting as molecular chaperones to stabilize or refold proteins damaged by heat, and by blocking apoptosis by preventing cytochrome c release from mitochondria during the early stages of apoptosis [73]. Moreover, these authors postulated that the *HSPA14* during embryo development with the presence of antibodies to HSP70 significantly decreases progression to the hatched blastocyst stage in murine embryos. Correspondingly, antisense oligonucleotides complementary to HSP70 mRNA had a similar effect on embryo development, which was amplified ninefold by arsenic exposure at a subtoxic dose. Hence, the embryos that did reach the blastocyst stage despite the inhibition of HSP70 expression, with and without the presence of arsenic, were characterized as degenerate with cell death accompanied by membrane blebbing. Thus, suggested that the requirement for HSP70 during embryo development is amplified by exposure to adverse environmental conditions [12]. *In vitro* matured bovine oocytes, 2-cell and 8-cell embryos, and day 9 hatched blastocysts subjected to control and elevated temperature conditions were analyzed by semiquantitative reverse transcription polymerase chain reaction methods for HSP70 mRNA expression. In the cytoplasm of 8-cell embryos that were inferred under control conditions, HSP70 was evenly disseminated in the cytoplasm but appeared as aggregates in some embryos exposed to elevated temperature. The hatched blastocysts show a competence to react to elevated temperature that is shown in the increased distributions noted after heat stress [74]. As described before, several authors pointed out that heat shock protein can be induced by bovine embryos exposed to heat shock. Those bovine embryos, presented to heat shock, also produce other cellular changes to make cell more impervious to a subsequent heat shock. The 2-cell bovine embryos can deliver HSP70 in response to raised temperature although it is sensitive to heat shock. Therefore, to test for induced thermotolerance, 2-cell bovine embryos were first exposed to a mild heat shock 40°C, allowed to recover at 38.5°C and 5% CO_2. Subsequently, the way in which HSP70 take part in embryonic development was examined at two different temperature, 38.5 and 40°C, culturing embryos with a monoclonal immunoglobulin to the inducible form of HSP70 experiment, a reduction of the proportion of 2-cell embryos ($p < 0.05$) by adding anti-HSP70 to the culture medium. Thus, bovine 2-cell embryos appear incapable of thermotolerance owing to the increased sensitivity of 2-cell embryos to heat shock as compared to embryos at later stages of development. The results also implicated a role for HSP70 in normal development of bovine embryos. Studies developed by Mayer and Bukau [75] showed that bovine 2-cell embryos appear incapable of thermotolerance owing to the increased sensitivity of 2-cell embryos to heat shock as compared to embryos at later stages of development. The results also implicated a role for HSP70 in normal development of bovine embryos. The same authors [75] pointed out that one of the central components of the cell network of molecular chaperones are HSP70 proteins. An abundant array of protein folding processes are assisted by HSP70 proteins in the cell through association transiently of segments of short hydrophobic peptide—within substrate proteins—with their substrate binding area. When substrate binding, it releases cycle which is driven by exchanging of HSP70 between the high-affinity ADP bound state and low-affinity ATP bound state. Hence, the chaperone activity of HSP70 proteins need hydrolysis and binding if ATP *in vivo* and *in vitro*. Cochaperones of the J-domain proteins family control this ATPase, which make their substrates targeted by nucleotide exchange factor and by HSP70s, decide the lifetime of the HSP70 substrate complex. This chaperone cycle is tweaked by additional cochaperones. The HSP90 and HSP100 among other chaperones couple with the HSP70 cycle for specific tasks. As a different understanding, Kampinga stated that several assortments of cellular internal and external cases of the stress can be distributed as proteotoxic stresses, which can be described as stresses that raise the main fraction of proteins that are in an unfolded state, thereby promoting the possibility of the formation of intracellular aggregates. These accumulations of assemble, whether not disposed, may lead to the apoptosis. In response to the appearance of denaturation and damaged proteins, cells promote the expression of heat shock proteins. These can have fundamental function as molecular chaperones to avoid protein from the assembling and to maintain the proteins in a state competent for either refolding or degradation. As *Bos indicus* cows usually have better reproductive performance in tropical and subtropical regions than *Bos taurus* cows, presumably due to their better adaptation to tropical environments, Camargo et al. [76] evaluated the developmental competence and expression of the HSP70 gene in immature oocytes from *Bos taurus* (Holstein) and *Bos indicus* (Gyr) dairy cows raised in a tropical region. The total RNA extracted from Holstein and Gyr oocytes and the HSP70 transcripts was conducted, which was formed by real-time PCR after reverse transcription. Cleavage and blastocyst rates were ultimately greater ($p < 0.05$) for Gyr breed ($n = 390$ oocytes) than for the Holstein ($n = 505$) breed (66.7% vs. 53.1% of cleavage and 19.6% vs. 10.8% of blastocysts, respectively), showing an adaptation of these two breeds to the environmental conditions. Studies developed by Virenque et al. [77] hypothesized that the high structural and functional conservation of HSP during evolution suggests crucial roles in fertilization, embryo development, and thus, fertility in cattle. Also, some HSP are considered housekeeping genes that are essential for many cell functions, such the HSP40 combined with HSP70 acting as chaperones to protect cells from apoptosis [78]. All HSP isoforms are ATP-dependent molecular chaperones as they protect nascent or denatured proteins from aggregation and assist their folding or refolding into native conformation and regulation of heat shock response.

8.2. The *Cx43* gene

Connexins (CXs) are a family of transmembrane proteins with molecular masses varying from 26 to 60 kD; *Cx43* has a molecular mass of 43 kD. In vertebrates, CXs are the building blocks of gap junction channels, intercellular channels that connect the cytoplasm of two neighboring cells. Wrenzycki et al. [79] examined the presence of the mRNA encoding connexin 43 (*Cx43*) in bovine embryos derived *in vivo* and *in vitro* and in the bovine embryos through morula and blastocysts grown *in vivo*, the transcription of the *Cx43* were disclosed. Conversely, when the early *in vitro* stages from cumulus oocyte complexes (COCs) to morula expressed *Cx43*, blastocysts and hatched blastocysts cannot have disclosed concentrations of mRNA from this gene as because it is not activated or if embryonic gene expression had been active, it terminated prematurely. The differences in transcription between bovine embryos derived *in vivo* or *in vitro* indicate that culture conditions affect gene expression. Melton et al. [80] reported that the gap junction is a major form of cell–cell communication and aggregations of intercellular channels composed of connexins (CXs), which are responsible for exchange of low molecular weight (<1200 Da) cytosolic materials. In ovarian tissue of mammals, investigators have established that the presence of *Cx43* is to determine the ontogeny of early stages of follicular development of embryos. Additionally, it has been found that the preovulatory LH surge caused a decrease in *Cx43* mRNA in granulosa cells of rat ovarian follicles. Therefore, the results reported indicated that increased expression of *Cx43* temporally correlates with the activation of follicular development and early differentiation of granulosa cells in follicles of prepubertal pig ovaries. Vozzi et al. [81] indicated that in ovarian follicles, oocyte is provided by cumulus cells with small molecules that license control maturation and growth. The germinal cell gets these nutrients through gap junction channels, present between the oocyte and cumulus cells. Goldberg et al. [82] reported that the gap junctions, composed of proteins from the connexin family, are the only channels that directly connect the cytoplasm of the adjacent cells to allow for the intercellular transfer of small hydrophilic molecules, essential for proper development and health in animals and humans. Kidder and Mhawi [83] showed that the gap junctions are a group of intercellular membrane channels which leads to adjacent cells to participate in small molecules (<1 kDa). Gap junction channels are composed of connexins, a homologous family of more than 20 proteins. For developing of follicles, the gap junction is coupled with the developing oocyte and its besetment of the follicle cells into an essential functional syncytium. Among the gap junctions and cumulus cells includes the majority connexin 43, and this connexin has also been detected utilizing immunoelectron microscopy in a small minority of gap junctions at the surface of the oocyte. The significance of connexin 43 for granulosa cell having fundamental function is demonstrated by the fact that follicles lacking this connexin arrest in early prenatal stages and produce incompetent oocytes. Connexin 37 is shown to be the only connexin participate by oocytes to the gap junctions coupling them with granulosa cells, and loss of this connexin interferes with the development of the secondary follicle. The expression of multiple connexins in growth follicles probably indicate the multiple functions served by gap junctional correspondence in folliculogenesis. In the absence of *Cx43*, granulosa cells block growing in an early preantral stage. To illustrate the fundamental role function of *Cx43*, dye injection experiments detected that granulosa cells from *Cx43* knockout follicles are not coupled, and this was confirmed by ionic current injections. However, electron microscopy detected that gap junctions are quite rare in mutant granulosa cells. Conversely, mutant granulosa cells were eligible to form gap junctions with wild-type granulosa cells in a dye preloading assay. It was accomplished that mutant granulosa cells comprise a population of connexins, composed of nonrecognized connexins that cannot contribute regularly to participate in gap junctions. Additionally, despite *Cx43* being the only gap junction protein existing in granulosa cells of early preantral follicles, it is the only one that makes a significant contribution to intercellular coupling [84]. Research conducted by Veitch et al. [85] uncovered that studies of mammalian animals with targeted disruption of specific connexin genes have revealed that at least two connexins, connexin 37 (*Cx37*) and connexin 43 (*Cx43*), play essential roles in ovarian follicle development. Immunofluorescence microscopy located *Cx37* within gap junction plaques between granulosa cells and the oocyte, and *Cx43* between surrounding granulosa cells. Gittens et al. [86] reviewed that the intercellular communication is required for ovarian folliculogenesis. Yogo et al. [87] reported that the connexin 43 (*Cx43*)-intermediate gap junctional communication in granulosa cells is crucial for germ line development and postnatal folliculogenesis. These authors showed that follicle-stimulating hormone (FSH) induced the phosphorylation of *Cx43* in primary granulosa cells and then further specified to identify Ser365, Ser368, Ser369, and Ser373 in the carboxy terminal tail as the major sites of phosphorylation by FSH, and found that the phosphorylation of these remains was substantial for channel activity. Furthermore, Borowczyk et al. [88] evaluated the role of gap junctions in the regulation of progesterone secretion. The changes in *Cx43* mRNA expression were positively correlated with changes in progesterone concentration. They demonstrated a relationship between gap junctions and progesterone secretion that was supported by (1) the positive correlations between progesterone secretion and *Cx43* mRNA expression and gap junctional interacelluer communication (GJIC) of luteal cells and (2) the inhibition of *Cx43* mRNA expression resulted in decreased production of progesterone by luteal cells. This suggested that gap junctions may be involved in the regulation of steroidogenesis in the corpus luteum. Gershon et al. [89] reported that the gap junctions that allow the direct communication between cytoplasmic compartments of neighboring cells are present in a variety of tissues and organs, allowing thus the rapid exchange of ions and metabolites. Besides in the bovine, follicles express *Cx43*, which is localized to granulosa cells from the primary follicle and increases upon antrum formation being necessary for follicle development and oocyte growth. The expression specificities of *Cx43* in ovary are still in discussion by several groups. During folliculogenesis, the granulosa cells give physical support and mediate signal between different types of follicular cells. Rhett et al. [90] reviewed that the *Cx43* is the most ubiquitous connexin, with expression in at least 46 different cell types being a gap junction protein widely expressed in mammalian tissues that mediates cell-to-cell coupling. Intercellular channels comprising GJ aggregates form from docking of paired connexons, with one each contributed by opposing cells. The regulation of gap junction coupling is a necessary component of cellular function and response to physiological and pathological stimuli. The cells can modify the expression, phosphorylation state, and protein interactions of *Cx43* throughout the cell cycle. Because of the short half-life of *Cx43*, which is as little as 1–2 h, regulation appears to exist on both short and long time scales through phosphorylation and protein interaction, and gene expression, respectively. Currently, there is a great deal of data on phospho- and transcriptional regulation of *Cx43* but less is known about the mechanistic basis and function of *Cx43* protein–protein interactions. Furthermore, concerning the *Cx43*, normally low expression of *Cx43* in different development stages of embryos has been associated with low quality and reduced survival capacity of embryos [91, 92].

9. Methods for studying differential gene expression

Several techniques have been developed for the screening of genomic alterations at the mRNA level, including subtractive hybridization, differential display-PCR, expressed sequence tag (EST), serial analysis of gene expression (SAGE), and microarray hybridization. Some of these techniques have been used to investigate changes in gene expression at oocyte cell development and differentiation [93]. In addition, the effective and simple methods for identifying and isolating those genes that are differentially expressed in various cells or under altered conditions. Advantages of the technique include the ability to isolate genes with no prior knowledge of their sequence or identity and the use of common molecular biology techniques that do not require specialized equipment or analyses, its abilities to compare multiple experimental samples for any number of treatment conditions, phenotypes, or genotypes simultaneously, and to identify genes that are either up- or downregulated in one sample relative to another [94]. The differential display include as first step is reverse transcription of mRNA to cDNA using one of anchor primers (which is usually poly T oligonucleotide with one or two additional bases, e.g., T_{12}AC) designed to anneal to the 3′ poly-A tail of messenger RNA (mRNA). The resulting of cDNA species is subsequently used as templates in a PCR, utilizing the same anchor primer from reverse transcription (RT) reaction in combination with an arbitrary primer. The PCR products may be labeled by incorporation of a radiolabeled nucleotide fluorescently labeled primer. Electrophoresis pattern can be then evaluated by comparing the relative intensities of bands produced from different treatment samples. Bands that are present in one sample and absent in another or bands that are present at different relative intensities, across different treatment, represent potentially differentially expressed mRNA transcripts. The final phase of differential display is excising and purification of the band of interest from the polyacrylamide gel and reamplification by PCR, and eventually subjected to sequencing.

Acknowledgements

The authors thank Dr. Sofia Quadros and Mr. Filipe António for their precious collaboration in this review. CITA-A is also fully acknowledged. The second author is partially supported by the Azorean Agency for Science and Technology, grant BD M3.1.2/F/044/2011.

Author details

Aya K. H. Mahdy, Krishna C. Pavani, Erica Baron and Fernando Moreira da Silva*

*Address all correspondence to: jsilva@uac.pt

Department of Animal Reproduction, Faculty of Agrarian Sciences and Environment, CITA-A (Research Centre for Agricultural and Environmental Sciences and Technology of the Azores), University of the Azores, Angra do Heroismo, Portugal

References

[1] Sherwin, A., Montgomery, I. and Lundy, G. The impact and implications of climate change for bats. Mammal Rev. 2012;**43**:1–18. DOI: 10.1111/j.1365-2907.2012.00214.x.

[2] Luo, J., Koselj, K., Zsebok, S., Siemers, M. and Goerlitz, R. Global warming alters sound transmission: differential impact on the prey detection ability of echolocating bats. J R Soc Interface. 2013;**11**(91):20130–20961. DOI: 10.1098/rsif.2013.0961.

[3] Vermaa, K., Prasadb, S., Mohantyb, T., Kumaresanb, A., Layekb, S., Patbandhac, T., Dattad, T. and Chandb, S. Effect of short-term cooling on core body temperature, plasma cortisol and conception rate in Murrah buffalo heifers during hot-humid season. J Appl Anim Res. 2016;**44**(1):281–286. DOI: 10.1080/09712119.2015.1031782.

[4] Badinga, L., Thatcher, W., Diaz, T., Drost, M. and Wolfenson, D. Effects of environmental heat stress on follicular development and steroidogenesis in lactating Holstein cows. Theriogenology. 1993;**39**:797—810. DOI: 10.1016/0093-691X(93)90419-6.

[5] Al-Katanani, M., Paula-Lopes, F. and Hansen, J. Effect of season and exposure to heat stress on oocyte competence in Holstein cows. J Dairy Sci. 2002;**85**(2):390–396. DOI: 10.3168/jds.S0022-0302(02)74086-1.

[6] Al-Katanani, M. and Hansen, J. Induced thermotolerance in bovine two cell embryos and the role of heat shock protein 70 in embryonic development. Mol Reprod Dev. 2002;**62**(2):174–180. DOI: 10.1002/mrd.10122.

[7] Ahmed, A., Tiwari, R., Mishra, G., Jena, B., Dar, M. and Bhat, A. Effect of environmental heat stress on reproduction performance of dairy cows. A review. Int J Livest Res. 2015;**5**(4):10–18. DOI: 10.5455/ijlr.20150421122704.

[8] Roth, Z. Physiology and Endocrinology Symposium: cellular and molecular mechanisms of heat stress related to bovine ovarian function. J Anim Sci. 2015;**93**(5):2034–2044. DOI: 10.2527/jas.2014-8625.

[9] Pavani, K., Carvalhais, L., Faheem, M., Chaveiro, A., Reis, F. and da Silva, F. Reproductive performance of Holstein dairy cows grazing in dry-summer subtropical. Asian-Australas J Anim Sci. 2015;**28**(3):334–342. DOI: 10.5713/ajas.14.0480.

[10] Nandi, S., Raghu, M., Ravindranatha, M. and Chauhan, S. Production of buffalo (Bubalus bubalis) embryos in vitro: premises and promises. Reprod Domest Anim. 2002;**37**(2):65–74. DOI: 10.1046/j.1439-0531.2002.00340.x.

[11] Wrenzycki, C., Herrmann, D. and Niemann, H. Messenger RNA in oocytes and embryos in relation to embryo viability. Theriogenology. 2007;**68**(1):77–83. DOI: 10.1016/j.theriogenology.2007.04.028.

[12] Matwee, C., Kamaruddin, M., Betts, H., Basrur, K. and King, A. The effects of antibodies to heat shock protein 70 in fertilization and embryo development. Mol Hum Reprod. 2001;**7**(9):829–837. DOI: 10.1093/molehr/7.9.829.

[13] Cushman, A. Physiology and Endocrinology Symposium: the current status of heat shock in early embryonic survival and reproductive efficiency. J Anim Sci. 2013;**91**(3):1141–1142. DOI: 10.2527/jas2013-6231.

[14] Miova, B., Dinevska-Kjovkarovska, S., Esplugues, V. and Apostolova, N. Heat stress induces extended plateau of hsp70 accumulation-a possible cytoprotection mechanism in hepatic cells. J Cell Biochem. 2015;**116**(10):2365–2374. DOI: 10.1002/jcb.25187.

[15] Li, H., Pang, Q., Qin, L., Jin, S., Zeng, X., Bai, Y. and Li, W. HSP70 overexpression may play a protective role in the mouse embryos stimulated by CUMS. Reprod Biol Endocrinol. 2015;**16**(13):125. DOI: 10.1186/s12958-015-0123-z.

[16] Sharma, T., Nath, A., Prasad, S., Singhal, S., Singh, N., Gade, E., Dubey, K. and Saikumar, G. Expression and characterization of constitutive heat shock protein 70.1 (HSPA-1A) gene in in vitro produced and in vivo- derived buffalo (Bubalus bubalis) embryos. Reprod Domest Anim. 2012;**47**(6):975–983. DOI: 10.1111/j.1439-0531.2012.02002.x.

[17] Kidder, G. Roles of gap junctions in ovarian folliculogenesis: implications for female infertility. In: "Gap Junctions in Development and Disease."Springer-Verlag Berlin Heidelberg. 2005, pp. 223–237. DOI: 10.1007/3-540-28621-7_10.

[18] Eppig, J. Intercommunication between mammalian oocytes and companion follicle cells. Bioessays. 1991;**12**:569–574. DOI: 10.1002/bies.950131105.

[19] Pointis, G., Fiorini, C., Defamie, N. and Segretain, D. Gap junctional communication in the male reproductive system. Biochim Biophys Acta. 2005;**1719**(1–2):1–16. DOI: 10.1016/j. bbamem.2005.09.017.

[20] McGee, A. and Hsueh, J. Initial and cyclic recruitment of ovarian follicles. Endocr Rev. 2000;**21**(2):200–214. DOI: 10.1210/edrv.21.2.0394.

[21] Senbon, S., Hirao, Y. and Miyano, T. Interactions between the oocyte and surrounding somatic cells in follicular development: lessons from in vitro culture. J Reprod Dev. 2003;**49**:259–269. DOI: 10.1262/jrd.49.259.

[22] De Felici, M., Klinger, G., Farini, D., Scaldaferri, L., Iona, S. and Lobascio, M. Establishment of oocyte population in the foetal ovary: primordial germ cell proliferation and oocyte programmed cell death. Reprod Biomed Online. 2005;**10**(2):182–191. DOI: 10.1016/S1432-6483(10)60939-X.

[23] Brunet, S. and Verlhac, H. Positioning to get out of meiosis: the asymmetry of division. Hum Reprod Update. 2011;**17**(1):68–75. DOI: 10.1093/humupd/dmq044.

[24] Fair, T. Follicular oocyte growth and acquisition of developmental competence. Anim Reprod Sci. 2003;**78**:203–216. DOI: 10.1016/S0378-4320(03)00091-5.

[25] Barnett, R., Schilling, C., Greenfeld, R., Tomic, D., and Flaws, A. Ovarian follicle development and transgenic mouse models. Hum Reprod Update. 2006;**12**(5):537–555. DOI: 10.1093/humupd/dml022.

[26] Mermillod, P., Dalbies-Tran, R., Uzbekova, S., Thélie, A., Traverso, M., Perreau, C., Papillier, P. and Monget, P. Factors affecting oocyte quality: who is driving the follicle? Reprod Domest Anim. 2008;**43**(2):393–400. DOI: 10.1111/j.1439-0531.2008.01190.x.

[27] Young, M. and McNeilly, S. Theca: the forgotten cell of the ovarian follicle. Reproduction. 2010;**140**(4):489–504. DOI: 10.1530/REP-10- 0094.

[28] Georges, A., Auguste, A., Bessière, L., Vanet, A., Todeschini, L. and Veitia, A. FOXL2: a central transcription factor of the ovary. J Mol Endocrinol. 2013;**52**(1):17–33. DOI: 10.1530/JME-13-0159.

[29] Hansen, P. Antecedents of mammalian fertility: lessons from the heat-stressed cow regarding the importance of oocyte competence for fertilization and embryonic development. Animal Front. 2014;**3**(4):34–39. DOI: 10.2527/af.2013-0031.

[30] Kakkassery, M., Vijayakumaran, V. and Sreekumaran, T. Effect of cumulus oocyte complex morphology on in vitro maturation of bovine oocytes. J. Vet.Anim.Sci. 2010;**41**:12–17.

[31] Stricker, A., Escalona, R., Abernathy, S. and Marquardt, A. Pharmacological analyses of protein kinases regulating egg maturation in marine nemertean worms: a review and comparison with Mammalian eggs. Mar Drugs. 2010;**8**(8):2417–2434. DOI: 10.3390/md8082417.

[32] Homer, H. New insights into the genetic regulation of homologue disjunction in mammalian oocytes. Cytogenet Genome Res. 2011;**133**(2–4):208–222. DOI: 10.1159-000324118.

[33] Kwon, S. and Lim, J. Small GTPases and formins in mammalian oocyte maturation: cytoskeletal organizers. Clin Exp Reprod Med. 2011;**38**(1):1–5. DOI: 10.5653/cerm.2011.38.1.1.

[34] Blanco, R., Demyda, S., Moreno, M. and Genero, E. Developmental competence of in vivo and in vitro matured oocytes: a review. Biotechnol Mol Biol Rev. 2011;**6**(7):155–165.

[35] Da Broi, G., Malvezzi, H., Paz, C., Ferriani, A. and Navarro, A. Follicular fluid from infertile women with mild endometriosis may compromise the meiotic spindles of bovine metaphase II oocytes. Hum Reprod. 2014;**29**(2):315–323. DOI: 10.1093/humrep/det378.

[36] Dumesic, A., Meldrum, R., Katz-Jaffe, G., Krisher, L. and Schoolcraft, B. Oocyte environment: follicular fluid and cumulus cells are critical for oocyte health. Fertil Steril. 2015;**103**(2):303–316. DOI: 10.1016/j.fertnstert.2014.11.015.

[37] Ferreira, M., Vireque, A., Adona, R., Meirelles, V., Ferriani, A. and Navarro, A. Cytoplasmic maturation of bovine oocytes: structural and biochemical modifications and acquisition of developmental competence. Theriogenology. 2009;**71**(5):836–848. DOI: 10.1016/j.therionology.

[38] Wang, Y., Wang, H., Zou, Y. and Xu, M. Mitochondrial functions on oocytes and preimplantation embryos. J Zhejiang Univ Sci B. 2009;**10**(7):483–492. DOI: 10.1631/jzus.B0820379.

[39] Kalo, D. and Roth, Z. Effects of mono (2-ethylhexyl) phthalate on cytoplasmic maturation of oocytes – the bovine model. Reprod Toxicol 2015;**53**:141–151. DOI: 10.1016/j.reprotox.2015.04.007.

[40] Sirard, A. Resumption of meiosis: mechanism involved in meiotic progression and its relation with developmental competence. Theriogenology. 2001;**55**(6):1241–1254. DOI: 10.1016/S0093-691X(01)00480-0 PMID: 11327682.

[41] Eichenlaub-Ritter, U. and Peschke, M. Expression in in-vivo and in-vitro growing and maturing oocytes: focus on regulation of expression at the translational level. Hum Reprod Update. 2002;**8**(1):21–41. DOI: 10.1093-humupd/8.1.21 PMID: 11866238.

[42] Tomek, W., Torner, H. and Kanitz, W. Comparative analysis of protein synthesis, transcription and cytoplasmic polyadenylation of mRNA during maturation of bovine oocytes in vitro. Reprod Domest Anim. 2002;**37**(2):86–91. DOI: 10.1046/j.1439-0531.2002.00336.

[43] Sirard, A., Richard, F., Blondin, P. and Robert, C. Contribution of the oocyte to embryo quality. Theriogenology. 2006;**65**(1):126–136. DOI: 10.1016/j.theriogenology.2005.09.020.

[44] Niemann, H., Carnwath, W. and Kues, W. Application of DNA array technology to mammalian embryos. Theriogenology. 2007;**1**(68 Suppl 1):S165–S177. DOI: 10.1016/j.theriogenology.2007.05.041.

[45] Demirtas, E., Holzer, H., Son, W., Chain, R. and Tan, S. In-vitro maturation of human oocytes. In: "Reproductive Endocrinology and Infertility" (Carrell, E. and Peterson, C.). Springer New York. 2010. vol. **5**, pp. 633–646. DOI: 10.1007/978-1-4419-1436-1_42.

[46] Gasparrini, B. In vitro embryo production in buffalo species: state of the art. Theriogenology. 2002;**1**:237–256. DOI: doi:10.1016/S0093-691X(01)00669-0.

[47] Ramos, F., Rumpf, R., Câmara, U., Mollo, R., Pivato, I., Marques, R. and Sartori, R. Effect of follicular wave synchronization on in vitro embryo production in heifers. Anim Reprod Sci. 2010;**117**(3–4):201–207. DOI: 10.1016/j.anireprosci.2009.04.009.

[48] Kathy, N., Niakan, H., Pedersen, R., Simo, C., Renee, A. and Pera, R. Human preimplantation embryo development. Development. 2012;**139**(5):829–841. DOI: 10.1242/dev.060426.

[49] Wolfenson, D., Roth, Z. and Median, R. Impaired reproduction in heat-stressed cattle: basic and applied aspects. Anim Reprod Sci. 2000;**61**:535–547. DOI: 10.1016/S0378-4320(00)00102-03.

[50] Rensis, F. and Scaramuzzi, R. Heat stress and seasonal effect on reproduction in the dairy cow – a review. Theriogenology. 2003;**60**:1139–1151. DOI: 10.1016/S0093-691X(03)00126-2.

[51] Payton, R., Romar, R., Coy, P., Saxton, A., Lawrence, J. and Edwards, J. Susceptibility of bovine germinal vesicle-stage oocytes from antral follicles to direct effects of heat stress in vitro. Biol Reprod 2004;**71**:1303–1308. DOI: 10.1095/biolreprod.104.029892.

[52] Hansen, J. Exploitation of genetic and physiological determinants of embryonic resistance to elevated temperature to improve embryonic survival in dairy cattle during heat stress. Theriogenology. 2007;**68**:242–249. DOI: 10.1016/j.theriogenology.2007.04.008.

[53] Roth, Z. Heat stress, the follicle, and its enclosed oocyte: mechanisms and potential strategies to improve fertility in dairy cows. Reprod Domest Anim. 2008;**2**:238–244. DOI: 10.1111/j.1439-0531.2008.01168.x.

[54] Hansen, J. Stress in dairy animals | heat stress: effects on reproduction. Phil Trans R Soc Lond B Biol Sci. 201109;**360**:3341–3350. DOI: 10.1098/rstb.2009.0131.

[55] Belhadj, I., Najar, T., Ghram, A. and Abdrrabba, M. Heat stress effects on livestock: molecular, cellular and metabolic aspects, a review. J Anim Physiol Anim Nutr (Berl). 2015;**100**(3):401–412. DOI: 10.1111/jpn.12379.

[56] Nguyen, T., Bowman, J., Haile-Mariam, M., Pryce, E. and Hayes, J. Genomic selection for tolerance to heat stress in Australian dairy cattle. J Dairy Sci. 2016;**99**(4):2849–2862. DOI: 10.3168/jds.2015-9685.

[57] Dash, S., Chakravarty, K., Singh, A., Upadhyay, A., Singh, M. and Yousuf, S. Effect of heat stress on reproductive performances of dairy cattle and buffaloes: a review. Vet World. 2016;**9**(3):235–244. DOI: 10.14202/vetworld.2016.235-244.

[58] Hansen, P. Effects of heat stress on mammalian reproduction. Phil Trans R Soc Lond B Biol Sci. 2009;**27-364**(1534):3341–3350. DOI: 10.1098/rstb.2009.0131.

[59] Paes, M., Vieira, A., Correia, H., Sa, A., Moura, A., Sales, D., Rodrigues, P., Magalhaes-Padilha, M., Santos, W., Apgar, A., Campello, C., Camargo, S. and Figueiredo, R. Effect of heat stress on the survival and development of in vitro cultured bovine preantral follicles and on in vitro maturation of cumulus-oocyte complex. Theriogenology. 2016:86(4);994–1003. DOI: 10.1016/j.theriogenology.2016.03.027.

[60] Waiz, A., Raies-Ul-Haq, M., Dhanda, S., Kumar, A., Goud, S., Chauhan, S. and Upadhyay, C. Heat stress and antioxidant enzyme activity in bubaline (Bubalus bubalis) oocytes during in vitro maturation. Int J Biometeorol. 2016;**60**(9):1357–66. DOI:10.1007/s00484-015-1129-0.

[61] Jones, T. Turning it on and off: M-phase promoting factor during meiotic maturation and fertilization. Mol Hum Reprod. 2004;**10**(1):1–5. DOI: 10.1093/molehr/gah009.

[62] Brunet, S. and Maro, B. Cytoskeleton and cell cycle control during meiotic maturation of the mouse oocyte: integrating time and space. Reproduction. 2005;**130**(6):801–811. DOI: 10.1530/rep.1.00364.

[63] Haccard, O. and Jessus, C. Oocyte maturation, Mos and cyclins--a matter of synthesis: two functionally redundant ways to induce meiotic maturation. Cell Cycle. 2006;**5**(11):1152–1159. DOI: 10.4161/cc.5.11.2800.

[64] Dumollard, R., Levasseur, M., Hebras, C., Huitorel, P., Carroll, M., Chambon, P. and McDougall, A. Mos limits the number of meiotic divisions in urochordate eggs. Development. 2011;**138**(5):885–895. DOI: 10.1242/dev.057133.

[65] Zhang, Y., Duan, X., Cao, R., Liu, L., Cui, S., Kim, H., Rui, R. and Sun, C. Small GTPase RhoA regulates cytoskeleton dynamics during porcine oocyte maturation and early embryo development. Cell Cycle. 2014;**13**(21):3390–3403. DOI: 10.4161/15384101.2014.9529.

[66] Coticchio, G., Dal, M., Mignini, M., Guglielmo, C., Brambillasca, F., Turchi, D., Novara, V. and Fadini, R. Oocyte maturation: gamete-somatic cells interactions, meiotic resumption, cytoskeletal dynamics and cytoplasmic reorganization. Hum Reprod Update. 2015;21(4):427–454. DOI: 10.1093/humupd/dmv011.

[67] Park, T., Seo, M., Lee, Y. and Lee, A. Lin28 regulates the expression of neuropeptide Y receptors and oocyte-specific homeobox genes in mouse embryonic stem cells. Clin Exp Reprod Med. 2012;**39**(2):87–93. DOI: 10.5653/cerm.2012.39.2.87.

[68] Rajkovic, A. and Matzuk, M. Functional analysis of oocyte-expressed genes using transgenic models. Mol Cell Endocrinol. 2002;**22;187**(1-2):5–9. DOI: 10.1016/S0303-7207(01)00710-9.

[69] Rajkovic, A., Yan, C., Yan, W., Klysik, M. and Matzuk, M. Obox, a family of homeobox genes preferentially expressed in germ cells. Genomics. 2002;**79**(5):711–717. DOI: 10.1006/geno.2002.6759.

[70] Kim, M., Ahn, J., Lee, S., Lee, A., Lee, M., Kim, H., Kim, S. and Park, S. Obox4 regulates the expression of histone family genes and promotes differentiation of mouse embryonic stem cells. FEBS Lett. 2010;**584**(3):605–611. DOI: 10.1016/j.febslet.

[71] DeJong, J. Basic mechanisms for the control of germ cell gene expression. Gene. 2006;**366**(1):39–50. DOI: 10.1016/j.gene.2005.10.012.

[72] Chandolia, K., Peltier, R., Tian, W. and Hansen, J. Transcriptional control of development, protein synthesis, and heat-induced heat shock protein 70 synthesis in 2-cell bovine embryos. Biol Reprod. 1999;**61**(6):1644–1648. DOI: 10.1095/ biolreprod61.6.1644.

[73] Mosser, D., Caron, W., Bourget, L., Meriin, B., Sherman, Y., Morimoto, I. and Massie, B. The chaperone function of hsp70 is required for protection against stress-induced apoptosis. Mol Cell Biol. 2000;**19**:7146–7159. DOI: 10.1128/MCB.20.19.7146 7159.2000.

[74] Kawarsky, J. and King, A. Expression and localisation of heat shock protein 70 in cultured bovine oocytes and embryos. Zygote. 2001;**9**(1):39–50. DOI: 10.1017/S0967199401001058.

[75] Mayer, P. and Bukau, B. Hsp70 chaperones: cellular functions and molecular mechanism. Cell Mol Life Sci. 2005;**62**(6):670–684. DOI: 10.1007/s00018-004-4464-6.

[76] Camargo, S., Viana, H., Ramos, A., Serapião, V., de Sa, F., Ferreira, M., Guimarães, F. and do Vale, R. Developmental competence and expression of the Hsp70.1 gene in oocytes obtained from Bos indicus and Bos taurus dairy cows in a tropical environment. Theriogenology. 2007;**68**(4):626–632. DOI: 10.1016/j.theriogenology.2007.03.029.

[77] Virenque, A., Camargo, S., Serapião, V., Rosa, A., Watanabe, F., Ferreira, M., Navarro, A., Martins, P. and Ferriani, A. Preimplantation development and expression of Hsp-70 and Bax genes in bovine blastocysts derived from oocytes matured in alpha MEM supplemented with growth factors and synthetic macromolecules. Theriogenology. 2009;**71**(4):620–627. DOI: 10.1016/j.theriogenology.2008.09.028.

[78] Zhang, B., Peñagaricano, F., Driver, A., Chen, H. and Khatib, H. Differential expression of heat shock protein genes and their splice variants in bovine preimplantation embryos. J Dairy Sci. 2011;**94**(8):4174–4182. DOI: 10.3168/jds.2010-4137.

[79] Wrenzycki, C., Herrmann, D., Carnwath, W. and Niemann, H. Expression of the gap junction gene connexin43 (Cx43) in preimplantation bovine embryos derived in vitro or in vivo. J Reprod Fertil. 1996;**108**(1):17–24. DOI: 10.1016/0093-691X(96)84724-8.

[80] Melton, M., Zaunbrecher, M., Yoshizaki, G., Patiño, R., Whisnant, S., Rendon, A. and Lee, H. Expression of connexin 43 mRNA and protein in developing follicles of prepubertal porcine ovaries. Comp Biochem Physiol B Biochem Mol Biol. 2001;**130**(1):43–55. DOI: 10.1016/S1096-4959(01)00403-1.

[81] Vozzi, C., Formenton, A., Chanson, A., Senn, A., Sahli, R., Shaw, P., Nicod, P., Germond, M. and Haefliger, A. Involvement of connexin 43 in meiotic maturation of bovine oocytes. Reproduction. 2001;**122**(4):619–628. DOI: 10.1530/rep.1.004.

[82] Goldberg, S., Moreno, P. and Lampe, D. Gap junctions between cells expressing connexin 43 or 32 show inverse sperm selectivity to adenosine and ATP. J Biol Chem. 2002;**277**(39):36725–36730. DOI: 10.1074/jbc.M109797200.

[83] Kidder, M. and Mhawi, A. Gap junctions and ovarian folliculogenesis. Reproduction. 2002;**123**(5):613–620. DOI: 10.1530/rep.0.1230613.

[84] Gittens, E., Mhawi, A., Lidington, D., Ouellette, Y. and Kidder, M. Functional analysis of gap junctions in ovarian granulosa cells: distinct role for connexin 43 in early stages of folliculogenesis. Am J Physiol Cell Physiol. 2003;**284**(4):880–887. DOI: 10.1152/ajpcell.00277.2002.

[85] Veitch, I., Gittens, E., Shao, Q., Laird, W. and Kidder, M. Selective assembly of connexin37 into heterocellular gap junctions at the oocyte/granulosa cell interface. J Cell Sci. 2004;**117**(13):2699–2707. DOI: 10.1242/jcs.01124.

[86] Gittens, E., Barr, J., Vanderhyden, C. and Kidder, M. Interplay between paracrine signaling and gap junctional communication in ovarian follicles. J Cell Sci. 2005;**118**(1):113–122. DOI: 10.1242/jcs.01587.

[87] Yogo, K., Ogawa. T., Akiyama, M., Ishida-Kitagawa, N., Sasada, H., Sato, E. and Takeya, T. PKA implicated in the phosphorylation of Cx43 induced by stimulation with FSH in rat granulosa cells. J Reprod Dev. 2006;**52**(3):321–328. DOI: 10.1677/JOE-06- 0076 PMID: 16474210.

[88] Borowczyk, E., Johnson, L., Bilski, J., Bilska, A., Redmer, A., Reynolds, P. and Grazul-Bilska, T. Role of gap junctions in regulation of progesterone secretion by ovine luteal cells in vitro. Reproduction. 2007;**133**(3):641–651. DOI: 10.1530/REP-06-0178.

[89] Gershon, E., Plaks, V. and Dekel, N. Gap junctions in the ovary: expression, localization and function. Mol Cell Endocrinol. 2008;**282**(1–2):18–25. DOI: 10.1016/j.mce.2007.11.001.

[90] Rhett, M., Jourdan, J. and Gourdie, G. Connexin 43 connexon to gap junction transition is regulated by zonula occludens-1. Mol Biol Cell. 2011;**22**(9):1516–1528. DOI: 10.1091/mbc.E10-06-0548.

[91] Lonergan, P., Rizos, D., Gutierrez-Adan, A., Moreira, M., Pintado, B., de la Fuente, J. and Boland, P. Temporal divergence in the pattern of messenger RNA expression in bovine embryos cultured from the zygote to blastocyst stage in vitro or in vivo. Biol Reprod. 2003;**69**:1424–1431. DOI: 10.1095/biolreprod.103.018168.

[92] Rizos, D., Gutierrez-Adan, A., Perez-Garnelo, S., De La Fuente, J. and Boland, L. P. Bovine embryo culture in the presence of serum: implication for blastocyst development, cryotolerance, and messenger RNA expression. Biol Reprod. 2003;**68**:236–243. DOI: 10.1095/biolreprod.102.007799.

[93] Hamatani, T., Yamada, M., Akutsu, H., Kuji, N., Mochimaru, Y., Takano, M., Toyoda, M., Miyado, K., Umezawa, A. and Yoshimura, Y. What can we learn from gene expression profiling of mouse oocytes?. Reproduction. 2008;**135**(5):581–592. DOI: 10.1530/REP-07-0430.

[94] Liang, P. and Pardee, B. Differential display of eukaryotic messenger RNA by means of the polymerase chain reaction. Science. 1992;**257**(5072):967–971. DOI: 10.1126/science.1354393.

Chapter 4

Cells: Segway for Genetically Desired Cattle through Embryotic Development Sequencings and Genetic Mapping

Marleen C. Dinis and Joaquim F. Moreira da Silva

Additional information is available at the end of the chapter

http://dx.doi.org/10.5772/65642

Abstract

Cells have a direct relation to understanding cattle genetic information aside from the cell's main role of housing genetic material. Gene presence being visible through phenotypic characteristics of living organisms allows for researchers to pinpoint specific genetic markers to access and evaluate the genetic information for desired visible traits. On a molecular level, through the interaction between cattle embryos and bovine cells, researchers can pair this information with current technological innovation to better understand on how genetics are manipulated naturally by environmental elements, which can have a direct effect on countries where cattle milk and meat production are the major contributors to economic stability. This overview of past, current, and potential future research involving cells can provide an understanding of the importance in cells and their relationship with biotechnology innovation. Through techniques involving cells and genetic analysis, various methods can be utilized to overcome limitations of cattle reproduction and increase the presence of desirable cattle traits, which in turn not only aid in the economic success of countries dependent on cattle products, but can also open the door to human therapeutics.

Keywords: genetics, cattle, cell, granulosa, embryo

1. Introduction

Since the age of primitive man and of the hunter-gatherer, cattle has been the source of nutrition, clothing, culture, and innovation of tools to improve man's existence. As seen in **Figure 1**, an early view of animals through the eyes of cave dwellers in prehistory time allows today's modern citizens to witness the existence of cattle (such as the ox) not only as a creatures of coexistence, but also as means of survival. As early as 8000 BC, the bovine species was domesticated as a means of a secure meat supply before becoming an essential object for clothes, tents, and even later becoming the main component in creating drums. Throughout history, cattles have been valuable not only as means of self-survival, but also played a major role in the art of agriculture and the conception of community. As the idea of growing food sources in one area (farming) grew more and more attainable the lifestyle of hunters and gathers phased into established communities with the help of cattle. The use of cattle as work tools for plowing fresh soil, as depicted in **Figure 2**, and the importance of manure for crop fertilization allowed the human race to settle and create civilized communities.

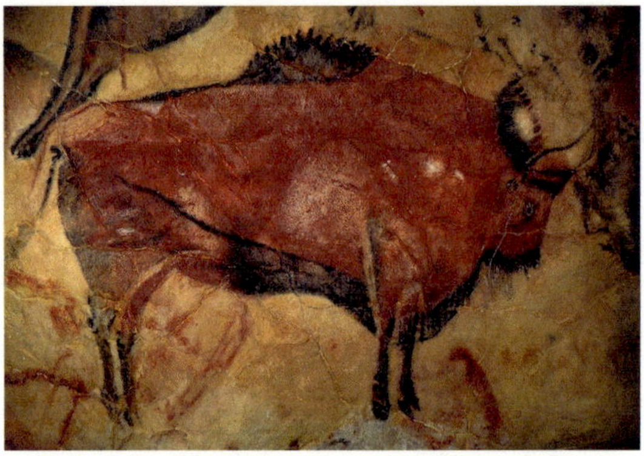

Figure 1. Untitled painting of ancient cave art. Retrieved from https://en.wikipedia.org/wiki/Bison_priscus.

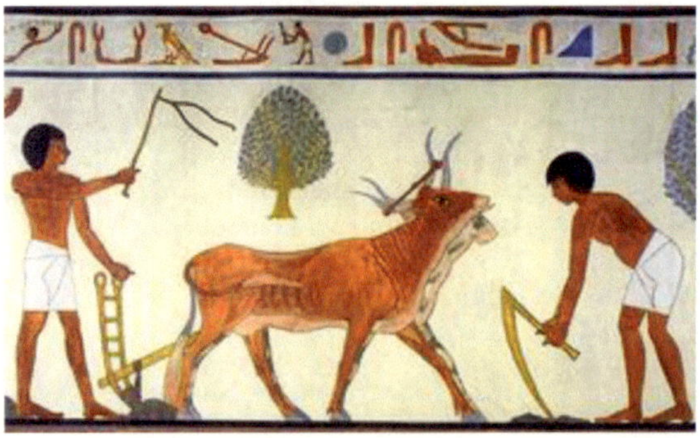

Figure 2. Untitled Egyptian art. Retrieved from https://ucfant3145f09-04.wikispaces.com/Ancient+Egyptian+Food+%26+Agriculture.

Today cattle remains a vital part in mankind's socio and economic progression through the same deliverables attained by their ancestors: food, clothing, and innovative tools. What worries the majority of cattle owners today is the pressure of supply and demand of meat and dairy products, which comes from sustaining high populations of cattle. Past and current techniques for increasing cattle population include nutritional management and health practices to maintain or increase cattle production. As technological advancements and understanding of cattle genetics progress, methods including cell activity, genetic practices, and bioinformatics tools have been utilized to increase a deeper understanding of the cattle genetics not only to increase livestock numbers, which increase the production of desirable cattle that yields high economic profit, but also open new opportunities for novel human therapeutics.

2. Breeding

One of the oldest methods for desirable cattle production involves breeding both close breeding and outbreeding (**Figure 3**). A popular and effective method of outbreeding, known as crossbreeding, involves breeding animals of pure breeds within each generation to produce desired animals. There are two main categories that fall under the crossbreeding umbrella: terminal- and rotational-crossing. Terminal-crossing is utilized more for meat animals and not dairy animals as it does not involve the progeny of breeding, but rather is slaughtered for commercialized meat. Whereas rotational-crossing involves the breeding of two breeds and utilizing the female offspring to breed with a sire of a different bred. The female offspring of this breeding sequence is introduced to one of the two breeds used in the original breeding scheme [1]. These techniques are particularly important when seeking heterosis. Heterosis is the improvement or enhancement of a specific trait that involves three types of improvement with respect to fertility: individual affecting the calf, maternal affecting the dam, and paternal affecting the sires. Individual heterosis increases live births and postnatal calf survival, while maternal increases conception rate, birth rates, and other economic traits such as milk product [2].

Close breeding
•Inbreeding
•Line breeding
Outbreeding
•Crossbreeding
•Outcrossing
•Backcrossing
•Topcrossing
•Granding up
•Mating likes
•Mating unlikes

Figure 3. Types of cattle breeding methods.

These techniques are important in producing genetically desirable cattle to improve economic stimulating traits, but novel techniques are being studied to further the progression and overcome variables in increasing cattle. As previously stated nutritional management has been a means of sustaining current cattle numbers, but what if the nutrition in itself becomes an issue of calf abortions and still borns? This is an issue that is not new to those who raise cattle in the archipelago of the Azores. The Azores are made up of nine volcano-derived islands centered in the Atlantic Ocean roughly 2454 km from the coast of the United States and 1600 km from Portugal [3]. Bovine population and production are a vital source of economic stability for the archipelago with products ranging from butter, milk, and cheese to meat supplies for commercial fast food chains. Unfortunately, the Azores face two debilitating periods within the year where animal product is limited due to lack of grass growth. Cattle owners are forced to supplement their cattle with a native invader plant as an alternative feed, of which contains *Pittosporum undulatum* [4]. The compound *Pittosporum undulatum* can have a negative effect on an animal's immune, endocrine, and reproductive system, thus becoming a problem with cattle production even though it is a means of sustaining the current cattle population. A recent study (2016) performed at the University of the Azores provided an in-depth understanding of how this compound can directly affect embryotic development through coculturing with bovine granulosa cells (**Figure 4**) [5].

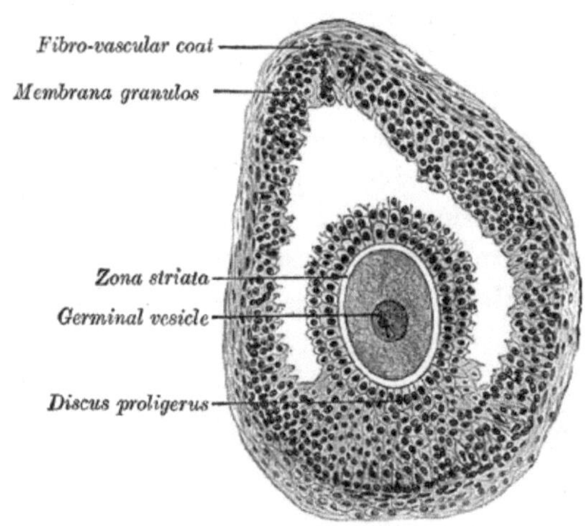

Figure 4. Depiction of ovarian follicle. The granulosa cells utilized in the previously discussed section of coculture utilized these cells that form the membrane granulose. Retrieved from: https://en.wikipedia.org/wiki/Ovarian_follicle#/media/File:Gray1164.png.

3. Coculturing

The idea behind coculturing cells with embryos allows for researchers to evaluate not only the progression of embryotic development, but also pinpoint interactions between the two entities to establish a better understanding of what cause and effects are taking place. Bovine granulosa

http://dx.doi.org/10.5772/65642

cells play a vital role in *in vitro* maturation (IVM) of coculture with oocytes as well as the development of embryos derived from *in vitro* fertilization (IVF) [6]. Granulosa cells express growth factor kit ligand (KL), which assist in follicular development and directly effects oocytes whenever gonadotropins, FSH- and LH-specific levels are present [7]. Through quantitative RT-PCR and specific primers one can analyze the gene expression level of KL. In the case involving *Pittosporum undulatum* previously mentioned, the study did not utilize RT-PCR, but rather relied on the expression of blocked embryo development. The idea behind the study at the University of the Azores stems from this hopeful possibility of understanding how and when embryotic development is affected when *Pittosporum undulatum* is present, which can have a relationship with KL production of the granulosa cells. The study showed that embryos cocultured with granulosa cells collected from cattle that were fed *Pittosporum undulatum* demonstrated higher embryo blocking when cocultured granulosa cells as opposed to the control group that were not exposed to the same feed (**Figures 5** and **6**).

Treatment	Nº of ovaries	No. of collected oocytes	No. of oocytes for maturation	Rate of		
				Maturation	Cleavage	Developed Embryo
Experimental	8	136	119	78.27±5.81[a]	29.92±4.31[a]	7.30±3.11[a]
Control	8	186	148	90.46±3.02[a]	41.86±5.58[b]	21.88±6.85[a]

Numbers in the same column with different letters (a, b) differ significantly at $P< 0.05$.

Data are expressed in percentage (%) as mean ± SEM, standard error of means.

% of developed embryos classified as morula, early blastocyst and blastocyst stages.

Figure 5. Rates of development embryonic *in vitro* of experimental and control groups.

3.1. Cells and transgenic techniques

Another interesting factor in applying cocultures with cells involves genetics directly by creating transgenic animals. A transgene is a genetic material that is naturally transferred from one organism to another through genetic engineering, which can change the genotype and phenotype of the transgenic organism. This process utilizes newly fertilized cells that are isolated and injected with specific DNA, the egg is then transferred into a host mother where it is able to develop into an embryo. Currently, a new method involves the removal of the nucleus from one egg and replaces with the nucleus of another cell; this is commonly known as nuclear transfer. This allows for complete transfer of genetic information of the donor cell into the recipient. Further yet the cells may be genetically modified with a laboratory before being transferred to the host. This type of cellular genetic transfer was conducted at the University of Georgia (Athens, Georgia) focused on the production of transgenic bovine embryos through a granulosa cell theater [8]. This allows for the development of genetically desirable cattle through selection of genetic enhancement which can increase specific phenotypes of economically pleasing cattle. The study conducted at the University of Georgia showed that bovine granulosa cells can transfect desirable genes *in vitro* without negatively affecting embryo viability; essentially bovine granulosa cells are potentially useful passage cells to establish nuclear transfer of gene cloning [8]. Transgenic animals can add an advantage to the human therapeutic industry by providing preclinical theatres for vaccine production and tissue growth for human use.

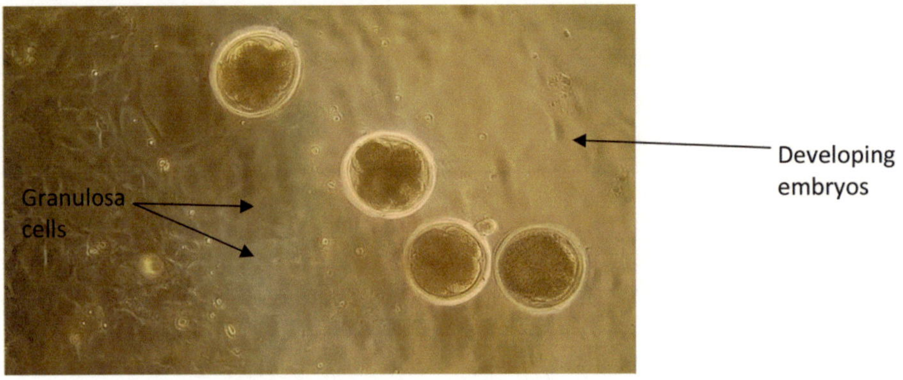

Figure 6. Picture of bovine granulosa cells utilized at the University of the Azores. Photograph taken by Dr. Helder Nunes at the University of the Azores.

3.2. Cells and cryopreservation advancement

Further evidence suggests that the use of various bovine cell lines can assist in the cryopreservation of bovine embryos. This becomes essential when one applies genetically desirable crossbreeding *in vitro* to create embryo offspring in numbers, especially with the current technique of offspring sex selection. Studies show that cell culture systems with bovine oviduct epithelium cells (BOECs) can be utilized *in vitro* to increase embryo robustness [9]. BOECs are comprised of ciliated and nonciliated (secretory) cells. The ciliated cells aid in moving the ovum away from the ovary and toward the uterus, while the nonciliated cells release secretions needed to lubricate, provide nourishment, and protection for traveling ovum. Furthermore, it has been proven that BOEC can have a direct effect on embryo development when present during the first 4 days or the last 4 days of development by accelerating blastocyst development [10]. Prior to cryopreservation the bovine oocytes are matured and fertilized *in vitro* in culture medium supplemented with serum, as its presence provides a beneficial environment, such as energy substrate, amino acids, vitamins, and growth factors. The serum has a biphasic effect on embryonic development, on the one hand by inhibiting the first division, and on the other, by encouraging the development of blastocysts [11]. Thus, the use of BOECs and its metabolic entities with bovine embryos in simple medium can aid in furthering the embryo environment into a rich maturation media. The use of BOECs in a culture system with embryos has not been exhausted and has not been studied in the comparison of "fresh" embryos and cryopreserved embryos. Second, according to Jang et al., it is highly recommended that BOECs be studied to investigate the specific mechanism of their actions with the development of embryos as well as provide a complete analysis of the somatic cell coculture system that supports high development rates *in vitro* as well as a potential increase in viability rates *in vivo* in both fresh and frozen embryos [12]. According to Schmaltz-Panneau et al., the mechanisms of BOECs have not been clearly clarified, but evidence shows that *in vitro* coculture of bovine embryos with BOECs can mimic the maternal environment which can improve the developmental quality of the embryo [15].

Previous studies suggest that tissue inhibitor of the enzyme metalloproteinase-1 produced in BOECs possess embryogenesis-stimulating activity, while another study demonstrated that BOECs contained luteinizing hormone (LH) receptors that are functional in increasing the synthesis of oviductal glycoprotein, which can increase the development of early embryos [13]. BOECs also control oxygen levels within the embryo environment, which is a vital factor is embryo success. To assist with embryo and maternal communication oviduct-secreted proteins (OSP) create a pathway for this communication as well as the maintenance of environment for successful embryo development [14]. There has been a progression in identifying many OSP, but two antioxidant enzymes seem to play a major part in continued embryo development: copper, zinc superoxide dismutase (Cu, Zn-SOD), and phospholipid hydroperoxide glutathione peroxidase (GPx-4) [14]. The metabolic exchange between SOD and GPx-4 maybe the explanation for the increase in the blastocyst rate of embryos when BOEC is present due to the gas regulation during development. BOECs also regulate the secretion of embryotrophic factors such as growth factors, component C3, oviduction, and osteopontin. The osteopontin protein is believed to have a direct effect on spermatozoa, oocytes, and embryos [15]. Osteopontin was first identified in the mineralized matrix of bovine bone, but it is also present in the testis and epididymis in males as well as within the female reproductive tissues including the oviduct. Further investigation of osteopontin determined that this protein is capable of enhancing bovine cleavage and blastocyst rates in culture [15]. This information sparks the question if a better genetic understanding of this occurrence is understood could researchers essentially pinpoint and modify this communication between embryo and its maternal surrounding (whether natural or synthetic) to aid in the fight against bovine miscarriages and to progress in successful postcryopreserved embryo development rates once they are introduced into carrying host. One way of using this information regarding cellular interaction is to understand the genetic phenomena that occur during specific phases of cellular expression. Another is to utilize this advancement in embryo cryopreservation in order bank transgenic embryos.

4. Genetic mapping

Improving genetic understanding and innovative techniques have long evolved since the first recorded line of breeding performed by Robert Bakewell and the first freezing of semen in 1949. In 2001, genomic selection and genetic mapping became a popular method in improving livestock genetics. Identifying and cloning genetically desirable traits can create a robust mapping of bovine genes. Genetic mapping is essential for researchers to identify where genes are located and how they function within cells and overall how it effects the phenotype of cattle. Genetic mapping of humans and cattle alike plays crucial roles in understanding chromosomal rearrangement through evolutionary progression. The understanding of cattle genome can shine a light on evolutionary changes but can also illuminate a path to pinpointing and selecting desirable and marketable phenotypes. Since it can be extremely costly to select specific desirable animals, it is beneficial to start the process as early as possible which makes embryo production of selective cattle not only more cost efficient, but also effective in ensuring that the trait is carried within the genetic information of the embryo.

4.1. Synteny mapping

A common approach to developing a genetic map is that of synteny mapping which utilized somatic cells. Synteny refers to two or more genomic regions within a set of chromosomes within a species that show evidence of deriving from one ancestral genomic region [16]. Synteny mapping consists of a method utilizing a generated list of well conserved genes, known as *syntentic blocks*, which are associated with the same chromosome for a specific species; whereas conserved synteny describes the location of homologous genes on the same chromosome, but for two different species [17]. Somatic cells are the primary component of synteny mapping, and they are living mammalian cells that are not gamete cells (i.e., ova and sperm cell) such as those that make up bones, organs, and blood cells. Theoretically, any gene product or sequence can be successfully mapped using the synteny method as long as the presence (or absence) of the gene of the species in question can be challenged against the fully retained rodent genomic background (through hybrid somatic cells) to confirm whether a concordance or discordance for the location of two genes is located on the same chromosome [17].

4.2. Bioinformatics and genomic selection targets

Today bioinformatics friendly programs such as BLAST are used to identify specific regions with similar genetic sequences for better understanding of characterizing organism and biological discoveries. Specific sites such as bovinegenome.org provide search and annotation tools to support bovine genome and those researchers seeking to expand bovine genetic mapping . Studies such as those conducted by Homer et al. touch upon genetic solutions to the increasing problem with milk production. Poor expression of estrus is considered to be a contributing factor to poor dairy cow fertility; by identifying where the genetic issue lies, Homer and his team believe that they can identify which cows display higher expressions of estrous, as well as identify the genetic issue associated with this lack of expression [18].

From a traditional standpoint, dairy cows are bred based on simple breeding selection, which primarily depends on the sire-side with the aid of worldwide semen distribution through artificial insemination. The use of genomic selection is used in dairy cattle to overcome limitation of traditional selection due to health and fertility problems. Genomic selection for dairy cattle owners becomes beneficial when comparing costs, reproduction, and generation cycles associated with traditional breeding using progeny testing. There are two ways one can use genetic selection for breeding: one way is by preselecting young bulls to test or the other option involves selecting the bull based on already available genomic information, thus the use of genetic selection for future dairy cow reproduction can have a major positive impact on the dairy industry [19]. As for beef, cattle selection of desired animals is based on the targeted market, and due to the large population of beef cattle and lower accuracy of beef cattle genetic markers, the idea of using genetic selection is not as desirable and economically pleasing as it is for dairy cows [20].

5. Conclusion

Conventional breeding involves hundreds of unidentified genes, which require continued advancement in modern molecular biology with gene mapping. By identifying and isolating specific genes to create transgenic animals, as well as with the aid of cells to advance the understanding of environmental influences and their ability to improve cryopreservation of genetically desired embryos. Through better understanding of cellular interaction and genetic traits, researchers seeking answers for issues regarding animal reproduction can ultimately find solutions to not only maintain stable offspring numbers, but also produce genetically desirable progenies.

As mentioned, new phenotype genetic selection along with easier transfer of genetics can answer the social demand of meat and dairy products through preferable phenotype production. In the future, the dairy and meat industry will be faced with higher populations and not enough cattle products to sustain the increasing populace, as such the need for faster reproduction cycles and robust dairy cows will be necessary to meet demands. Future researchers are urged to expand their knowledge of the cattle genetic map, which allows for a better understanding not only of possible genetic selection for breeding purposes, but also aids in understanding the human genome itself. This is especially true when focusing on reproduction, when considering both human female and a cow, the only difference between the two is the length of the estrus cycle. Further studies on genetic relation to estrous expression can not only aid cattle owners in effectively increasing cattle head but also can aid in human infertility-related research as well.

A future capability of cellular participation in innovation is endless. Here a very small number of potential uses of cells for genetic selection are briefly introduced. There are numerous uses of cells to expand our knowledge of veterinary genetics. Even though cells house the information that makes everything what it appears to be, research progression in biotechnology has opened a portal to understanding how these fragments of information function and (to an extent) how to manipulate them to better understand their capabilities in creating their natural end product. A global perspective cells are minuscule in size but hold an enormous amount of information and material for researchers to utilize the information for animal and human therapeutic innovation.

Acknowledgements

The authors would like to thank the University of the Azores for allowing me to be a scientific collaborator, specifically Professor Joaquim F. Moreira da Silva, PhD and Dr. Helder Patricio Barcelos Nunes for allowing me to help and for introducing us to the amazing capabilities of the granulosa cells.

Author details

Marleen C. Dinis* and Joaquim F. Moreira da Silva

*Address all correspondence to: marleencook@gmail.com

The University of the Azores, Angra do Heroismo, Azores, Portugal

References

[1] FAO. Chapter 6 Crossbreeding [Internet]. 1982 [Updated: 2016]. Available from: http://www.fao.org/docrep/004/X6536E/X6536E06.htm

[2] Greiner, S. Crossbreeding Beef Cattle [Internet]. May 1, 2009. Available from: https://pubs.ext.vt.edu/400/400-805/400-805.html

[3] Visit Azores. The Archipelago [Internet]. 2016. Available from: http://www.visitazores.com/en/the-azores/the-9-islands/the-archipelago/geography

[4] Nunes, H., Faheem, M., Dinis, M., Borba, A., da Silva, F.M. Effect of feed with Pittosporum undulatum in vivo on bovine progesterone levels and embryo produced in vitro. Canadian Journal of Animal Science. Forthcoming. DOI: CJAS2

[5] Nunes, H.P., Furnas, S., Dinis, M., Borba, A., Da Silva, F.M. Maturation, fertilisation and culture of bovine oocyte using chlorogenic acid in media. Animal Science. Forthcoming. DOI:

[6] Pinkert, C.A., editors. A Laboratory Handbook. 3rd ed. Waltham, MA: Elsevier; 2014; p. 696. DOI: 978-0-12-410490-7

[7] Parrot, J.A., Skinner, M.K. Thecal cell-granulosa cell interactions involved a positive feedback loop among keratinocyte growth factor, hepatocyte growth factor, and kit ligand during ovarian follicular development. Endocrinology. 1998;139(5):2240–2245.

[8] Sezen, A., Rzucidlo, S.J., Gibbons, J., Kazuchika, M., Stice, S.L. Production of transgenic bovine embryos by transfer of transfected granulosa cells into enucleated oocytes. Molecular Reproduction and Development. 2001;(60):20–26.

[9] Abe, H., Hoshi, H. Bovione oviductal epithelial cells: Their cell culture and applications in studies for reproductive biology. Cytotechnology. 1997;(23):171–183.

[10] Cordova, A., Perreau, C., Uzbekova, S., Ponsart, C., Locatelli, Y., Mermilloid, P. Development rate and gene expression of IVP bovine embryos cocultured with bovine oviduct epithelial cells at early or late state of preimplantation development. Theriogenology. 2014;(81):1163–1173.

[11] Jonge, C., Barratt, C., editors. Assisted Reproductive Technology. New York: Cambridge University Press; 2002. 435 p.

[12] Jang, H.Y., Jung, Y.S., Cheong, H.T., Kim, J.T., Park, C.K., Kong, H.S., et al. Effects of cell status of bovine oviduct epithelial cell (BOEC) on the development of bovine IVM/IVF embryos and gene expression in the BOEC used or not used for the embryo culture. Asian Australasian Journal of Animal Science. 2008;21(7):980–987.

[13] Ian Gordon. Laboratory Production of Cattle Embryos. 2nd ed. Cambridge, MA: CABI; 2003. 549 p.

[14] Mermillod, P., Schmaltz, B., Perreu, C., Tslkis, G., Martinot, E., Cordova, A., et al. Early development of ruminant embryos, autonomous process or the result of a positive dialog with surrounding maternal tissues. Acta Scientiae Veterinariae. 2010;38(2):521–533.

[15] Schmatz, B., Cordova, A., Dhorne, S., Hennequet, C., Uzbekova, S., Martinot, E., et al. Early bovine embryos regulate oviduct epithelial cell gene expression during in vitro co culture. Animal Reproduction Science. 2014;149:103–116.

[16] Cogepedia. Synteny [Internet]. July 24, 2014. Available from: https://genomevolution.org/wiki/index.php/Synteny

[17] Womack, J.E. The cattle gene map. ILAR Journal. 1998;39(2):153–159.

[18] Homer, E., Derecka, K., Webb, R., Garnswothy, P. Mutations in genes involved in oestrous cycle associated expression of oestrus. Animal Reproduction Science. 2013;142:106–112.

[19] Jonas, E., Koning, D. Genomic selection needs to be carefully assessed to meet specific requirements in livestock breeding program. Frontiers in Genetics. 2015;6(49):1–8.

[20] Johnston, D., Tier, B., Graser, H. Beef cattle breeding in Australia with genomics: opportunities and needs. Animal Production Science. 2012;52:100–106.

Section 3

Conservation and Basic Genetics

Chapter 5

Beyond Fifty Shades: The Genetics of Horse Colors

Adriana Pires Neves, Eduardo Brum Schwengber,
Fabiola Freire Albrecht, José Victor Isola and
Liana de Salles van der Linden

Additional information is available at the end of the chapter

http://dx.doi.org/10.5772/65848

Abstract

Since the dawn of horse domestication, coat colors have always fascinated humankind. In the last century, knowledge of genetics and development of scientific tools have become powerful enough so that the effects of many DNA mutations could be critically studied. Coat color nomenclature varies according to countries and breed associations; in addition, many factors can modify the color of the coat, such as sun exposure, age, sex, and nutritional status of the animal. Nevertheless, horses are capable of producing only two pigments. Several genes have been indicated as putative to coat color modification, altering the basic color by dilution, redistribution, or lacking of pigments.

Keywords: horse, genetics, coat color, alleles, DNA

1. Introduction

Nearly 6000 years ago, an extraordinary event would change the course of human history: the domestication of horse, which began in the region known today as Kazakhstan [1], in Central Asia. Initially looking for food and materials for making clothes and tools, the primitive man had also found an ally that would provide relatively fast transport, and later an important instrument of war, agriculture, and trade. Still later, this partnership would inaugurate a new concept in supportive therapy for people with special needs, limited physical abilities [2, 3], and scientific research.

The horse ancestor, *Hyracotherium* (also known as *Eohippus*), dates from the Eocene period [1] (about 55–35 million years BP=before present, for modern archaeologists) and lived in the northern hemisphere; the genus *Equus* appeared later in North America and migrated to Asia in the Pleistocene [1] (about 2.6–0.12 million years BP). It is believed that the wild coat color (more frequently from occurring in nature; "general rule") of the first horses was a light brown body (ranging from yellowish to light brown) with dark mane, tail, and limbs plus a dominant dilution called dun (characteristic marks and dilution of the body color); this phenotype apparently provided satisfactory camouflage against predators. At the end of the Pleistocene and early Holocene, appaloosa and black coats were already existent [4] in primitive herds.

Throughout horse's history, appearances of different phenotypes were promoted by genetic mutations. Such different phenotypes became more frequent when equine populations faced climatic and geological events of major proportions. For example, appearance of black horses at the beginning of Holocene in Europe (eastern and central regions) and Siberia could mean that there was a postice age migration and subsequent selection due to increasing foresting of areas. Reducing the space occupied by a given population would have led to departing from Hardy-Weinberg equilibrium (principle of gene balance) [5, 6] and the chances of mating between individuals carrying mutations increased, providing the birth of homozygotes for features that were previously not expressed in the phenotypes. But it was only with domestication, and later, when horse breeding was established in primitive societies (confinement of an equine population in smaller spaces with restricted matings; slaughter of undesirable individuals, as male offsprings and other stallions) that an explosion of new colors began. Black and chestnut horses became more frequent in the Copper Age, and it was not until 3000 years BP, at the beginning of the Bronze Age, that today's most widespread-diluted coats appeared [4].

It is also important to mention that at the time the horse was the main means of transport by land, different colors draw the attention of people holding some kind of power (political, financial, or religious) such that many understood that riding striking-looking animals would also represent the power those people possessed. As the Australian poet Pamela "Pam" Brown wrote:

"The horse is the projection of people's dreams about themselves—strong, powerful, beautiful, and it has the capability of giving us escape from our mundane existence."

Thus, kings, tribal chiefs, senior military ranked officers, noblemen, emperors, and the great conquerors were generally seen mounting horses of exquisite colors, which distinguished them from the common people. Those powerful ones usually rode stallions, and so it becomes easy to understand the spread of these mutations in relatively reduced timespan: a mare produces, even considering the advances in reproductive biotechnologies of today, much less offspring per year than a single stallion can produce by the same time.

Nowadays, various breeds are known to have impressive looking animals (although aiming a performancer), either through changes in the hair structure (such as the magnificent metallic sheen of the Akhal-Teke or the curly hairs of the Curly breed), or through different meshes and patches scattered over the horse's body. Usually, the colors with greater visual appealing are those originating from the combination of several mutations that lead to the localized

http://dx.doi.org/10.5772/65848

absence of pigment producing cells, contrasting with areas of intense and darker colors. Some of these mutations deliver somewhat unpredictable effects but still have great visual appeal.

2. Basic concepts

Since the dawn of horse domestication, coat colors have always fascinated mankind. However, it was not before a century ago that the knowledge of genetics and the development of scientific tools have become powerful enough so that major changes could be identified and their effects better understood.

Much of the confusion arising when the purpose is naming a coat color refers to the fact that not always this classification is in accordance with the genetic origin of the color or colors in question. For example, a very dark stallion mistakenly registered as dark brown, could be, in fact, a very dark chestnut. Another extreme example would be the presumed occurrence of a third allele at the Extension locus (other candidate locus might be the beta defensin locus [7]), relatively rare, called dominant black (represented as E^D) [8]; considering expression of only Extension and Agouti loci, such allele, when present, would determine an entirely black phenotype, regardless of the existence of the dominant allele agouti (A^A) on the ASIP locus (which encodes a bay phenotype in eumelanic horses). The important information about dominant black here is, no matter the intensity of the black (some could display even a near-black brown) color on a dominant black horse, it completely overrules the ASIP locus expression.

Another example would be the genetic difference between roaned (sparse white hairs intermingled with the basic color) and the true roan (sparse white hairs intermingled with the basic color, while maintaining solid mane, tail, limbs, and head): While no specific locus (or loci) has yet been determined for the roaned trait—in fact, it may even be not an inheritable characteristic [9]—the true or genetic roan is clearly documented as a dominant mutation in the KIT (KIT^R) [10] gene.

Additional difficulties on identification arise when considering:

Different classifications according to each breed standard. Different nomenclatures for the same coat color are not rare, depending on different countries, or regions within the same country. For example *alazão sopa de leite* (Southeastern Brazil), *baio ruano* (Southern Brazil, Uruguay, Argentina, and other Spanish-speaking countries), and *palomino* (USA and other English-speaking countries) are different names standing for the same genotype, which in time codes for a yellowish coat color with lighter mane and tail.

Subjective perception of a particular shade—for example, mahogany bay, dark bay, light bay, blood chestnut, liver chestnut, chocolate palomino, and jet black.

In fact, for some colors the expression of many genes plus external influences and individual factors (such as animal's age, time of year, insolation, and nutritional status) can make it somewhat difficult to identify a horse's color. A classic example is a black horse kept outdoors all summer long, which causes a "fading" effect on coat color, making it easily confounded with a dark brown horse to the eyes of an unaware observer.

To really understand the genetic basis of coat color in horses, it is necessary to first understand some basic precepts. Because of empirical observations and secular traditions, it is not always easy to accept some of these key concepts:

Even though a wide range of nuances are noticeable in coat colors, and even considering the different classifications according to racial standards and individual assessments, the melanocytes of the horses are able to produce only two types of pigments [11]: eumelanin (black pigment) and pheomelanin (reddish pigment). Melanocytes are cells with dendritic extensions, originated from the embryonic neural crest and in which melanogenesis takes place in specialized organelles called melanosomes [12]. From these two pigments and the influence of several other genes [13], all variations of colors observed in the horse coat color are produced. For melanogenesis to happen, specific enzymes are required in melanocytes, being tyrosinase the one responsible for the initial step in the melanogenesis process, converting the amino acid tyrosine into a compound called dopaquinone [11].

The important matter herein is the definition of "points" of a horse. These mean manes, tail, and lower part of limbs and to some scholars, the inner line of the ear. For the identification of coat color it is very important to understand the concept of "points," as this is the first step to identify the color genetics: horses may have black points or points of the same color of the rest of the body (in some cases there can be variation on shade, though the color is the same), in the case of a nonblack horse. By points of the same body color we mean they are usually yellowish or reddish, but may also be dark brown (if the horse is brown). Knowing the horse's points color will provide the differentiation between horses producing eumelanin (black, dark pigment) from those producing only pheomelanin (reddish pigment). That is, horses with black points, independent of the rest of the body color, have at least one dominant allele at the Extension locus: E^E. Animals with points of the same color as the rest of the body (except in cases of entirely white horses) have a double dose (homozygous) of the recessive allele at the Extension locus: E^eE^e, meaning it is impossible to them to produce the black pigment eumelanin [14, 15].

The white in the coat of a horse is always superimposed on the basic coat color. The horses are primarily colored, being capable of producing pigment all over the body, and any and every white in the equine species is derived from a genetic directive that prevents color development due to the absence of melanocytes in that part of the body [16], and not to the lack of pigment production by melanocytes. Whether it is the meshes of a tobiano, or the entirely white body of an extensive expression of a white spotted, this means that in these areas there are no melanocytes. The same goes for the common white marking seen on the face and lower portion of horse's limbs (e.g., markings commonly found on the head as "star," "stripe," and on the limbs as "socks"). Such common marking is also due to the absence of melanocytes in the white hairs regions and has polygenic origin influenced by other random factors [13].

Once understood these fundamental concepts, one may proceed to the study of the genetic basis of the several coat colors.

http://dx.doi.org/10.5772/65848

3. The three basic colors

Three basic colors, built from the two pigments produced by horses, are derived from the interaction of two genes: melanocortin-1 receptor (MC1R) and agouti signaling protein (ASIP) [14]. These colors are *bay, black,* and *chestnut*. The influence of other genes (for example, dilution genes) determines the variations of each of the three basic colors [13].

-MC1R gene: The dominant allele (E^E) determines the production of eumelanin; the recessive allele (E^e) determines the production of pheomelanin. The MC1R gene encodes the production of a protein called melanocortin-1 receptor, which plays a pivotal role in the pigment production process. This receptor is located on the surface of melanocytes. When activated by melanocyte stimulating hormone (MSH), it triggers a series of chemical reactions within the melanocytes, leading to production of eumelanin. In fact, melanocytes are capable of producing both eumelanin and pheomelanin, but when the animal has the E^eE^e genotype, what happens is that the receptor is defective, making it unable to properly transmit the information passed by MSH, thus leading to production of pheomelanin only. The net result of the forms of this gene is therefore an animal with a black coat when there is at least one dominant allele (E^EE^E or E^EE^e), or a *chestnut* horse (reddish color) when homozygous to the recessive allele (E^eE^e). The recessive allele (E^e) is a mutation of the wild form (E^E), which occurred about 7000 years BP [1].

-ASIP gene: the dominant allele (A^A) encodes production of a protein called agouti signaling protein—hence the gene's name—which has the ability to block the melanocortin receptor 1 in existing melanocytes in the body (but not in the points) of the horse. When the receptor is blocked, there is no stimulus for the production of eumelanin (as explained above), and only pheomelanin synthesis occurs. Therefore, an eumelanic horse (E^EE^-) with a dominant allele at the Agouti locus (A^AA^-) yields a *bay* horse—a horse with a reddish to brownish body color and black points. About 8000 years BP [1], a recessive mutation occurred in the ASIP locus, yielding black color throughout the entire body of the horse. For this to happen; however, two doses (homozygosity) of the recessive allele are required: A^aA^a. An interesting fact is that the agouti signaling protein is effective only in eumelanin-producers horses (i.e., whose genotype is E^EE^E or E^EE^e). As in *chestnuts* (whose genotype is E^eE^e) melanocortin-1 receptor is defective, the protein has no effect.

As a net result of the interaction of MC1R and ASIP genes, we have:

Genotype E^EE^- A^aA^a = *black* horse. It is a very common color in the Percheron breed, and valued when having white markings in some other breeds. Some breeds, such as Friesian admit only black animals. Note that a superscript dash character (-) along with the locus letter (as in E^E E^-) does not mean "negative," this dash means that the allele occupying that locus is unimportant to the phenotype.

Genotype E^EE^- A^AA^- = *bay* horse, comprising all its variants regarding shades: *Light bay, dark bay, blood bay, mahogany bay,* etc.; in South American countries, a bright red bay is called *colorado;* a faded shade of colorado is called *douradilho*. There are two more alleles (so far) possible to exist at this locus: A^+ for *wild bay* (a bay where black on the limbs is restricted to the region below the fetlocks) and A^t, which would be responsible for the near black coat color with conspicuous lighter regions. These lighter areas are tan or reddish, and should not be confused with the mealy modifier (Pa^+), a dominant trait that affects all the basic coats, causing paler areas around the eyes, muzzle, distal part of limbs, and underside the body. In Latin America countries, this variant is known as *zaino* (causing many mistakes by the time of breed registry); in English-speaking countries they are called *seal browns*.

Genotypes E^eE^e A^AA^- *or* E^eE^e A^aA^a = *chestnut* horse. This means that *bay* is, in fact, hypostatic to *chestnut*, that is, the dominant allele in the locus Agouti (A^A) is masked by the homocigosis of the recessive allele in the Extension locus (E^eE^e). In other words, E^eE^e results in chestnut horses regardless that alleles are present in the ASIP locus.

Although recessive homozygous alleles at the MC1R locus encode always pheomelanic animals, each country (and regions within the same country) has its own designation based solely on phenotypic shade of red in the coat. For example, in Spanish and Portuguese-speaking countries, there is the *alazán, tostado,* and *ruano,* each one becoming even more detailed when more variants are perceived on the basic shade. Examples: *Tostado negro, tostado requeimado, alazán sangre,* and *alazán tostado*. In some English-speaking countries, the term *chestnut* defines a darker red horse, while *sorrel* would be a lighter colored red horse. Some breed associations, such as the American Quarter Horse Association (AQHA) use this distinction as a rule. Some breeds, namely the Suffolk Punch and the Haflinger admit only chestnut or sorrel animals.

As for breeders of draft horses, *sorrel* would be applied to a chestnut horse carrying the mealy modifier.

Once determined which pigment(s) is (are) produced by the horse and understood the relationship between all possible alleles in genes MC1R and ASIP, it is possible to understand the effects that other alleles, at other loci, yield over the three basic colors.

4. Diluted colors

Occur when proteins encoded by specific genes alter amount of pigment or deposition of pigment in receiver structures (keratinocytes and hairs). The effect is a dilution in the intensity of the original color.

4.1. Dun

(*gateado,* in Latin American countries): This is perhaps the oldest dilution, better known by the so-called *primitive marks.* It is believed that it was present in the primitive herds, being an effective camouflage against predators (**Figures 1** and **2**). Thus, the genotype notation would be the wild-type D^+ D^-. It is a consistent coat color in the Tarpan (*Equus ferus ferus*), Przewalski (*Equus przewalski*), and breeds like Konik (only *grullos,* black animals with the dun dilution), Sorraia, Fjord, and Dülmen.

The first mutation encoding a nondun phenotype occurred about 45,000 years BP, that is, predating domestication of horse. This phenotype retains the primitive marks, though a little lighter than the wild type. Evidences suggest a second nondun mutation originating from a chromosome

http://dx.doi.org/10.5772/65848

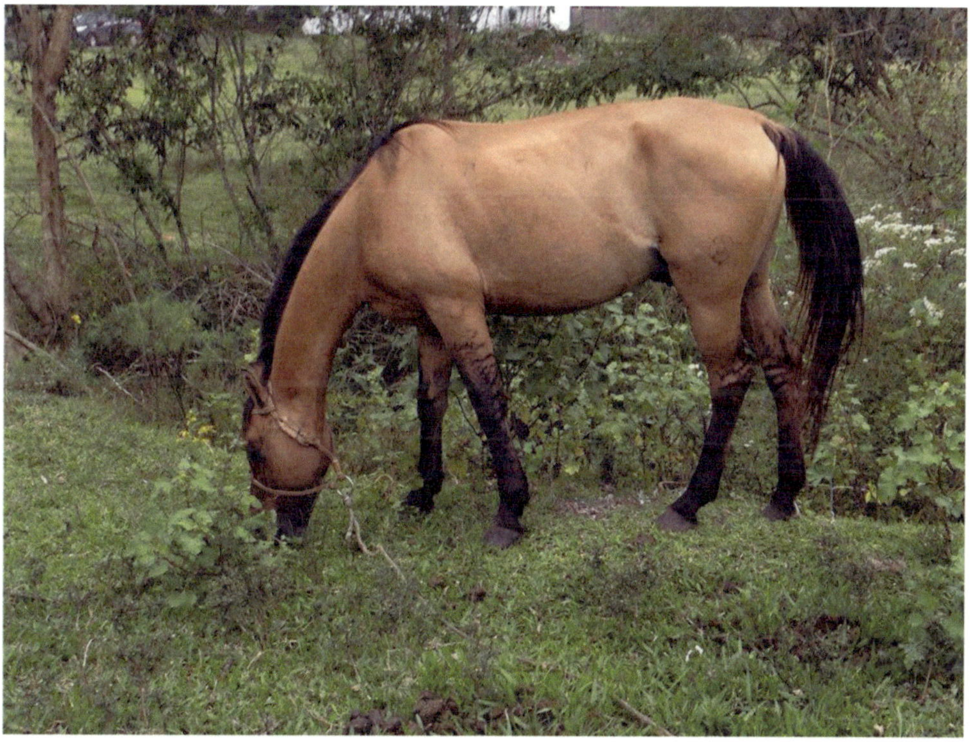

Figure 1. Dun (gateado, in Latin American countries): the oldest dilution factor.

carrying the first nondun mutation and that would have happened only a few thousand years ago; this is consistent with selection to colors with no camouflage at the time of domestication [17]. The dun effect over the basic colors—no matter how many dominant alleles are present—is a dilution of body color but not of head and points color, and the primitive marks, being the *dorsal stripe* the more consistent and best observed one. Primitive marks vary in extent and intensity. They are called so because are displayed in breeds considered primitive, though not limited to. They consist in darkening of coat on some body parts, forming recognizable patterns:

- *Cob webbing*: These are thin darker stripes on the horse's front. It has radial orientation, hence the name *cob webbing* or *spider webbing*. It is not visible in all duns, being more visible in *grullos* (black animal carrying the dun dilution).
- *Shoulder stripe*: A shadow or stripe of darker hairs running distally from (and over) the withers. It may vary in color intensity, shape, and extent.
- *Zebra stripes, stripped legs* or *leg bars*: Horizontal stripes appearing on the carpi and hocks, varying in number and color intensity. These are not always seen. In *grullos* they are usually black or very dark colored.
- *Dorsal stripe*: This is the most common mark on the dun dilution carriers. If a horse lacks the dorsal stripe, then it does not have the dun factor. It is a dark stripe clearly distinct from the rest of the coat, extending from the poll to the dock of the tail on the

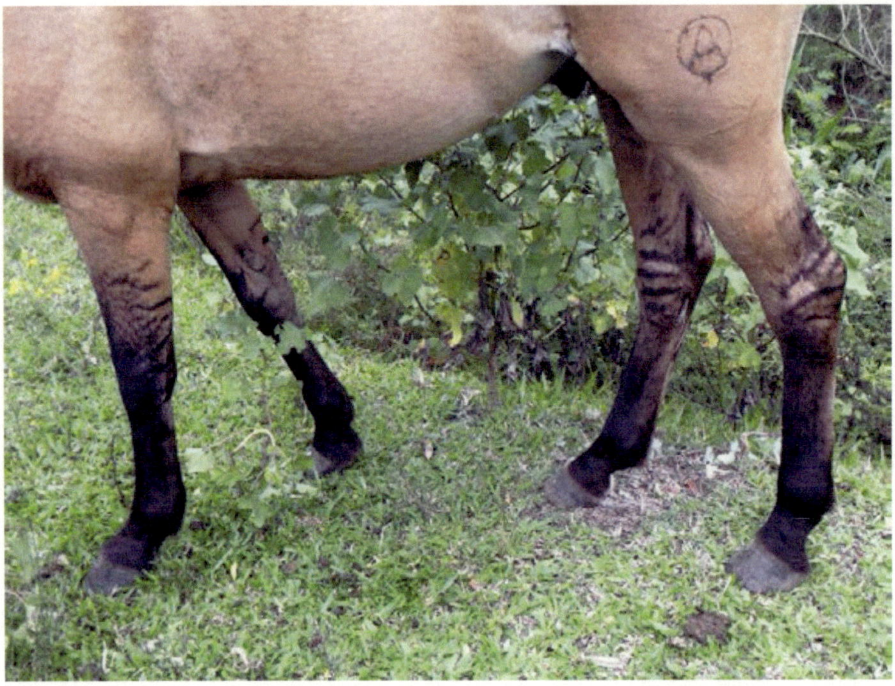

Figure 2. Dun markings as zebra and shoulder stripes are shown in more detail. *Source 1 and 2*: Mr. Jose Victor Isola.

dorsal line. Some horses not carrying the dun dilution may display a dorsal stripe, though this is less clear and lighter, and often subject of controversy. Whether this type of dorsal stripe is due to the first of mutations in wild-type allele [17], remains to be cleared by future researches.

- *Facial mask*: It is the undiluted color on the head coat. It varies in size, from a small band over the bridge of the nose or forehead to an entire undiluted head coat.

- *Guard hairs* (sometimes called *frosting*) are lighter colored hairs growing on the edges of the mane and at the tail base. A good example is the Fjord breed. Despite having different characteristics, care should be taken to not confuse guard hairs with those found on the tails of *roans* (genetic roans or not) and *rabicanos*.

There are some primitive marks that are not observed in all horses carrying dun, or slightly observed, or observed only during the first months of life. Such marks are not characteristic nor they attest the presence of the dun factor by themselves; often they are not even present in all duns. These appear as:

- *Dark bands* perpendicular to the dorsal stripe (barbs off the dorsal stripe) that may extend variably toward the ribs;

- *Shading on the neck (neck shadow)*, which can vary from a well-defined mark to only a shadowing;

http://dx.doi.org/10.5772/65848

- Small dark marks (roughly the size of a pea) called *mottling*, on the stifle, legs, shoulders, and arms;
- *Dark bars on the ears*, occurring below a dark tip of the ears (upper third of the ear, caudal view), which are observed in most duns;
- *Zippers*, a thin longitudinal line of lighter hairs along the shins;
- *Bider marks*—a dark band or shadowing varying in shape and extent on the shoulder, identified so far only in some horses from Mongolia [18].

The nomenclature question when it comes to dun dilution colors, is somewhat complex due to different countries and breed registries where it is permitted. In Latin America countries these animals are called *gateados* preceded or succeeded by a term that identifies the underlying coat. In North America they are called *linebacked duns*, a clear reference to the typical dorsal stripe of the dun dilution. A wide range of terms is assigned to the various nuances caused by dun on basic coats and other dilutions. Interestingly, often two or more nuances, despite having different names, actually have the same genetic signature.

Until a few years ago, the gene responsible for the phenotype dun was unknown; it was known only about its autosomal mode of inheritance and complete dominance. Thus, it has been represented by the capital letter D, and the possible alleles as + (wild) and nd (mutant allele, not dun); with the recent release of the locus responsible for dun dilution, and possibly new genetic tests that will determine the type of mutation (nd1 or nd2) [17], this notation might be amended.

The net effects of dun on the basic coats are as follows:

- *Genotype* E^EE^- A^aA^a D^+D^- That means a *black* horse with dun dilution becomes a *grullo* (female: *grulla*). *Grullos* are animals of yellow-grayish coat and black points and head. Like all carriers of this dilution, the primitive markings are present. In Latin countries they are called *lobuno*, a clear allusion to the wolf color ("lobo" is the Spanish and Portuguese word for wolf). This is one of the most susceptible to seasonal variations phenotypes: During winter months, when the coat is denser with longer hairs, the body presents an almost uniform and lighter cream color compared to summer months when the color can come to a grayish color similar to a mouse color. Obviously, cream and gray tones vary individually according to other genes in action, as well as the factors already mentioned, such as nutritional status and age. Thus, the lighter shades of this variant in North America are designated *silvery grullo*, *olive dun*, or *slate grullo*; the darker shades are called *wolf dun*.
- *Genotype* E^EE^- A^AA^- D^+D^- This is a *bay* with dun dilution: In Latin America countries, it is called *gateado*; in North America nomenclature varies greatly, richly describing the intensity of the underlying color. Thus we have the *golden duns* and *silvery duns* (dun on *light bay*), *zebra dun* (dun on *medium bay*), *dark dun* (dun on *dark bay*), and *coyote dun* (dun on *sooty bay*); *dusty dun* (dun on lighter shades of *seal brown*), *shaded mealy grullo* (dun on intermediate shades of *seal brown*—note that *mealy* and *grullo* here are solely

phenotypic definitions, that hold no genetic match with the real (genetic) *mealy* and *grullo*), *shaded wolf dun* (dun on darker shades or sooty variant of *seal brown*). Sooty is the presence of very dark hairs spread over the coat, especially on the dorsal region. Many theories offer explanations for its origin and genetic mechanisms, but none has yet been adequately proven.

- *Genotype* E^eE^e A^-A^- D^+D^- *Chestnut* carrying dun: In Latin America countries it is called *gateado ruivo* (something like "auburn dun" or "ginger dun"). In North America, the dun on lighter *chestnuts* (and *sorrels*) is called *apricot dun* or *sooty apricot dun* (for sooty variant of *sorrel*), while dun on *tostado* (*chestnut*) ranges from *apricot dun* or *claybank dun* (lighter shades) to *red dun* for intermediary and sooty shades of *chestnut*.

4.2. Cream

Another widespread dilution; results from a dominant mutation in the membrane-associated transporter protein gene (MATP) [19]. The effect over the coat color depends on the allelic zygosity—what is called *incomplete dominance*. It means that homozygosity or heterozygosity of the dominant allele affect differently the phenotype. In the case of cream dilution, it happens that homozygosity of the dominant allele affects the phenotype more aggressively than heterozygosity. The MATP gene is represented by the C letter by convention; this comes from a time when it was thought that a "C" gene (with "C" standing for "color") was responsible for the color over the body, so that double-diluted cream horses lacked the "color gene" and were regarded as albinos. Obviously, the cream dilution had not yet been postulated at that time. Additionally, there are different effects of the cream dilution over feomelanic and eumelanic horses. Thus, the genotype $C^{Cr}C$ acting over pheomelanin will produce cream-colored hairs, varying from a very light cream color to a dark caramel, while genotype $C^{Cr}C^{Cr}$ will dilute hairs color to an off-white shade and will dilute also the skin color (which will become pinkish); the eyes will have a bluish color. On the other hand, the genotype $C^{Cr}C$ will have little (if much) effect over eumelanin (*black* horses with one copy of the mutated allele may display a faded black color or, in some cases, a very dark brown color), while homozygosity will produce a horse with off-white-colored hairs, pinkish skin, and bluish eyes. Therefore, we have the following net effect of cream dilution on the basic colors:

- One gene cream on *chestnut* = *Palomino*, a valued coat color especially when the body holds a golden sheen. The body is yellowish ranging from pale yellow/cream to dark caramel. Palominos can vary in shade, though manes and tails are usually lighter like the horse in the picture. The genetic representation is as follows:

  E^eE^e A^-A^- $C^{Cr}C$ Note that when the Extension locus presents both recessive alleles, any combination of alleles at the Agouti locus (A) will not produce any effect on the phenotype: *Chestnut* horses can only produce pheomelanin.

- Two genes cream on *chestnut* = *Cremello* (*cremello* is the definition given to the horse with very pale cream coat color, pink skin, and blue eyes). These animals usually have

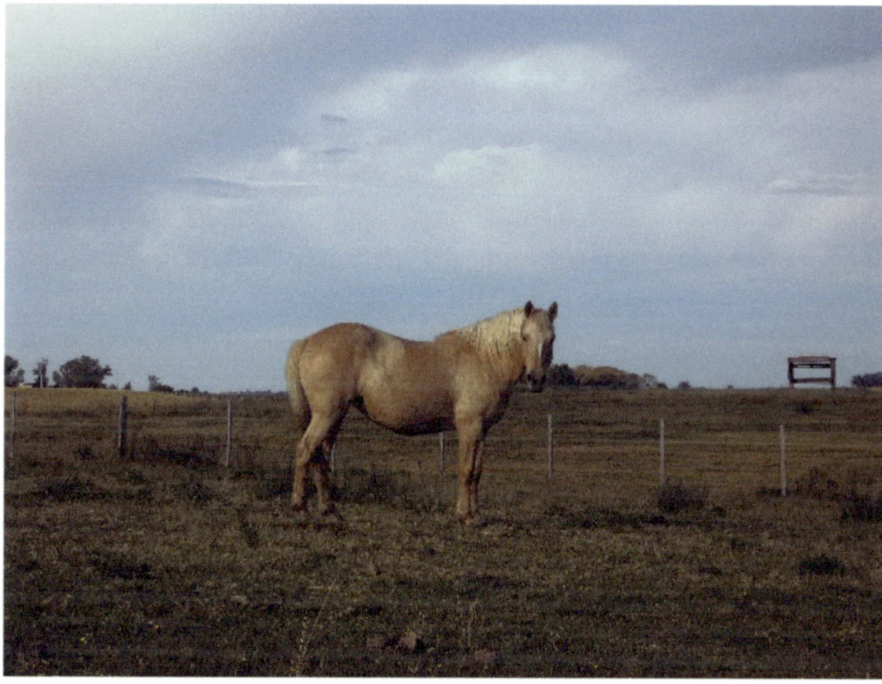

Figure 3. Palominos may vary in shade from a very light cream color like the horse in the picture. *Source*: Mrs. Albrecht.

eye and skin problems when not protected from continuous sun exposure (**Figure 3**). These horses are called *salgo* (because of the light-colored eyes) or *melado* in Spanish and Portuguese-speaking countries. The genetic representation is:

$E^eE^e\ A^-A^-\ C^{Cr}C^{Cr}$ Again, any combinations of alleles in the Agouti locus do not produce any effect on the phenotype, because E^eE^e horses are capable of producing only pheomelanin.

- One gene cream on *black* = *Smoky Black* (the coat color is usually faded black). In some Brazilian regions it is called *preto macaco*. The genetic representation is:

  $E^EE^-\ A^aA^a\ C^{Cr}C$ Note that in the Extension locus, only one of the alleles must be dominant to produce eumelanin. For the horse to display a black coat over the entire body (i.e., with melanocortin-1 receptors present and responsive to MSH in all melanocytes), it is necessary homozygosity of the mutant allele at the Agouti locus.

- Two genes cream on *black* = *Smoky Cream*, a very pale cream coat, with pinkish skin, and blue eyes; however, usually some areas still retain dark pigment—seen like dark hairs scattered over the entire body. The genetic representation is:

  $E^EE^-\ A^aA^a\ C^{Cr}C^{Cr}$ Note that, at the Extension locus, only one dominant allele is needed to produce eumelanin.

- One gene cream on *bay* = *Buckskin* is the name of the animal with black points and yellowish body, ranging from light cream to dark caramel. In Spanish and Portuguese-speaking countries it is called *baio*. The genetic representation is:

  $E^E E^-$ $A^A A^-$ $C^{Cr} C$ Note that, at the Extension locus, only one dominant allele is needed to produce the agouti signaling protein.

- Two genes cream on *bay* = *Perlino* (very pale cream coat with pinkish skin and blue eyes; some areas still retain dark pigment, mainly on the points. Also called melado and salgo in Spanish/Portuguese-speaking countries. The genetic representation is:

  $E^E E^-$ $A^A A^-$ $C^{Cr} C^{Cr}$ In Extension and Agouti loci, it is necessary only one dominant allele to produce eumelanin and agouti signaling protein, respectively.

Cream-diluted coats are highly valued by some breed associations, for example, the American Cream Draft Horse.

Because dun and cream loci operate separately, it is possible for a horse to carry both dilutions. In this case, the colors become even more diluted and an identification based solely on the visual aspect becomes more difficult and prone to mistakes.

4.3. Silver or silver dapple

It is a mutation at PMEL17 gene [20] (premelanosomal protein 17), which encodes a transmembrane protein involved in melanosomal production of eumelanin. The mutation produces a defective protein, causing a dilution effect on that pigment. Hence, the black color is diluted to shades of sepia or chocolate (called *silver chocolate* in some locations; in Australia it is known by *taffy*) and the manes, tails, eyelashes, and tactile hairs of face and muzzle show a grayish to whitish, sometimes silvered color. Limbs can be either whitish or near black colored. Usually the coat is dappled, and the more heavily dappled, the more valued it is. It is a dominant trait represented as Z^Z; the recessive allele (wild, normal, and nonsilver) is represented by Z^+. The variants are named according to the intensity of dilution; so we have the *blue silvers, black silvers, silvers chocolate, and silver dapples*. In the case of bay horses carrying the silver dilution, only eumelanic regions are affected, and so they are called *red* or *bay silvers* (in Rocky Mountain Horse breed, these are called *red chocolate*). It is a highly valued coat in some countries and quite common in breeds such as the Rocky Mountain Horse, Mountain Pleasure Horse, Kentucky Mountain Saddle Horse, and the Icelandic breed. It also appears in Quarter Horses, Morgans, and Miniatures. In horses homozygous for the condition it has been observed different combinations of symptoms affecting the anterior and posterior segments of the eye; such condition is known as multiple congenital ocular abnormalities (MCOA) [21–23].

In the same way, the cream and dun dilutions can act together, so when Z^Z Z^- occurs on a diluted coat color (by any other diluting gene) the degree of difficulty of color identification increases, and cases of mistaken registration due to several concurrent dilutions are not rare. For example, a *silver buckskins* can be easily confused with a *Palomino* due to the golden color of the body and pale points; *silver buckskins* usually have lighter skin, which can make them superficially similar to some *champagnes* (another dilution).

4.4. Champagne

A dominant mutation in the SLC36A1 gene (Solute Carrier 36 family A1) showing complete dominance [24]. It causes dilution of coat color, sometimes giving it a metallic sheen; it also makes the skin to dilute to a light brown color (with many small and darker splotches like freckles) and amber eyes. The dilution is represented as Ch^{Ch} (mutant allele) and Ch^{+} stands for the wild-type allele, nonchampagne. The net effect on the basic coat colors completely changes the original names. Sometimes very clear *champagnes* are confused with some cream-related coats colors due to a very light shade presented in some variants; however, the striking characteristics of skin and eyes colors should avoid confusion. Champagne dilution causes dilution of the coat color ranging from a very light yellowish to a light chocolate shade with varying points colors. The genetic representations are:

$E^{E}E^{-}$ $A^{a}A^{a}$ $Ch^{Ch}Ch^{+}$ it is called *classic champagne*. The color varies from dark beige to light chocolate, with points slightly darker than body.

$E^{E}E^{-}$ $A^{A}A^{-}$ $Ch^{Ch}Ch^{+}$ Champagne on a *bay* coat. It is called *amber champagne*. The body color is light tan brown or light yellowish brown and the points are usually light chocolate colored. Champagne on a *seal brown* coat ($E^{e}E^{e}$ $A^{t}A^{t/a}$ $C^{Ch}C^{+}$) or on darker shades of *bay* is called *sable champagne*.

$E^{e}E^{e}$ $A^{-}A^{-}$ $Ch^{Ch}Ch^{+}$ This is a *gold champagne*, often confused with *palominos* due to the golden glisten and lighter color. The combination of champagne with a cream allele causes an even lighter color, with greenish blue eyes with a hint of amber—these horses are called *ivory champagnes*.

4.5. Other dilutions

There are other dilutions found hitherto in some breeds (some not yet fully characterized from a genetic point of view). Examples are the *pearls* (dilution similar to champagne), *mushrooms* (dilution similar to silver, though it affects pheomelanin instead of eumelanin; so far found only in Miniatures). Some of these alleged dilutions/mutations have not yet been critically studied on a scientific basis. A dilution known as the lavender foal syndrome occurs in the Arabian breed and is due to a defective Myosin Va protein, coded by a recessive mutation in the gene MYO5A [25], causing severe neurological disorders and very light reddish, almost lilac hairs and skin in the neonate. These and other dilutions are an interesting and extensive subject, which could easily be the subject of an entire chapter.

5. Coat color modifiers

These genes impose areas of different colors on the basic coat color, modifying the original aspect.

5.1. Pangaré or mealy

This is a modifier whose genetic origin is unclear. It makes some areas paler than the rest of the body. These are around the eyes, muzzle, underside the body, flanks, and inner part of limbs [13]. The name pangaré derives from the observation made in horses of Spanish-speaking countries, and is translated into English as mealy. Apparently it is a dominant trait and is considered a wild trait, i.e., likely to be present in the original color of primitive horses. It is represented by the notation Pa^{+}, with the recessive mutation represented by Pa^{np} (standing for nonpangaré). It affects all coat colors, with its most dramatic effect seen on the *sorrel* coat color. Generally mealy *chestnuts* or *sorrels* (in Spanish and Portuguese, only *pangaré*) present a mane very lighter than the rest of the coat. The body color becomes slightly lighter, although pangaré is not considered a dilution factor. In *black* horses, it renders the coat to a slightly lighter or brownish color, easily leading to confusion with the *seal brown* color; it differs from the *seal brown* primarily due to the shade of the light areas: while in *seal brown* the lighter areas are tan and less extensive, in the *pangaré* those areas are more extensive and pale.

5.2. Rabicano

Its mechanism of action and genetic control are still unknown [13]. It causes the appearance of white hairs scattered on the coat over the rib cage (indeed following the direction of the bones), flanks, and tail base. It varies in intensity of expression and may appear as only a few white hairs on the base of the tail and sides of the rib cage, to a large amount of white hairs over these regions, in this case being easily confused with roaned or a true roan.

5.3. Flaxen

It is a recessive trait with variable expression; when homozygous determines a lighter shade (than the body) of the manes and tails (**Figure 4**). Acts only on chestnuts and sorrels. Its mechanism of action and genetic control are unclear, and it is even accepted to be of polygenic nature [13].

5.4. Brindle

Brindle is a very rare color, referred to as vertical dark stripes on any background color [13]. Usually, points and head are unaffected and may occur in any breed. It was suggested two causes for the brindle in horses [13]: either it is a reorganization of sootiness into vertical stripes instead of the usual sooty variant, or it is a chimera; in fact, some animals have been proven to be chimeras, resulting from the fusion of two embryos early during pregnancy.

6. The gray case

Gray is a dominant mutation in the gene STX17 [26], Syntaxin 17, represented by the capitalized letter G. It consists in a gradual and progressive whitening of all hairs on the horse's body, but the skin may remain dark for many years. In some cases, such as the Lipizzaners, the skin becomes gradually unpigmented as well. When this mutation is present, at every shedding time the original color of the horse will be replaced by white-colored hairs, even if the underlying coat is determined by dominant alleles. Thus, the gene that causes the graying of the coat is epistatic, which occurs when a gene at one locus masks the effect of another gene at another locus.

The dominant nature of the mutation implies that any gray horse is required to have at least one of its parents being a gray too. Gray horses, especially homozygotes (G^G G^G) tend to develop a type of tumor called the melanoma of the gray horse [27].

Animals are born colored (the color of the original coat) and graying starts around the eyes, already during the first months of life. However, total whitening can take years, ranging individually from horse to horse. This mutation leads to an excess of melanin production, and that is the reason why gray-carrying horses are born with vivid darker colors; such a characteristic is well observed in the foals whose coat is a jet black, unlike the black foals without the mutation, who are born a grayish color. This is the reason because some breeders say "blacks are born grays and grays are born blacks."

Many denominations are applied according to different stages of the graying process, varying by country: *Tordilho medalhado* or *apatacado* (*tordilho/tordillo* stands for gray in Portuguese and Spanish; respectively, the word is derived from "tordo," a bird whose plumage has a similar color) is the same of *dapple gray*; *branco/blanco porcelana* is the Portuguese/Spanish equivalent of *white porcelain/porcelain gray* (older grays with depigmented skin contrasting with the white hairs of body), *tordilho/tordillo vinagre* (*rose gray*), *tordilho/tordillo negro* (*iron gray*), and *tordilho/tordillo*

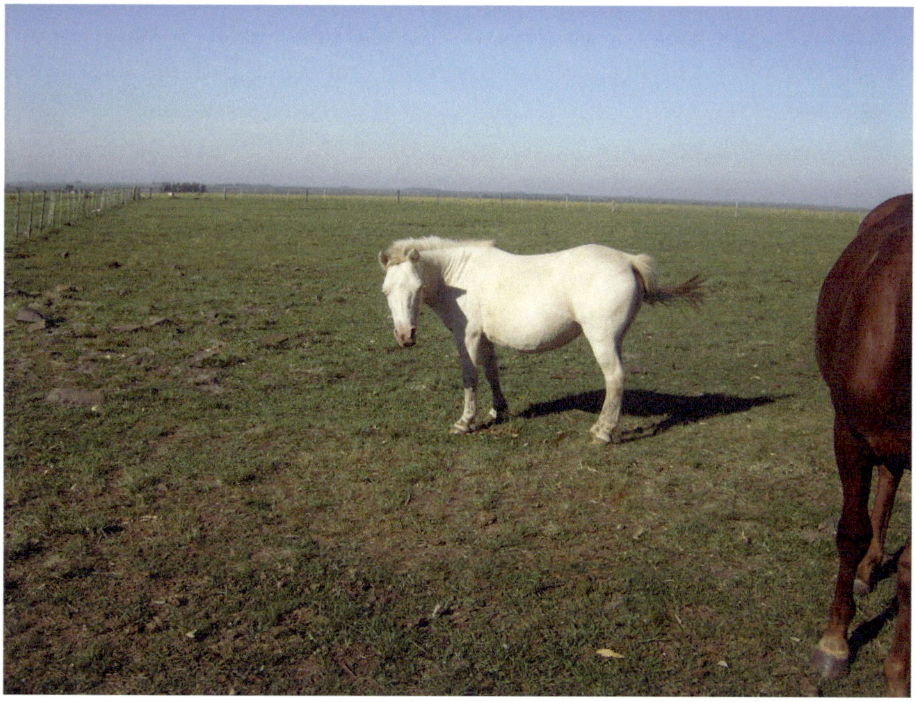

Figure 4. A cremello horse has pinkish skin, blue eyes, and a coat of a very light shade of cream. *Source*: Mrs. Albrecht.

pedrês (fleabitten gray). It is a widespread color between various breeds such as Thoroughbred, Purebred Arabian, Percheron, Andalusian, and it is the only color seen in Lipizzaners.

7. White patterns

Consist of white hairs mixed by or arranged in white spots overlapping the underlying coat; it has dominant or polygenic nature and arises from mutations in several genes. The phenotypic appearance can vary from one extreme to another, often being impossible to say how many and which mutant genes are present without genetic testing. These white patterns should not be confused with common white marks present on the face and the lower portion of limbs (white markings of small size, limiting white to small patches in the forehead, and white lower limbs not reaching carpi and hocks).

7.1. Overo

Overo frame is the name of a mutation in the gene EDNRB [28] (endothelin receptor B), represented by the letter O with superscript lw (lethal white). Much confusion has been caused due to this gene. Because it does not manifest phenotypically in all horses carrying the mutation, it was mistakenly understood as a recessive trait. For this reason, it is known as the "ninja gene" or "007 gene." What happens though, is that O^{lw} has highly variable expression, depending on the action of other genes, which makes confusing its mechanism of action—It can even crop out in a foal from parents with apparently solid-colored coats—in these case, hiding the gene ("ninja gene!"). What is known for sure is that it is a dominant mutation capable of amplifying the expression of other white patterns such as Splashed White and Sabino.

To breeders and horse enthusiasts, *overo* is the general empirical name given to animals showing many asymmetrical white spots of relatively reduced size and jagged edges distributed throughout the body (**Figure 5**); however, only with genetic testing one can be sure that the frame gene is present.

Usually limbs are solid (i.e., do not have any white marking) and the head is largely marked with white (sometimes called "baldface"). Irregular white spots appear on the sides of the body and neck (whence the name "frame"); many *overos* has the upper lip solid colored and blue eyes are common, even when the coat around the eyes is pigmented. *Overos* minimally marked can show only the baldface.

The problem with overo frame is that it is lethal when homozygous, causing the lethal white foal syndrome [28]. The medical condition is called ileocolonic aganglionosis and requires euthanasia of the foal by the first days of life for humanitarian reasons. It is a pleiotropic effect of the mutant gene EDNRB, resulting in faulty areas of intestinal innervation and a foal completely (or near so) white colored. Pleiotropy is a genetic condition in which a gene causes more than one effect [29]. That is why breeding programs discourage mating of two *overos*. Making use of the Punnet square, a tool that allows simple calculation of outcome probabilities out of a given mating, the possibility of obtaining a homozygous overo frame (O^{lw} O^{lw})—a

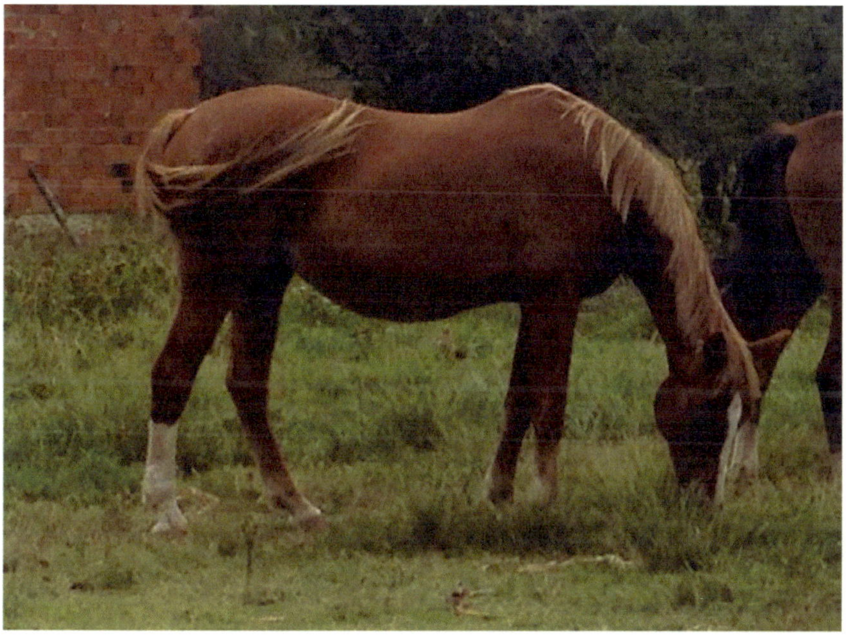

Figure 5. Flaxen. *Source*: Mrs. Albrecht.

lethal white foal—from the mating of two *overos* is 25% which is an unacceptable risk both for ethical and economical issues.

7.2. Splashed White

At least two loci are identified as having mutant alleles for Splashed White [30]: microphtalmia transcription factor (MITF) and paired box-3 (PAX3). Three mutations have been identified hitherto, SW1 (dominant mutation in MITF gene), SW2, and SW3 (dominant mutations in the PAX3 gene). Splashed White causes white spots in a horizontal pattern on the horse's body coat, and these white spots always cross the ventral line. The head is extensively marked (the white mark on the forehead and muzzle is quite wide and round and the muzzle is usually all white; this is called a "blaze") and the limbs are white above carpi and hocks. In extreme-marked horses, the head may be entirely white and the body may keep color only on the dorsal line. The more copies of mutant genes, the greater the amount of white. Splashed Whites minimally marked can display only an extensively marked forehead, nose, and muzzle; limbs can have white only below shins, and usually in the forelimbs.

In Latin America countries, it is called *bragado* preceded by the name of the main coat (i.e., *colorado bragado*). In English-speaking countries, it is used *splash* after the name of the main coat, as in *bay splash*.

Splashed White is widespread among several breeds, including Welsh Pony, Icelandic, Finnish Draft, and Paints. It is present in some other breeds, although the respective stud books do not recognize and does not register it as a specific characteristic.

Accordingly to the extent of depigmentation on the animal's head, it may have blue eyes and/or congenital deafness. A problem of embryonic death occurs when both PAX3 alleles are mutated.

7.3. Roan

It is characterized by white and colored hairs intermingled over the coat in different proportions only on the horse's body, not affecting points and head. Sometimes when there is very little amount of white, it is confused with *roaned*, which does not have the same genetic origin of the true or genetic *roan*. Some confusion may also occur between *roans* and *rabicanos*. Roan is a dominant mutation in the KIT gene [10] (mast/stem cell growth factor receptor; v-kit Hardy-Zuckerman 4 feline sarcoma viral oncogene homolog), represented by KIT^R. Contrary to what was once believed, homozygosity is possible in living animals and does not cause embryonic death. It can occur on any basic coat colors, diluted or modified. The nomenclature varies according to the country of origin: in Latin America countries, the word *rosilho* (*rosillo* in Spanish) is used with the name of the main coat, as in *rosilho gateado* (a roan dun horse), *rosilho prateado* (*chestnut* with large amount of white hairs intermingled with the basic color; does not means the presence of the silver dilution); *mouro* is the roan horse whose basic color is black. In English-speaking countries the word roan is used after the main color:

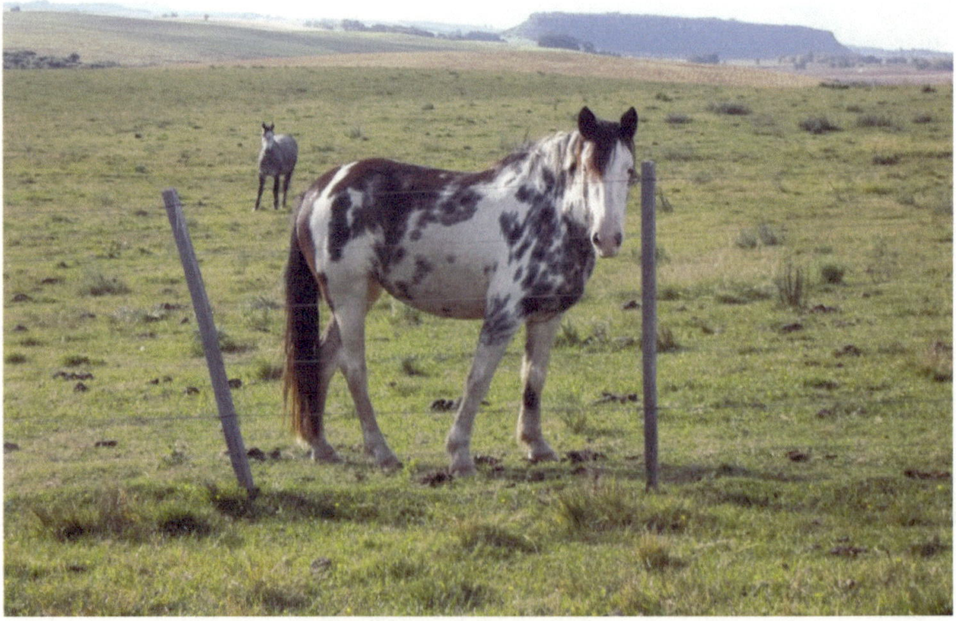

Figure 6. Overo. *Source*: Mr. Isola.

http://dx.doi.org/10.5772/65848

red roan (a *chestnut* or *sorrel roan*), *blue roan* (the roan black), *bay roan*, *strawberry roan*, and so on (**Figure 6**).

7.4. Tobiano

Tobiano spotting is another mutation in the KIT gene [31], characterized by white spots in a vertical pattern crossing the dorsal line (unlike Splashed White, wherein the spots have a horizontal pattern and cross the ventral line). It has dominant nature and is represented by KIT^{To}. Usually the head is solid or has minimal white marking, the limbs have high socks (white mark that reaches the carpi and hocks), and the tail and manes are usually bicolored. The maximally marked *tobiano* may have the body almost completely white (especially if Splashed White is present), but keep solid-colored ears, what is called "Medicine Hat." On the other hand, minimally marked *tobianos* may display only high socks. In these cases, only a genetic test can demonstrate the presence of this mutant gene.

A frequent feature in homozygous *tobianos* (KIT^{To} KIT^{To}) is the so-called "paw prints," "cat tracks," "bear paws" (English), "marcas do perdigueiro" (Portuguese): colored small rounded spots arranged in small groups spread over white areas on the horse's body. Despite the presence of these marks be of great help when one wants a *tobiano* foal, the absence of these marks does not mean the *tobiano* parent is heterozygous.

Tobiano derives its name from Tobias, a Brazilian general who came to Argentina in the mid 1800s bringing with him soldiers mounted in very odd-spotted horses. The nomenclature varies according to country. Moreover, in Latin countries it varies also among countries' regions. *Tobiano* is used, in North and South America, including Southern Brazil, along with the main coat name: *tobiano colorado* (Portuguese and Spanish), *bay tobiano*, and *black tobiano* (English); in other regions of Brazil, *pampa de baio* (or other coat color) is used to designate a *buckskin tobiano* animal with large proportion of white spotting, or *baio pampa* (or other coat color) for the animal with little white spotting.

7.5. White spotted

Formerly known as Dominant White, it is another dominant mutation in the KIT gene [16] that holds extensive phenotypic variation. It is characterized by large amounts of sparse white hairs with no set pattern, overlapping the adjacent coat. The horses also have depigmented skin and dark eyes, and in extreme cases the animal can be completely white being easily confused with an older gray. When the eyes have colors other than dark brown, there is another gene (or genes) acting. White spotted is represented by the capitalized letter W followed by a number, which corresponds to the mutation variant [32] (for example, KIT^{W1} and KIT^{w19}). There are by now 20 known mutations, some of which are derived from spontaneous mutations in the gene. It occurs even in the Thoroughbred breed, and some countries such as Australia, New Zealand, and Japan recognize and do list these horses as authentic Thoroughbreds.

It has long been discussed the issue of lethal homozygosity (KIT^{W-} KIT^{W-}), taken as true for a long time. This is a debatable question considering that there are living animals whose genetic tests confirmed the presence of two alleles W [9, 33].

7.6. Sabino

Sabino is a common term originated from Spanish-speaking countries, to designate a coat speckled with white hairs that do not form a specific pattern [13]. This definition is based only on the phenotype and is generally used to define a white patterned coat that not necessarily has the genetic basis of the same name gene.

Sabino (genetic) occurs in two forms: a dominant mutation in the KIT gene named Sabino-1 (KIT^{Sb1} KIT^{-}) [34]. This variant, when homozygous, causes much more white on the body (incomplete dominance). The second form has a polygenic mode of inheritance [13] and results in horses completely white or near so. The eyes may be blue or dark brown. A typical sabino feature is the roaned edges of the white spots. White spots with these characteristics are common in the belly and intermandibular space. The appearance of *sabinos* may vary greatly from only common white marks on the limbs with roaned edges, to a whole white animal with very little pigmentation, whence it is called "the everything gene." This renders identification of the underlying coat color, whether or not there is expression of other white patterns, practically impossible without genetic testing or at least, extensive knowledge of the genealogy of the animal in question.

Usually the coat name is followed or preceded by the word "sabino:" *Colorada sabina* (Portuguese and Spanish); *bay sabino* (English).

An interesting fact about KIT mutations is that only two mutations can be presented in the KIT gene in a particular animal, since there are only two copies of the gene in every horse; that being understood, it becomes easy to see why we will never have one "white-spotted red roan tobiano" (it would require three KIT gene copies) or a homozygous tobiano roan.

7.7. Appaloosa

Characteristic coat color of the homonymous breed and frequent color in breeds like Knabstrupp, Miniatures, Noriker, and others. It is a white pattern with symmetric white patches. *Appaloosa* is the generic name of the leopard complex; "complex" because all patterns in this color are genetically related, and "leopard" because of the most distinctive feature observed: the round-colored spots on a white area, varying in extent over the animal's body. It is caused by a mutation in the gene TRPM1 (transient receptor potential cation channel, subfamily M, member 1) [35]. It shows incomplete dominance, represented by Lp^{Lp}. The most common appearance is a variable solid-colored anterior part of the body and the remainder covered by white (which is called *white cap blanket* or *snow cap blanket*), which may or may not display spots, depending on the genetic makeup (homozygous vs. heterozygous). The animals called "leopards," highly valued, present a white body (including the head) covered with white round spots (leopard spots). The leopard complex can be split into several patterns, and usually at least two of these patterns are expressed in the same animal. These patterns relate to quantity and arrangement of white areas on the animal's coat:

- *Frost* describes a roaning pattern that consists of scattered white hairs over the entire body of the horse.

- *Varnish roan* is like frost, though areas over bony prominences are darker than the remainder of the coat.
- *Snowflake* occurs as small round patches of white hairs spread over the entire body. As well as frost and varnish roan, it is progressive from birth to maturity; that is why animals that have the leopard complex will present, year after year, an increasingly white-covered coat, although many horses end up stabilizing at some point in their lifes, contrary to what happens in the case of gray.
- *Speckled* describes a pattern of extensive roaning with numerous small dark spots are placed on a white background.
- *Blanket* is a white covering extending variably over the horse's body (**Figure 8**); it can be as small as only a few white patches on the hips, or extensive enough to cover the entire body. When the animal is heterozygous for Lp (Lp^{Lp} Lp) the blanket is covered by colored round spots that can vary in size (**Figure 7**). Homozygous (Lp^{Lp} Lp^{Lp}) horses show no spots, no matter the extent of the white blanket. In case of an extensive white blanket, the entire body will display white, while maintaining some color at the points and head and some very small-scattered spots on some regions of the body. These horses are called *few spots* (**Figure 8**).

The extent of the white blanket is a function of other loci, known to exert modifying action on the extent of white in the body [13, 35]. One of these modifiers is named Pattern-1, a domi-

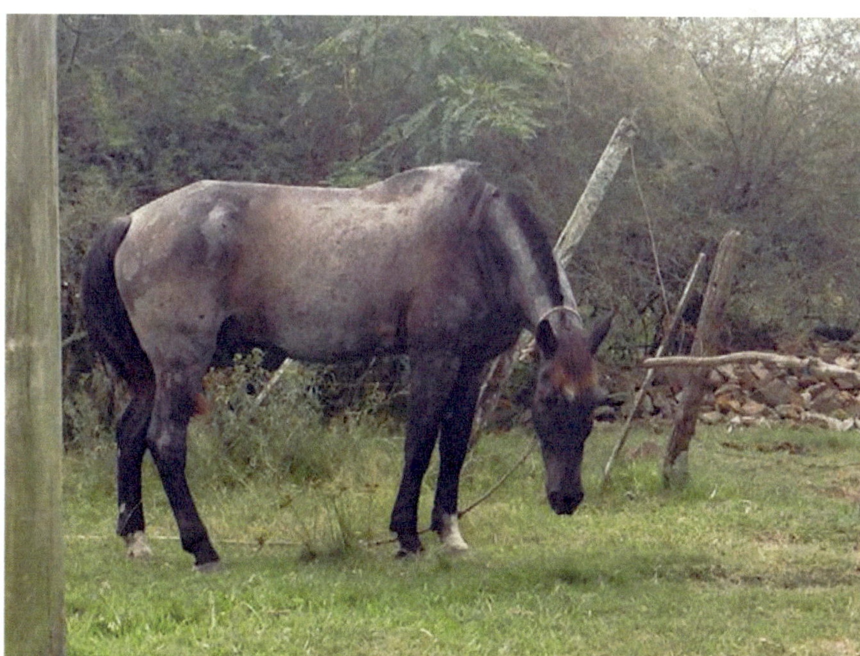

Figure 7. Blue roan. *Source*: Mr. Isola.

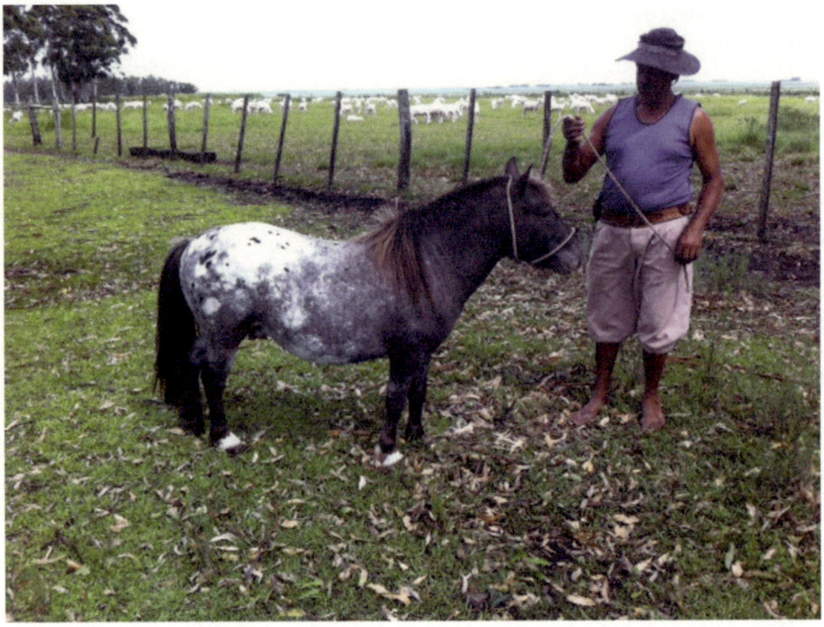

Figure 8. A white blanket may vary in extension. *Source*: Mrs. Albrecht.

nant trait ($PATN^{P}$) that regulates the extent of the white blanket and acts when at least one copy of the leopard gene is present. Horses that do not have the dominant gene ($PATN^{+}$) can be solid-colored coats without white cover, displaying only the patterns of white hairs and depigmented skin described below.

Some characteristics occur independently of other manifestations of the leopard complex, being present in all animals carrying the mutation, whether they are homozygous or not. These characteristics are shown as small spots on the skin of the nose, genitalia, anus, mouth, and eyelids, called *mottled;* when the skin is dark these spots are pink and when it is clear, the spots are dark. Also there are changes in the sclera, which is white, resembling a human eye to many people.

The limbs may display the common white marks like in any other coat color. In leopard complex carriers lacking these common marks, a blend of white and dark regions may be presented on the lower limbs. These are called *lightning strikes* or *lightning marks,* and the coronary band is generally colored. The hooves can be striped. An interesting feature of the leopard complex are sparse manes and tails, often called "rat tailed" and more strongly expressed in dark-colored hairs.

A common problem found in homozygous horses (Lp^{Lp} Lp^{Lp}) is the congenital stationary night blindness (CSNB) [36].

The "appaloosa" mutation appeared about 25,000 years ago, according to drawings found in the Perch Merle caves in southwestern France. In the modern era, it was developed by Indians

http://dx.doi.org/10.5772/65848

of the Nez Perce tribe, from horses brought by Europeans in the sixteenth and seventeenth centuries; these tribes lived in the northwestern United States, at the banks of the Palouse River, from where the name Appaloosa is originated and consequently the name by which the leopard complex became known worldwide.

8. Conclusion

The colors of horses are determined by genetic factors and influenced by factors such as insolation, season, nutritional status, age, sex, and health. The naming of colors varies according to individual perceptions of shades and colors, countries (regional classifications), and breed standards. A wide variety of colors appeared after the domestication of horse, with more impressive-looking phenotypes preferred since antiquity. The cells responsible for pigment production are the melanocytes, where melanogenesis takes place in specialized organelles called melanosomes. Two pigments are produced by horses (eumelanin and pheomelanin) and the interaction of the MC1R and ASIP genes determines the three basic colors of horses (bay, chestnut, and black). These pigments can be influenced by dilution genes and modifier genes, resulting in a variety of colors. Observing the color of a solid-colored horse's points, one can say which pigment is produced. Any white in the coat of a horse derives from the absence of melanocytes in the depigmented area. The exception is the process of graying, a depletion of pigment production, and leading to the gradual appearance of white hairs instead of colored hairs. Pleiotropic effects arise from the expression of some genes related to coat colors, affecting physiological systems of the horse and may even lead to death. Many colors have not been critically related to specific genes yet. Genetic tests are available to check the presence of many alleles, and without such testing is often difficult to pinpoint exactly that genes are at work to produce the color.

Acknowledgements

The authors hereby declare, that all the pictures of horses in this chapter were taken by Mrs. Albrecht and Mr. Isola, especially on purpose to insert here, and the animals belong to them.

Author details

Adriana Pires Neves[1]*, Eduardo Brum Schwengber[1], Fabiola Freire Albrecht[2], José Victor Isola[1] and Liana de Salles van der Linden[2]

*Address all correspondence to: adripneves@yahoo.com.br

1 Pampa Federal University, Dom Pedrito, RS, Brazil

2 Federal University of Rio Grande do Sul, Porto Alegre, RS, Brazil

References

[1] Bowling AT, Ruvinsky A, editors. The Genetics of the Horse. 1st ed. London: CABI Publishing; 2000. 538 p.

[2] Ajzenmann HF, Standeven JW, Shurtleff TL. Effect of hippotherapy on motor control, adaptative behavior, and participation in children with autism spectrum disorder: A pilot study. American Journal of Occupational Therapy. 2013; 67: 653–663. DOI 10.5014/ajot.2013.008383

[3] Araujo TB, Silva NA, Costa JN, Pereira MM, Safons MP. Effect of equine-assisted therapy on the postural balance of the elderly. Brazilian Journal of Physical Therapy. 2011; 15: 414–419. DOI 10.1590/S1413-35552011005000027

[4] Ludwig A, Pruvost M, Reissman M, Benecke N, Brockmann GA, Castaños P, Cieslak M, Lippold S, Llorente L, Malaspinas AS, Slatkin M, Hofreiter M. Coat color variation at the beginning of horse domestication. Science. 2009; 324: 485.

[5] Hardy GH. Mendelian proportions in mixed population. Science. 1908; 28: 49–50.

[6] Weinberg W. On the demonstration of heredity in man. In: Boyer SH, editor. Papers on Human Genetics. Englewood Cliffs: Prentice Hall; 1963.

[7] Candille SI, Kaelin CB, Cattanach BM, Yu B, Thompson DA, Nix MA, Kerns JA, Schmutz SM, Millhauser GL, Barsh GS. A β-defensin mutation causes black coat color in domestic dogs. Science. 2007; 318: 1418–1423.

[8] Sponenberg DP, Weise MC. Dominant black in horses. Genetic Selection Evolution. 1997; 29: 403–408.

[9] Holl H, Brooks S, Bailey E. De novo mutation of KIT discovered as a result of a non-hereditary white coat colour pattern. Animal Genetics. 2010; 41: 196–198. DOI 10.1111/j.1365-2052.2010.02135.x

[10] Marklund S, Moller M, Sandberg K, Andersson L. Close association between sequence polymorphism in the KIT gene and the roan coat color in horses. Mammalian Genome. 1999; 10: 283–288.

[11] Cone RD. Studies on the physiological functions of the melanocortin system. Endocrine Reviews. 2006; 27: 736–749.

[12] Riley PA. Melanogenesis and melanoma. Pigment Cell Research. 2003; 16: 548–552.

[13] Sponenberg DP. Equine Color Genetics. 3rd ed. Iowa: Wiley-Blackwell; 2009.

[14] Rieder S, Taourit S, Mariat D, Langlois B, Guérin G. Mutations on the agouti (ASIP), the extension (MC1R) and the brown (TYRP1) loci and their association to coat color phenotypes in horses (Equus caballus). Mammalian Genome. 2001; 12: 450–455.

[15] Hearing VJ, Jiménez M. Mammalian tyrosinase: The critical regulatory control point in melanocyte pigmentation. International Journal of Biochemistry. 1987; 19: 1141–1147.

[16] Haase B, Brooks SA, Schlumbaum A, Azor PJ, Bailey E, Alaeddine F, Mevissen M, Burger D, Poncet PA, Rieder S, Leeb T. Allelic heterogeneity at the equine KIT locus in dominant white (W) horses. PLOS Genetics. 2007; 3: 2101–2108. DOI 10.1371/journal.pgen.0030195

[17] Imsland F, McGowan K, Rubin CJ, Henegar C, Sundström E, Berglund J, Schwochow D, Gustafson U, Imsland P, Lindblad-Toh K, Lindgren G, Mikko S, Millon L, Wade C, Schubert M, Orlando L, Penedos MC, Barsh GS, Andersson L. Regulatory mutations in TBX3 disrupt asymmetric hair pigmentation that underlies dun camouflage color in horses. Nature Genetics. 2016; 48: 152–160. DOI 10.1038/ng.3475

[18] Masuda M, Tsunoda J, Nomura H, Kimura N, Altangerel G, Namkhai B, Dolj U, Yokohama M. New primitive marking (Bider) in Mongolian native horses and Equus przewalskii. Journal of Equine Veterinary Science. 2007; 18: 145–151.

[19] Mariat D, Taourit S, Guérin G. A mutation in the MATP gene causes the cream coat color in the horse. Genetics Selection Evolution. 2003; 35: 119–133. DOI 10.1051/gse:2002039

[20] Brunberg E, Andersson L, Cothran G, Sandberg K, Mikko S, Lindgren G. A missense mutation in PMEL17 is associated with the silver coat color in the horse. BMC Genetics. 2006; 7. DOI 10.1186/1471-2156-7-46

[21] Ramsey DT, Ewart SL, Render JA, Cook CS, Latimer CA. Congenital ocular abnormalities of Rocky Mountain Horses. Veterinary Ophtalmology. 1999; 2: 47–59.

[22] Grahn BH, Pinard C, Archer S, Bellone R, Forsyth G, Sandmeyer LS. Congenital ocular anomalies in purebred and crossbred Rocky and Kentucky Mountain Horses in Canada. Canadian Veterinary Journal. 2008; 49: 675–681.

[23] Andersson LS, Wilbe M, Viluma A, Cothran G, Ekesten B, Ewart S, Lindgren G. Equine multiple congenital ocular anomalies and silver coat colour result from the pleiotropic effects of mutant PMEL. PLOS Genetics. 2013; 8: 1–8.

[24] Cook D, Brooks S, Bellone R, Bailey E. Missense mutation in Exon 2 of SLC36A1 responsible for champagne dilution in horses. PLOS Genetics. 2008; 4: 1–9. DOI 10.1371/jornal.pgen.1000195

[25] Brooks SA, Gabreski N, Miller D, Brisbin A, Brown HE, Streeter C, Mezey J, Cook D, Antczak DF. Whole-genome SNP association in the horse: Identification of a deletion in Myosin Va responsible for lavender foal syndrome. PloS Genetics. 2010; 6: 1–7. DOI 10.1371/journal.pgen.1000909

[26] Rosengren PG, Golovko A, Sundstrom E, Curik I, Lennartsson J, Seltenhammer MH, et al. A cis-acting regulatory mutation causes premature hair graying and susceptibility to melanoma in the horse. Nature Genetics. 2008; 40: 1004–1009.

[27] Sundstrom E, Imsland F, Mikko S, Wade C, Sigurdsson S, Pielberg GR, Golovko A, Curik I, Seltenhammer MH, Sölkner J, Lindblad-Toh K, Andersson L. Copy number expansion of the STX17 duplication in melanoma tissue from grey horses. BMC Genomics. 2012; 13.

[28] Santschi E, Purdy A, Valberg S, Vrotsos P, Kaese H, Mickelson J. Endothelin receptor B polymorphism associated with lethal white foal syndrome in horses. Mammalian Genome. 1998; 9: 306–309.

[29] Bellone RR. Pleiotropic effects of pigmentation genes in horses. Animal Genetics. 2010; 41: 100–110. DOI 10.1111/j.1365-2052.2010.02116.x

[30] Hauswirth R, Haase B, Blatte M, Brooks SA, Burger D, Drögemüller C, Gerber V, Henke D, Janda J, Jude R, Magdesian KG, Matthews JM, Poncet PA, Svansson V, Tozaki T, Wilkinson-White L, Penedo MCT, Rieder S, Leeb T. Mutations in MITF and PAX3 cause "splashed white" and other white spotting phenotypes in horses. PLOS Genetics. 2012; 8: 1–9. DOI 10.1371/journal.pgen.1002653

[31] Haase B, Jude R, Brooks SA, Leeb T. An equine chromosome 3 inversion is associated with the tobiano spotting pattern in German horse breeds. Animal Genetics. 2008; 39: 306–309. DOI 10.1111/j.1365-2052.2008.01715.x

[32] Haase B, Brooks SA, Tozaki T, Burger D, Poncet PA, Rieder S, Hasegawa T, Penedo C, Leeb T. Seven novel KIT mutations in horses with white coat colour phenotypes. Animal Genetics. 2009; 40: 623–629. DOI 10.1111/j.1365-2052.2009.01893.x

[33] Haase B, Obexer-Ruff G, Dolf G, Rieder S, Burger D, Poncet PA, Gerber V, Howard J, Leeb T. Haematological parameters are normal in dominant white Franches–Montagnes horses carrying a KIT mutation. The Veterinary Journal. 2010; 184: 315–317. DOI 10.1016/j.tvjl.2009.02.017

[34] Brooks SA, Bailey E. Exon skipping in the KIT gene causes a Sabino spotting pattern in horses. Mammalian Genome. 2005; 16: 893–902. DOI 10.1007/s00335-005-2472-y

[35] Sponenberg DP, Carr G, Simak E, Schwink K. The inheritance of the leopard complex of spotting patterns in horses. Journal of Heredity. 1990; 81: 323–331.

[36] Rebecca R, Bellone RR, Brooks SA, Sandmeyer L, Murphy BA, Forsyth G, Archer S, Bailey E, Grahn B. Differential gene expression of TRPM1, the potential cause of congenital stationary night blindness and coat spotting patterns (LP) in the Appaloosa horse (Equus caballus). Genetics. 2008; 179: 1861–1870. DOI 10.1534/genetics.108.088807

Further reading

[37] American Paint Horse Association Guide to Coat Color Genetics. Available from: http://apha.com

[38] Nicholas FW. Introduction to Veterinary Genetics. 3rd ed. Ames: Blackwell Publishing; 2010. 329 p.

[39] Scott DW, Miller WH. Equine Dermatology. 1st ed. St. Louis: Elsevier Science; 2003, 829 p.

Chapter 6

Major Histocompatibility Complex-Associated Resistance to Infectious Diseases: The Case of Bovine Leukemia Virus Infection

Silvina Elena Gutiérrez, Eduardo Néstor Esteban,
Claudia María Lützelschwab and
Marcela Alicia Juliarena

Additional information is available at the end of the chapter

http://dx.doi.org/10.5772/65804

Abstract

The major histocompatibility complex (MHC) is a polymorphic gene cluster of about 150 genes, present in all vertebrates. Many of these genes contribute to immunity. Particularly, MHC-encoded class I and class II molecules, which are typically highly polymorphic and polygenic, are central in defining the specificity of the adaptive immune response. Among the diversity of genes associated with disease resistance, MHC genes are particularly interesting as they are associated with resistance and susceptibility to a wide range of diseases, some of which produce important economic losses in livestock. Enzootic bovine leukosis is an infectious disease caused by the retrovirus bovine leukemia virus (BLV), with an important economic impact, mainly in dairy herds. In this chapter, MHC-associated genetic resistance to BLV is revised. Certain alleles of the bovine MHC (*BoLA*) class II locus have been found strongly associated with resistance to viral dissemination. Genetic selection of resistant animals emerges as a natural strategy for the control of infectious diseases, especially when there is no other alternative of control or prevention, as vaccines. Founded on this knowledge, a BLV control program based on selection of genetically resistant cattle was designed. The proof of concept indicates that this strategy is feasible to implement in dairy herds.

Keywords: major histocompatibility complex, BoLA, genetic resistance, infectious diseases, bovine leukemia virus, control, veterinary, livestock

1. Introduction

The immune system has evolved in vertebrates to protect them from invading pathogens. To attain this objective, it compromises an enormous variety of cells and molecules that interact with each other in a complex network to recognize, counteract, and, if properly regulated, eliminate the pathogen. The major histocompatibility complex (MHC), which is found to occur in all mammalian species, plays a central role in the development and function of the immune system. Genes encoding the MHC are highly polymorphic, and numerous associations between allelic variants and immune responsiveness and disease resistance are well documented. Hence, the MHC genes are attractive as candidate genes involved in susceptibility/resistance to various diseases.

Breeding for improved disease resistance has emerged as a major challenge for animal geneticists. The benefits of successfully improving the resistance of animals to an infectious disease are manifold, including animal welfare, increased efficiency and productivity, and hence a reduced environmental footprint, reduced reliance on other disease-control measures, and improved public perception [1].

Enzootic bovine leucosis is an endemic disease in many countries, causing important economic impact in the dairy industry. The fine characterization of the resistance phenotype, the strong association between certain MHC class II alleles with resistance, and the absence of preventive or therapeutic measures against the disease make the genetic selection of resistant animals a feasible approach to control bovine leukemia virus (BLV) infection.

2. The major histocompatibility complex

Vertebrates have the capacity to recognize, destroy, and develop immunological memory to invading microorganisms through the activation of cells and molecules of their immune system. In order to achieve these ends, the two arms of the immune system (i.e., the innate and the acquired immunity) have to interact with each other. The innate immune system comprises mainly cells from the myeloid lineage that recognize common structures on a broad spectra of microorganisms, known as the pathogen-associated molecular patterns (PAMPs) through their pathogen recognition receptors (PRRs). Some of these cells, like macrophages and dendritic cells, are also involved in the activation of the adaptive immune system, by capturing and processing the antigens and acting as antigen presenting cells (APC) for T lymphocytes.

The effector cells of the adaptive immune system, consisting of B and both helper T lymphocytes (LTH) and cytotoxic T lymphocytes (CTL), recognize a very large variety of self and nonself antigens in a more specific manner by their antigen receptors (BCR and TCR, respectively). The BCR can bind directly to free or soluble native antigen, while the TCR requires the protein antigen to be processed into small peptides. These peptides have to be associated within the endoplasmic reticulum with molecules encoded by a single genetic locus containing many polymorphic genes, the MHC. The assembled MHC molecule (mMHC)-peptide complex is then transported to and expressed on the surface of the APCs, where the antigen-loaded mMHC interacts with the TCR and initiates the activation of T lymphocytes [2]. The CTL and the LTH recognize antigen in the context of two different mMHCs: class I and class II, respectively. The class II mMHCs have a restricted expression, mainly on professional APCs, and expose peptides mainly derived from captured extracellular antigens for the recognition by the LTH. The class I mMHCs are displayed on the surface of every nucleated cell of the organism, presenting peptides essentially originated from intracellular proteins (i.e., intracellular microorganisms or cell-derived proteins) to be recognized by the CTLs. The class I mMHC does not only play a fundamental role in the recognition of foreign intracellular antigens but also in inducing self-tolerance and alloreactive immune responses.

2.1. Structure of class I and class II MHC molecules

Most of the current knowledge about these molecules arose from pioneer studies on the rejection of normal and malignant transplanted tissues in mice and rabbits [3–6]. The evidence produced by these studies indicated that the destruction of the grafted tissue was determined upon the existence of inherited antigenic differences between transplant and host, leading to the discovery of the mMHC and, later on, their genetic complexity.

The mMHCs have different domain organizations but similar structure. The variations are concentrated in three to four discrete hypervariable regions in the extracellular domains, while the rest of the molecule is highly conserved. The X-ray crystallography of the proteins demonstrated that the class I mMHC is a heterodimer consisting of a transmembrane α chain non-covalently linked to a small non-transmembrane chain, called β2-microglobulin (β2m). Besides a transmembrane and an intracellular region, the α chain has three extracellular globular domains ($\alpha 1$, $\alpha 2$, and $\alpha 3$). The $\alpha 1$ and $\alpha 2$ domains of the α chain form a groove that accommodates an 8- to 10-mer antigenic peptide [7, 8]. The class II mMHC is a heterodimer composed of an α and a β chain, both with an intracellular, a transmembrane, and two extracellular domains (**Figure 1A**). The pairing of the $\alpha 1$ and $\beta 1$ domains form an antigen-binding groove with open ends, allowing the allocation for a larger peptide (14-mer or more) extending out of both sides of the groove [9] (**Figure 1B**).

The polygenic and polymorphic features of the MHC grant these molecules with an enormous capability for antigen presentation. A single individual co-expresses several mMHCs from a large pool of alleles within a population. Moreover, each mMHC molecule can associate with a great amount of similar peptides, expanding even more the breadth of MHC-regulated immune responses to pathogens. The polymorphic residues in the mMHC antigen-binding groove are responsible for the different peptide specificities of the different alleles. The class I molecules require an allele-specific peptide length and a defined peptide motif that includes two anchor amino acids or residues with closely related side chains, which interact with both ends of the antigen-binding site of that particular mMHC [10]. The class II mMHCs have less stringency for size but also have allele-specific peptide motifs (or anchor residues) that reach into pockets within and on the sides of the groove of the class II mMHC [11] (**Figure 1B**). Moreover, conserved residues within the class II peptide-binding groove induce a conformational change, forcing bound peptides into a twisted configuration and exposing sites for external interactions [12].

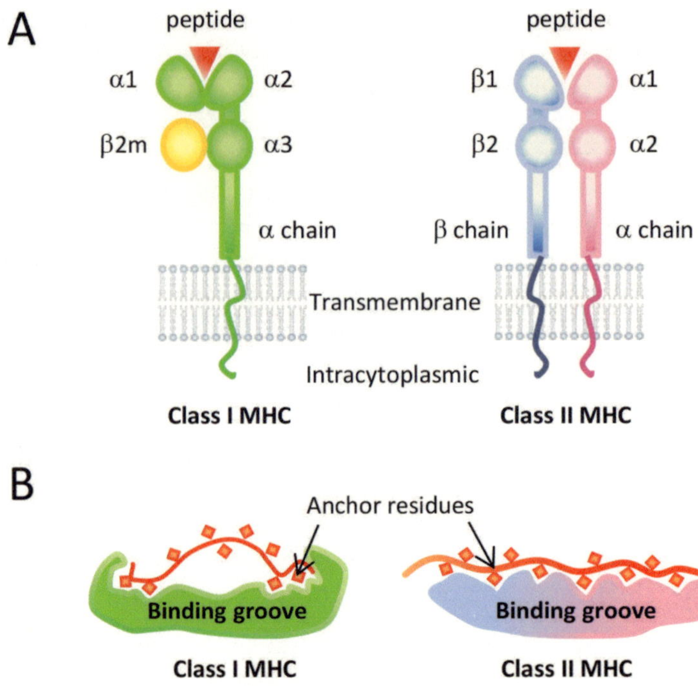

Figure 1. Structure of MHC molecules and its binding sites. Panel A: schematic representation of class I and class II mMHCs. Panel B. MHC peptide-binding sites. Amino acid positioning within the peptide-binding grooves of class I and class II MHC proteins is shown. Squares represent individual amino acids of the antigenic peptides binding in the groove of each class I and class II mMHC.

2.2. Organization of the Major Histocompatibility Complex

Since its first description in mice and humans [5, 13], the study of the MHC genetic architecture has expanded substantially, with the discovery and characterization of many class I and class II genes in different vertebrate species, except for jawless fish [14]. The collective name given to the proteins encoded by MHC genes depends on the species, except for mice and chickens, in which they were first described as transplantation antigens and maintain their original nomenclature H-2 and B, respectively. Hence, in humans, they are called human leukocyte antigen (HLA); in swine, SLA; in ovine, OLA; in equine, ELA; in dogs, DLA; in bovine, BoLA; and so on. The genetic structure of the MHC is best known for HLA and is relatively conserved among other mammalian species [15].

The HLA complex covers about 4 Mb of the short arm of chromosome 6 and contains three major regions with the confirmed presence of more than 260 loci, including over 160 protein-coding genes [16, 17].

The HLA locus is divided into three closely linked regions: class I, class II, and class III. The first two regions contain genes that control the specific immune response (so-called "classical" MHC genes), and the class III region, enclosing about 75 genes, encodes a variety of different proteins, some related to the innate immunity [18].

http://dx.doi.org/10.5772/65804

The class I region contains three classical genes, *HLA-A*, *HLA-B*, and *HLA-C*, and three non-classical genes: *HLA-E*, *HLA-F*, and *HLA-G* [19] (**Figure 2**). Each of the classical HLA is a single functional gene, encoding a class I mMHC α chain. The gene coding for the β2m is located outside the MHC, on chromosome 15. *HLA-H*, *HLA-J*, *HLA-K*, and *HLA-L* are nonfunctional pseudogenes, closely related in nucleotide sequence to the class I functional genes [18].

The class II HLA cluster comprises three classical class II genes: *HLA-DP*, *HLA-DQ*, and *HLA-DR*, each encoding one α and one or two β chains; three nonclassical, non-polymorphic class II genes; *HLA-DM*, *HLA-DN*, and *HLA-DO*; and some pseudogenes [19] (**Figure 2**). These nonclassical class II genes are not expressed on the cell surface, but form heterotetrameric complexes involved in catalytic peptide exchange and loading onto classical class II molecules [20, 21].

The class III region is located between the class I and class II regions and contains genes coding for molecules with diverse function. Among the most prominent are the complement factor genes coding for factors C2, C4, and B; genes coding for cytokines belonging to the tumor necrosis factor (TNF) superfamily, TNF-α, lymphotoxin-α and lymphotoxin-β, which are involved in various inflammatory pathways; heat shock protein genes; and many other genes encoding proteins not related to the immune system [19].

2.3. The major histocompatibility complex in cattle

In cattle, the first evidence for the existence of a MHC system was found by lymphocyte immunizations and by the generation of monospecific antilymphocyte antisera against skin grafts, followed by studies on the inheritance of the antigens they detected [22, 23]. As in the human, the *BoLA* locus is highly complex and contains about 154 predicted functional genes spanning about 4 centimorgan on chromosome 23 [24]. **Figure 2** shows the BoLA organization

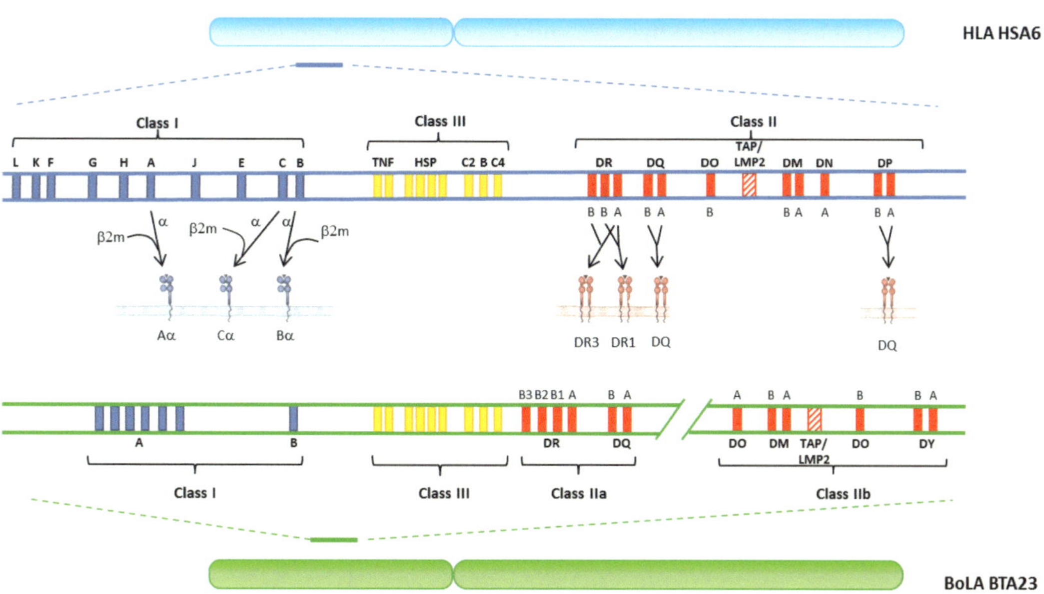

Figure 2. An abridge map of the genetic organization of HLA and BoLA.

compared to its human counterpart. Compared to the HLA system, the BoLA system differs in gene arrangement without compromising its functions. Class I genes are clustered in two regions: *BoLA-A* and *BoLA-B*. Only the *A* locus seems to be functional with at least six putative classical class I genes, named *genes 1–6* [25]. To date, 96 *BoLA-A* alleles are listed on the Immuno Polymorphism Database (IPD)-MHC database [26], and 29 different haplotypes have been identified, expressing between one and three combinations of these classical class I genes [27, 28]. The nonclassical BoLA class I genes include *NC1*, *NC2*, and *NC3*, encoding molecules with a relevant role during reproduction in dairy cows [29].

The main difference between BoLA and HLA gene organization is that in cattle the class II gene cluster is divided into two subregions, separated about 15 cM apart from each other: the class IIa, located near the class I/III regions, and the class IIb, resulting from a transposition, located close to the centromere on autosome 23 [30, 31]. This feature is shared by various ruminant species [32].

The subregion IIa incorporates the gene clusters *DR* and *DQ* but lack a *DP* gene [27]. This subregion expresses one DR molecule and one or two DQ molecules per haplotype [33]. Bovines have one monomorphic *DRA* gene. By contrast, there are three genes that encode for the β chain of the DR (*DRB*) molecule of which *DRB1* is a pseudogene and *DRB2* is poorly expressed, leaving the *DRB3* locus as the most polymorphic and strongly expressed gene from this group. To date, 130 alleles have been identified using different approaches in various breeds of cattle (listed in IPD-MHC database) [34].

The *DQ* cluster comprises five *DQA* (*DQA 1–5*) and five *DQB* (*DQB 1–5*) genes, which have arisen from gene duplication. From this cluster, at least 61 *BoLA DQA* and 81 *BoLA DQB* alleles have been described and listed in the IPD-MHC database, and 56 different haplotypes were described in Japanese Black and Holstein cattle [35]. The high number of different alleles, both on the *DR* and *DQ* loci, suggests that DR and DQ molecules complement each other for the presentation of a broad spectrum of antigens in cattle.

The BoLA class IIb locus is divided into two regions. The region known as "extended class II" region contains some genes involved in antigen processing and transport, i.e., LMP complex (low molecular mass polypeptide, *LMP2*, *LMP7*) and *TAP* genes (transporter associated with antigen processing: TAP2.1, TAP1, and TAP2) and also some non-MHC genes like *H2B* (histone H2B-like), among others [36–38].The second region is known as "classical class II" region and encloses genes of unknown function and unique to ruminants: *DSB (DRβ-like)*, *DYA*, and *DYB*. The *DYA* and *DYB* genes encode for proteins of 253 and 259 amino acids, respectively. DY molecule has been shown to be expressed by a subpopulation of afferent lymph dendritic cells, suggesting its involvement in the prominent antigen processing and presentation capability of these cells [39–41].

2.4. Association of the major histocompatibility complex to disease susceptibility and resistance

Although age, stress, and physiologic status are important factors influencing the outcome of infection, evidence for genetic control has been observed in many animal species. Based on data registered in the Domestic Animal Diversity Information System (DAD-IS) 2015 report [42], 483 mammalian breed populations are recorded as having resistance or tolerance to specific diseases or parasites, among which 236 correspond to breeds of cattle, 94 breeds of sheep, 56 breeds of chicken, 54 breeds of goats, and 36 breeds of pigs.

Not unexpectedly, the high degree of genetic polymorphism in the MHC has been associated with health status, vaccine responsiveness, and production traits in cattle [43–47]. Examples of some studies for which there is documented evidence of MHC association with resistance or susceptibility to disease include mastitis in cattle and sheep [44, 48], tick-borne disease [49–51], dermatophilosis in cattle [52], enzootic bovine leucosis in cattle and sheep [53–56], neosporosis in cattle [57], theileriosis in cattle [58], gastrointestinal parasites in sheep [59, 60], diarrhea in pigs [61, 62], Marek's disease in chicken [63, 64], coccidiosis in chicken [65], and coronavirus resistance in chickens [66], among others.

3. Enzootic bovine leukosis and the bovine leukemia virus

Enzootic bovine leukosis is one of the most frequent neoplastic diseases of cattle caused by an exogenous retrovirus designated BLV. BLV is the type species of the genus *Deltaretrovirus* in the Retroviridae family. This genus also includes pathogenic viruses from human and nonhuman primates (human and simian T-cell leukemia viruses) that share biological and molecular characteristics with BLV [67].

BLV infection is globally distributed in cattle-raising countries. An assessment of BLV infection in US dairy operations in 2007 showed that 83.9 % of them were seropositive for BLV [68]. A national study of BLV infection in Canada in 1980 showed that 40 % of its dairy herds and 11 % of its beef herds were infected [69]. On the other hand, BLV control programs have been established in member countries of the European Union since the 1980s, resulting in seroprevalence between 0.5 and 1.5 % in some countries, while others such as Belgium, Denmark, Germany, Estonia, Spain, France, Ireland, Austria, Finland, Sweden, the United Kingdom, and few others are considered officially free by the European Community [70–72].

In natural conditions BLV only infects cattle, zebus, buffalos, and capybaras, but other species such as sheep, goats, and rabbits can be experimentally infected [73]. Although both beef and dairy breeds are equally susceptible to BLV infection [74], the impact is higher in dairy herds, mainly because of differential management practices.

The major target of the virus is the B lymphocyte [75]. Although evidence of infection of other peripheral blood cell subpopulations has been reported [76], these results have not been confirmed by others. Soon after infection of a cell, the viral RNA is copied into DNA by the virus-encoded reverse transcriptase. The provirus then integrates into the cellular DNA at random sites, and the infection persists for the whole life of the animal, despite the presence of neutralizing and other antiviral antibodies.

3.1. Pathological and clinical features associated to BLV

BLV infection is characterized by the "iceberg principle," typical of many viral diseases. While the majority (approximately 70 %) of infected cattle remain asymptomatic, one third of infected cattle develop a permanent increase in the number of B lymphocytes termed persistent lymphocytosis (PL), which is considered a benign condition. The tip of the iceberg is represented by those animals that develop the neoplastic disease, which is usually less than 5 % of the infected cattle. The accumulation of transformed lymphocytes in one or more organs after a long latency period of 1–8 years leads to a multicentric lymphosarcoma. This condition is typically observed in cattle older than 3 years of age. In two thirds of the animals, the development of tumors is preceded by a phase of PL. Lesions can be localized in almost any organ, but the abomasum, heart, visceral and peripheral lymph nodes, spleen, uterus, and kidneys are most frequently affected. Lesions can be observed as white firm tumor masses or as a diffuse tissue infiltrate in any organ. Clinical signs are variable and depend on the affected organ, the speed of grow of tumors, and the degree of dissemination of the neoplastic process. In most cases the course of the illness is subacute to chronic, initiated by a marked loss of weight and appetite, and weakness. Clinical signs most often observed are decreased milk production, lymphadenopathy, and posterior paresis. Once the clinical signs of the illness are evident, the course is rapid and invariably culminate in death [77].

3.2. Transmission of BLV and economic impact of the infection

As cell-free virus is rarely detected in vivo, most susceptible cattle become infected by exposure to infected lymphocytes. Vertical transmission may occur in utero but is infrequent. The main biologic fluids that contain sufficient infected lymphocytes to transmit the infection are the blood, colostrum, and milk. Other fluids such as saliva, semen, urine, and nasal secretions, while potentially infectious, have not been demonstrated to transmit the infection in natural conditions [78].

Under general or standard production conditions, the risk of horizontal transmission is augmented by management practices or procedures involving blood transfer such as gouge dehorning, ear tagging or tattooing, blood extraction, and rectal palpation, using shared or not properly disinfected instruments [78]. This risk is augmented when contaminating blood comes from cattle with persistent lymphocytosis [79]. The use of natural service (i.e., bulls) to breed heifers was also identified as a risk factor for augmented prevalence of BLV infection compared to artificial insemination [80].

Evidence has been reported on the role of bloodsucking insects, such as stable flies, horn flies, and tabanids in the transmission of BLV [81]. Furthermore, the lack of insect control program has been recognized as a risk factor for BLV infection [82, 83]. In warm regions, the animals may be exposed to a high density of hematophagous insects that continuously fed on them; hence, the control of bloodsucking insects by pesticides has been reported to prevent the transmission in a model farm [84]. Both colostrum and milk from BLV-positive cows contain infected lymphocytes, and evidence exists for the transmission of BLV to calves by feeding bulk milk, a common practice in dairy herds [78, 85]. The rate of transmission attributable to this route has been estimated to be 6–16 % under natural conditions. On the other hand, feeding colostrum from infected dams, which contains high titers of antiviral antibodies, seems to have a protective role, being the susceptibility of calves dependent on the presence of specific antibodies obtained from the dam's colostrums and the age of the calf [78, 86, 87].

Enzootic bovine leucosis causes significant economic losses. The most obvious economic losses are due to culling or death due to lymphosarcoma, shortening of lifespan, and loss of production potential. Other indirect losses are related to the costs of control and eradication programs and restrictions in the international trade of cattle and their by-products. Annual economic losses to the US dairy industry associated with BLV are estimated to be $285 million for producers and $240 million for consumers [80]. The effects of subclinical BLV infection on milk production, reproductive performance, longevity, and culling rate are variable. Using data from the National Animal Health Monitoring System's 1996 dairy herd study, it was found that herds with test-positive cows produced 218 kg less milk per cow/per year than those with no test-positive cows [88].

There is no treatment for BLV infection or its associated disease. The possibility of a vaccine for protection against BLV has been explored (reviewed in [89]). A BLV vaccine would have to be noninfectious and non-oncogenic and should not interfere with the serological tests commonly used to detect infection [77].

3.3. Phenotypes associated with resistance and susceptibility in BLV infection

Studies from our laboratory have gone further into the characterization of BLV-infected, hematologically normal cattle (i.e., those animals that do not develop PL). Based on the proviral load in the peripheral blood and antibodies against BLV major proteins, we could describe two defined phenotypes in BLV-infected cattle. Proviral load was determined in DNA from peripheral blood leukocytes by a very sensitive nested PCR or a semiquantitative PCR [90], while antibody titers were measured against the BLV major antigens by ELISA [90, 91].

One group of animals is characterized by high proviral load (HPL) in peripheral blood (>100,000 BLV proviral copies/μg of DNA) and high antibody titers against the envelope protein of BLV of 51 kDa (BLVgp51). On the other hand, the remaining non-PL animals harbor an exiguous number of infected lymphocytes in the peripheral blood, almost undetectable by the molecular methods currently used (PCR and real-time PCR); we have termed this group low proviral load (LPL) cattle. These cattle develop low titers of antiviral antibodies against BLVgp51, while antibodies against BLVp24, the main core protein of BLV, are undetectable in the majority of LPL cattle or developed at very low titers. The follow-up of HPL and LPL cattle showed that each phenotype was maintained throughout, at least, a 1.5-year period. The characterization of PL cattle in terms of proviral load and titers of antibodies against BLV showed no significant differences with non-PL HPL cattle. Cattle with LPL profile represented about 60 % of hematologically normal cattle and 40 % of all BLV-infected cattle [92]. **Table 1** shows the main parameters that characterize both HPL and LPL infection phenotypes.

As virtually all cattle infected with BLV will continuously have antibodies against the virion proteins in their serum, serologic tests are commonly used for diagnosis of BLV infection in cattle > 6 months old. PL cattle and non-PL HPL cattle have high titers of antibodies against the major viral antigens, and then, they are easily classified as positive by means of the majority of serological tests in the market (mainly ELISAs or immunodiffusion tests). On the other hand, antibody titers against BLVgp51 are lower in most LPL animals compared to HPL cattle, and antibodies against BLVp24 are at very low titers or undetectable in most serum samples

BLV infection phenotype	Hematological status	Proviral load[a]	Antibody titer	
			BLVgp51	BLVp24
HPL	PL	≥100,000	400 to ≥ 6400	50–800
HPL	Non PL	≥100,000	400 to ≥ 6400	Seronegative to 400
LPL	Non PL	≤100	2–1600	Seronegative to 50

Proviral load was determined by semiquantitative PCR in DNA extracted from the peripheral blood. Antibody titers against BLVgp51 and BLV p24 were determined in plasma samples by ELISA.
[a] Proviral copies/μg DNA
Adapted from Juliarena et al. [92]

Table 1. Characterization of HPL and LPL phenotypes in terms of proviral load in the peripheral blood, hematological status, and antibody titer against BLVgp51 and BLVp24.

from LPL cattle. Hence, sensitivity of serological tests is decisive in their capacity to detect LPL animals. We have consistently detected LPL animals with a highly sensitive blocking ELISA developed in our lab, designated ELISA 108. This method detects antibodies against an immunodominant conformational epitope of the BLVgp51 at low titers. Other serological methods using BLVgp51 as antigen may also detect BLV-infected LPL animals, provided that they are sensitive enough. This is not the case of agar gel immunodiffusion (AGID) test commercialized in Argentina. On the other hand, serological tests using BLVp24 as antigen would not be able to detect LPL cattle in most cases.

We inoculated sheep with blood from LPL cattle to give further evidence of infection. This was an easily available alternative for the amplification and study of the BLV strain [93]. As the number of infected lymphocytes in peripheral blood from LPL cattle is extremely low, it was necessary to inoculate a large volume of blood to obtain the minimal quantity of infected lymphocytes to transmit the infection. The minimal dose necessary to infect sheep is about 926 BLV-infected lymphocytes [94]. One microliter of blood from a HPL cow was enough to infect lambs. In contrast, blood from LPL cattle also infected lambs, but 100 ml of blood was necessary to infect the ovine host. In order to determine if differences in the observed phenotypes could be attributable to differences at the nucleotide level between strains, a fragment of the *env* gene was amplified from infected lambs by nested PCR and sequenced. No mutations in the *env* gene that could be attributable to the passage from cow to lamb were detected. When comparing a 400-bp sequence from the *env* gene from six LPL and six HPL strains, no mutations were found that could be associated with any particular phenotype, strengthening the hypothesis that the development of each phenotype could be associated primarily with some genetic or epigenetic property of the host [95].

As LPL cattle maintained their phenotype for prolonged periods of time, without developing any hematologic or pathologic condition, it is proposed that these animals are naturally resistant to BLV replication.

3.4. Association of BLV phenotypes to polymorphisms at the major histocompatibility complex

Early observations on the aggregation of lymphoma/leukemia or PL in certain BLV-infected families, but not in others, suggested that host genetic factors were involved in the development of these conditions [96]. There were also indications that host genetic factors influenced the susceptibility to one condition or the other independently [97].

Studies on the relationship between BLV infection and bovine MHC (BoLA) revealed an association between serologically determined *BoLA-A* class I antigens and resistance and susceptibility to B-cell lymphocytosis in Shorthorn cattle [98], Holstein [99, 100], and other breeds [101]. However, these associations were relatively weak at the population level, and different *BoLA-A* alleles had significant effects in different breeds [102]. Subsequently, it was shown that resistance and susceptibility to PL map more closely to MHC class II *BoLA-DRB3* gene than to *BoLA-A* locus [56, 103]. A peptide motif named ER, which is present in *BoLA-DRB3* alleles **11, *23*, and **28*, was associated with resistance to PL in BLV-infected cattle. Resistance appears to be dependent upon the presence of the polar amino acids Glu-Arg at positions 70–71 within a highly polymorphic segment of the peptide-binding region [56]. This contributes to the putative peptide-binding specificity of the molecule at the β1 domain [11]. It is believed that the allelic differences influence the binding and orientation of viral peptides [104], thus determining allele specificity differences in the spectrum of peptides presented to the immune system. These differences may have important consequences for infection resistance [105]. Furthermore, it was shown that *BoLA-DRB3* alleles encoding Glu, Arg, and Val at positions 74, 77, and 78 of the BoLA-DRβ chain, respectively, might be related to tumor development resistance [106]. Moreover, evidence was presented that BLV-infected cattle selected for the presence of the *DRB3*11* allele carry less infected lymphocytes than other infected animals [107].

Based on these previous reports found in literature about the association of *BoLA* polymorphisms with PL development or the number of BLV-infected lymphocytes in peripheral blood up to 1998, we decided to evaluate the association between the BLV infection phenotypes described above and *BoLA-DRB3* genotype. Various molecular methods were used for the genotyping of *BoLA-DRB3* exon 2 (the only one expressed from *BoLA-DRB3* gene). In a first instance, we used the PCR-restriction fragment length polymorphism (PCR-RFLP) method, which can differentiate only 57 different alleles (designated by the nomenclature based on this method). The PCR-sequence specific oligonucleotides polymorphisms (PCR-SSOP) is an alternative method which is more specific, allowing the identification of 104 alleles from the 130 described by sequencing, and defines the alleles according to the nomenclature adopted by the International Society for Animal Genetics [34].

Xu et al. [56] described a correlation between *BoLA-DRB3*11* allele and PL in Holstein cattle. The allele **11* (identifiable by PCR-RFLP) can be differentiated into two variants: *BoLA-DRB3*0901* and *BoLA-DRB3*0902* by using PCR-SSOP or by sequencing. By studying the genotype of 230 BLV-infected cattle belonging to seven dairy herds, we found that allele *BoLA-DRB3*11* was significantly associated with the LPL phenotype (odds ratio (OR) = 5.82; p < 0.0001); however, the subtype *BoLA-DRB3*0902,* which is the most prevalent subtype of allele *11 in our population, showed a stronger association with the LPL phenotype (OR = 8.24; p < 0.0001) than allele **11* itself. Allele *BoLA-DRB3*1701* also showed significant association with LPL profile (OR = 3.46; p < 0.0055). The HPL phenotype was significantly associated (OR = 0.36; p < 0.0005) with only one allele: *BoLA-DRB3*1501* (allele **16* as determined by PCR-RFLP). According to these associations, the DRB3 alleles were assigned to three categories: resistant (R) if the allele was associated with LPL phenotype, susceptible (S) if the allele was associated with HPL phenotype, and neutral (N) if the allele was not associated with any phenotype [53].

It is concluded that the host genetic background influences BLV infection phenotype development and that allele *BoLA-DRB3*0902* appears to be, up to now, the best candidate marker of BLV resistance in Argentinean Holstein cattle. The penetrance of *BoLA-DRB*0902* allele for the LPL phenotype is notably high compared to the penetrance of MHC alleles in other systems which, in general, is much lower (about 10 %). More than 80 % of cattle carrying the *BoLA-DRB3*0902* allele develop LPL when naturally or experimentally infected with BLV [53, 108, 109]. However, only one third of LPL cattle harbors the *BoLA-DRB3*0902* allele [53]. This finding suggests that other genetic or epigenetic factors might be involved in the regulation of BLV proviral load.

3.5. Influence of resistance-associated alleles on specific immune response and infectivity of LPL cattle

Cattle with LPL phenotype were grouped according to the presence of alleles associated to the LPL phenotype (i.e., R alleles **0902* and **1701*) in their genotype. **Table 2** shows the average anti-BLVgp51 antibody titer for each group and the resulting classification of cattle according to the level of antibody response against the main envelope glycoprotein of BLV. The R alleles *BoLA-DRB3*0902* and *BoLA-DRB3*1701* were significantly associated with low antibody titers against both BLVgp51 and BLVp24 [110]. Important differences were observed in the infectivity of the blood from cattle in each group, as determined by the sheep bioassay. While all lambs inoculated with blood from LPL cattle not harboring any allele R or harboring one R allele (**0902* or **1701*) in heterozygosis were infected, only one from six lambs inoculated with 100 ml of blood from LPL cattle with R/R genotype acquired the infection. From these results, it seems that LPL cattle carrying two R alleles have an increased ability to restrict BLV replication [108].

It is unlikely that BLV-infected LPL cattle would be a source of infection for BLV-free animals, as large volumes of blood are never exchanged between animals under usual management practices and natural breeding in dairy farms.

***BoLA-DRB3* genotype**	**n**	**BLVgp51 antibody titer**[a]	**Classification**[b]	**Infectivity**[c]
Without allele R	54	662.3	Medium or high responders	6/6
Allele R in heterozygosis	34	344.3	Medium or low responders	4/4
Allele R in homozygosis	9	275.0	Extremely low responders	1/6

[a] Average
[b] Classification was done according to the level of antibody titer against BLVgp51.
[c] Infectivity was assessed by inoculating 100 ml of blood in lambs. Number of lambs infected/number of lambs inoculated

Table 2. Grouping of BLV-infected cattle with LPL phenotype, according to the presence of alleles associated with resistance (R) in their genotype.

3.6. Strategies to control BLV infection

BLV control and eradication programs based on culling infected animals have been accepted and implemented successfully in several western European countries. In dairy farms with low prevalence of BLV infection, the cost of implementing these programs is less than the total cost caused by BLV infection [111]. However, in herds where the prevalence of infection is high, the feasibility of implementation of these programs depends on the official compensation to producers for the removal of BLV-positive animals. In Argentina, not only there is no official BLV control program, but official apathy since the 1970s has been the best ally for the lush spread of BLV in all dairy regions, including Patagonia. By 1995, the failure of the voluntary control program of BLV proposed by the National Authority in Animal Heath (Resolution 337/94 from SENASA) was the indicator that Argentina had lost the opportunity to reduce the spread of BLV by means of serological testing and culling and to protect the scarce herds and regions that were still free of BLV.

To limit the spread of BLV, infected cattle are often eliminated on the basis of their risk of transmitting the infection to other cattle. Among BLV-infected cattle, those with PL are considered the most efficient transmitters because they harbor a high percentage of infected lymphocytes in peripheral blood [112] and consequently have HPL [107]. Furthermore, although not all PL animals develop lymphosarcoma, in approximately two thirds of cases, neoplasia is preceded by PL. The application of control plans based on hematological tests and elimination of PL animals has failed to control not only BLV infection but also the associated lymphosarcoma. In 1959, Denmark implemented an eradication program based on the occurrence of clinical lymphosarcoma and the identification of PL cattle by using the Bendixen hematological keys [113]. Affected herds were quarantined, and indemnity was offered to induce owners to have slaughtered their entire herd. This herd-slaughter policy was continued until 1982. However, when the serological tests were introduced, some herds which were classified as leucosis-free based on the hematological keys were found to be infected [77]. One of the major causes of this failure was probably due to the presence of HPL animals that do not present PL. These non-PL HPL animals are as efficient as PL cattle to transmit the BLV, and it is likely that the animals that develop lymphosarcoma without a previous stage of PL also belong to this group of cattle. Therefore, the corrective management based in classification of animals according to HPL and LPL phenotypes should be safer that the plan based on traditional hematological classification (PL and non-PL).

4. Genetic selection of resistant animals

The genetic selection of resistant animals would be an efficient strategy for controlling the spread of BLV in the host and, therefore, to reduce the occurrence of clinical lymphosarcoma. We have shown that, in the Holstein breed, the *BoLA-DRB3*0902* allele is the best molecular marker for the selection of resistant animals. The *BoLA-DRB3* gene is highly polymorphic, with 130 alleles described so far. The allele frequency of the **0902* allele is relatively high (5–10 %) at the population level; therefore, it is possible to easily increase its frequency by directed crossbreeding or artificial insemination. At the herd level, it is essential that these resistant animals disrupt the transmission of BLV to uninfected animals. Hence, the effectiveness of this procedure would depend on the accuracy of the premise that BLV-infected LPL cattle harboring *BoLA-DRB3*0902* marker do not transmit the virus to BLV-negative cattle under normal breeding conditions in commercial dairy herds.

4.1. The proof of concept

In order to test this premise, an experiment was carried out in a commercial dairy herd located in a subtropical region of Argentina, having extreme environmental conditions (experimental dairy herd). In the experimental dairy herd, BLV-free and BLV-infected LPL-*BoLA-DRB3*0902* animals cohabited for 20 months. This period included two summers during which BLV-infected and BLV-uninfected cattle were exposed to heat stress and to a high density and varied population of bloodsucking insects that continuously fed on the animals. As is usual in any commercial dairy herd, the cattle population was dynamic, and necessary replacements were made according to production needs and milk production requirements, which were within expected parameters in the region. Nevertheless, only previously characterized animals (BLV-free or BLV-infected LPL-*BoLA-DRB3*0902* animals) were introduced to the experimental herd. Normal management practices and production requirements were maintained in the herd. We examined the spread of BLV in the experimental herd and also in other four local commercial herds in which no selection of cattle was made. The incidence rates observed in these four herds were between 0.06 and 0.17 cases per 100 cattle-days. The observed incidence rate explains the increase of prevalence registered in the region from 2002–2003 to 2010–2011 [114, 115]. In contrast, in the experimental herd, no new BLV-infected animals were detected, and as a corollary, the incidence rate was zero. These results indicate that LPL-*BoLA-DRB3*0902* cattle do indeed disrupt the BLV transmission chain and that selection of cattle carrying this allele represents a promising approach to control the virus [116].

The results presented are the base of a BLV control strategy based on genetic selection of resistant animals, using *BoLA-DRB3*0902* allele as molecular selection marker. The idea is to gradually replace HPL cattle in high-prevalence herds with *BoLA-DRB3.2*0902* harboring cattle. The expected increase in herd resistance to BLV would block the transmission of BLV, thereby counteracting the main epidemiological advantage of BLV, i.e., its transmission.

4.2. Influence of resistance and susceptibility-associated alleles on other health and productive traits

Due to the relevant role of MHC genes in the immune response, a potential risk in expanding or segregating *BoLA*-selected populations of cattle is that it might increase susceptibility to other common viruses. A special concern is raised by the strong association found between *BoLA-DRB3*0902* and *BoLA-DRB3*1701* and low antibody titer against major BLV structural proteins. This phenomenon, which may depend on host genetic factors, might influence the host response to other viruses requiring, unlike BLV, strong and long-lasting humoral immune response in order to prevent infection. Therefore, we determined the association between antibody titer against three widespread bovine viruses and *BoLA-DRB3* gene polymorphism. These three viruses, the bovine viral diarrhea virus (BVDV), the bovine herpesvirus type 1 (BHV-1), and the foot and mouth disease virus (FMDV), which are spread in most or several countries all over the world, cause diseases and syndromes that negatively affect the economic performance of the dairy and beef cattle industries. Protection against these three viruses is achieved when high titers of neutralizing antibodies are raised. No association was found between neutralizing antibody titers against FMDV, BVDV, or BHV-1 and polymorphism of the *BoLA-DRB3* gene [110]. Therefore, increasing *BoLA*-selected BLV-resistant cattle or segregating *BoLA* alleles associated with BLV susceptibility would not affect the resistance or susceptibility to BVDV, BHV-1, or FMDV infection. Further studies involving other parameters, such as the persistence or viral load status concerning FMDV, BHV-1, and BVDV, and their association to *BoLA-DRB3* polymorphism, are needed. These parameters would probably represent a better indicator of resistance against the aforementioned viruses.

Preliminary data obtained from endemic areas showed that there is no association between the allele *BoLA-DRB3*0902* and infection with BVDV, bovine herpesvirus type 4 (BoHV-4), and *Neospora caninum* [117]. A recent study also showed no association of the aforementioned allele with infection by *Mycobacterium bovis (M. bovis)*, although this observation should be confirmed in a more extensive study. Moreover, it was shown that the ability of cattle carrying resistance-associated marker to control BLV and to progress to LPL phenotype was not altered by *M. bovis* coinfection [118].

Alleles *BoLA-DRB3*0902* (or *11 as determined by PCR-RFLP) and *BoLA-DRB3*1701* (or *12 as determined by PCR-RFLP) are associated with resistance to intramammary infection and higher production traits [119, 120]. Thus, expanding the population of cattle harboring these alleles in order to control BLV infection would also increase resistance to mastitis. When targeting BLV control by means of genetic selection, animals carrying alleles associated to susceptibility, such as *BoLA-DRB3*1501*, are not desired. This allele did not show association with antibody titer against FMDV, BHV-1, or BVDV [110] nor it affected productive traits [45]. *BoLA-DRB3*1501* has been previously associated with high somatic cell score (SCS) in milk [44, 121]. Thus, if we are to decrease the frequency of the *BoLA-DRB3*1501* allele in order to control BLV infection, the SCS of the cattle population would additionally be reduced. It has been reported that BLV infection is frequently associated with an increase in SCS [122–124]. It is conceivable that this association derives from host genetic susceptibility to both conditions, probably conferred by *BoLA-DRB3*1501* allele.

Up to date, the presence of *BoLA-DRB3*0902* allele in the genotype of Holstein cattle neither has it been associated with susceptibility to any infectious disease nor with negative effects on production or reproductive traits.

4.3. Concluding remarks

We have proposed a BLV control and eradication program based on genetic selection. This plan is based on two main premises: (1) the development of LPL phenotype (BLV-resistant cattle) can be predicted by a marker (*BoLA-DRB3*0902*) that is transmitted to the progeny by controlled crossbreeding, and (2) BLV-infected cattle with LPL phenotype do not transmit the virus.

The *BoLA-DRB3*0902* heterozygous animals comply these two premises. This marker has a penetrance of 82 % and its pattern of inheritance is codominant. *BoLA-DRB3*0902* animals with LPL phenotype did not transmit the infection at herd level in natural conditions, and under experimental conditions, it was required to inoculate a large volume of blood to infect sheep. Finally, up the date, the *BoLA-DRB3*0902* allele has not been associated with susceptibility to other infectious agents, nor has it affected production or reproduction traits.

The BLV control and eradication program has been designed in two steps: as the first step, HPL cattle should be replaced by cattle harboring the *BoLA-DRB3*0902* marker. Once culling of HPL animals has been completed, as the second step, LPL cattle should be replaced by BLV-negative cattle. The selected animals for the replacement in the first step should carry the *BoLA-DRB3*0902* allele in heterozygosis with other alleles not associated with any BLV phenotype [53]. Finally, it should be mentioned that a potential risk exists in expanding or segregating *BoLA* genotype-selected populations, which might increase susceptibility to other infectious agents.

5. Conclusions

Among the diversity of genes associated to disease resistance, MHC genes are particularly interesting as they are associated with resistance and susceptibility to a wide range of diseases. Some of these diseases produce important economic losses in livestock. Genetic selection of resistant animals emerges as a natural strategy for the control of infectious diseases, especially when there is no other alternative of control or prevention, as vaccines.

The control of BLV infection based on genetic selection of resistant cattle is presented as a model that may potentially be replicated in other infectious diseases affecting livestock.

Author details

Silvina Elena Gutiérrez[1*], Eduardo Néstor Esteban[1, 3], Claudia María Lützelschwab[1] and Marcela Alicia Juliarena[1, 2]

*Address all correspondence to: segutier@vet.unicen.edu.ar

1 Department of Animal Health and Preventive Medicine, Veterinary Research Center of Tandil (CIVETAN), CIC-CONICET, Faculty of Veterinary Science, National University of the Center of Buenos Aires Province, Tandil, Argentina

2 Department of Animal Production, Veterinary Research Center of Tandil (CIVETAN), CIC-CONICET, Faculty of Veterinary Science, National University of the Center of Buenos Aires Province, Tandil, Argentina

3 Director of BIOALPINA Program (GENIAL/COTANA), Colonia Alpina, Santiago del Estero, Argentina

References

[1] Bishop SC, Axford RFE, Nicholas FW, Owen JB Principles and Methods. In: Bishop SC, Axford RFE, Nicholas FW, Owen JB, editor. Breeding for Disease Resistance in Farm Animals. Wallingford: CAB International; 2010. p. 1-54.

[2] DeFreitas EC, Chesnut RW, Grey HM, Chiller JM. Macrophage-dependent activation of antigen-specific T cells requires antigen and a soluble monokine. Journal of Immunology. 1983;131(1):23-9.

[3] Tyzzer EE. A study of inheritance in mice with reference to their susceptibility to transplantable tumors. The Journal of Medical Research. 1909;21(3):519-73.

[4] Little CC, Tyzzer EE. Further experimental studies on the inheritance of susceptibility to a transplantable tumor, carcinoma (J. W. A.) of the Japanese waltzing mouse. The Journal of Medical Research. 1916;33(3):393-453.

[5] Gorer PA. The genetic and antigenic basis of tumour transplantation. The Journal of Pathology and Bacteriology. 1937;44(3):691-7.

[6] Medawar PB. The behaviour and fate of skin autografts and skin homografts in rabbits: A report to the War Wounds Committee of the Medical Research Council. Journal of Anatomy. 1944;78(Pt 5):176-99.

[7] Bjorkman PJ, Saper MA, Samraoui B, Bennett WS, Strominger JL, Wiley DC. Structure of the human class I histocompatibility antigen, HLA-A2. Nature. 1987;329(6139):506-12.

[8] Bjorkman PJ, Saper MA, Samraoui B, Bennett WS, Strominger JL, Wiley DC. The foreign antigen binding site and T cell recognition regions of class I histocompatibility antigens. Nature. 1987;329(6139):512-8.

[9] Brown JH, Jardetzky TS, Gorga JC, Stern LJ, Urban RG, Strominger JL, et al. Three-dimensional structure of the human class II histocompatibility antigen HLA-DR1. Nature. 1993;364(6432):33-9.

[10] Falk K, Rotzschke O, Stevanovic S, Jung G, Rammensee HG. Allele-specific motifs revealed by sequencing of self-peptides eluted from MHC molecules. Nature. 1991;351(6324):290-6.

[11] Stern LJ, Brown JH, Jardetzky TS, Gorga JC, Urban RG, Strominger JL, et al. Crystal structure of the human class II MHC protein HLA-DR1 complexed with an influenza virus peptide. Nature. 1994;368(6468):215-21.

[12] Allen PM, Matsueda GR, Evans RJ, Dunbar JB, Jr., Marshall GR, Unanue ER. Identification of the T-cell and la contact residues of a T-cell antigenic epitope. Nature. 1987;327(6124):713-5.

[13] Dausset J. Iso-leuko-antibodies. Acta Haematologica. 1958;20(1-4):156-66.

[14] Flajnik MF, Kasahara M. Comparative genomics of the MHC: glimpses into the evolution of the adaptive immune system. Immunity. 2001;15(3):351-62.

[15] Vaiman M, Chardon P, Cohen D. DNA polymorphism in the major histocompatibility complex of man and various farm animals. Animal Genetics. 1986;17(2):113-33.

[16] Horton R, Gibson R, Coggill P, Miretti M, Allcock RJ, Almeida J, et al. Variation analysis and gene annotation of eight MHC haplotypes: the MHC Haplotype Project. Immunogenetics. 2008;60(1):1-18.

[17] Trowsdale J, Knight JC. Major histocompatibility complex genomics and human disease. Annual Review of Genomics and Human Genetics. 2013;14:301-23.

[18] Marsh SGE, Parham P, Barber LD. 3 - The Organization of HLA Genes Within the HLA Complex. The HLA FactsBook. London: Academic Press; 2000. p. 7-13.

[19] Shiina T, Hosomichi K, Inoko H, Kulski JK. The HLA genomic loci map: expression, interaction, diversity and disease. Jouranl of Human Genetics. 2009;54(1):15-39.

[20] Liljedahl M, Kuwana T, Fung-Leung WP, Jackson MR, Peterson PA, Karlsson L. HLA-DO is a lysosomal resident which requires association with HLA-DM for efficient intracellular transport. The EMBO Journal. 1996;15(18):4817-24.

[21] Alfonso C, Karlsson L. Nonclassical MHC class II molecules. Annual Review of Immunology. 2000;18(1):113-42.

[22] Amorena B, Stone WH. Serologically defined (SD) locus in cattle. Science. 1978;201(4351):159-60.

[23] Spooner RL, Leveziel H, Grosclaude F, Oliver RA, Vaiman M. Evidence for a possible major histocompatibility complex (BLA) in cattle. Journal of Immunogenetics. 1978;5(5):325-46.

[24] BGSA C, Elsik CG, Tellam RL, Worley KC, Gibbs RA, Muzny DM, et al. The genome sequence of taurine cattle: a window to ruminant biology and evolution. Science. 2009;324(5926):522-8.

[25] Birch J, Murphy L, MacHugh ND, Ellis SA. Generation and maintenance of diversity in the cattle MHC class I region. Immunogenetics. 2006;58(8):670-9.

[26] IPD. (Immuno Polymorphism Database). MHC Database. BoLA Nomenclature. Cattle: European Bioinformatics Institute; Available from: https://www.ebi.ac.uk/cgi-bin/ipd/mhc/view_nomenclature.cgi?bola.classi.

[27] Ellis SA, Ballingall KT. Cattle MHC: evolution in action? Immunological Reviews. 1999;167:159-68.

[28] Aida Y, Takeshima S, Baldwin CL, Kaushik AK. Bovine immunogenetics. In: Garrick DJ, Ruvinsky A, editors. The genetics of Cattle. 2nd ed. Croydon, UK: CAB International; 2015. p. 153-91.

[29] Shu L, Peng X, Zhang S, Deng G, Wu Y, He M, et al. Non-classical major histocompatibility complex class makes a crucial contribution to reproduction in the dairy cow. The Journal of Reproduction and Development. 2012;58(5):569-75.

[30] Andersson L, Lunden A, Sigurdardottir S, Davies CJ, Rask L. Linkage relationships in the bovine MHC region. High recombination frequency between class II subregions. Immunogenetics. 1988;27(4):273-80.

[31] McShane RD, Gallagher DS, Newkirk H, Taylor JF, Burzlaff JD, Davis SK, et al. Physical localization and order of genes in the class I region of the bovine MHC. Animal Genetics. 2001;32(5):235-9.

[32] Skow LC, Simples SN, Davis SK, Taylor JF, Huang B, Gallagher DH. Localization of bovine lymphocyte antigen (BoLA) DYA and class I loci to different regions of Chromosome 23. Mammalian Genome. 1996;7(5):388-9.

[33] Takeshima S-N, Aida Y. Structure, function and disease susceptibility of the bovine major histocompatibility complex. Animal Science Journal. 2006;77(2):138-50.

[34] IPD. Immuno Polymorphism Database—MHC Database. BoLA Nomenclature, Cattle, BoLA DRB3: European Bioinformatics Institute; Available from: https://www.ebi.ac.uk/cgi-bin/ipd/mhc/view_nomenclature.cgi?bola.drb3.

[35] Miyasaka T, Takeshima SN, Sentsui H, Aida Y. Identification and diversity of bovine major histocompatibility complex class II haplotypes in Japanese Black and Holstein cattle in Japan. Journal of Dairy Science. 2012;95(1):420-31.

[36] Shalhevet D, Da Y, Beever JE, van Eijk MJ, Ma R, Lewin HA, et al. Genetic mapping of the LMP2 proteasome subunit gene to the BoLA class IIb region. Immunogenetics. 1995;41(1):44-6.

[37] Behl JD, Verma NK, Tyagi N, Mishra P, Behl R, Joshi BK. The major histocompatibility complex in bovines: a review. ISRN Veterinary Science. 2012;2012:872710.

[38] Childers CP, Newkirk HL, Honeycutt DA, Ramlachan N, Muzney DM, Sodergren E, et al. Comparative analysis of the bovine MHC class IIb sequence identifies inversion breakpoints and three unexpected genes. Animal Genetics. 2006;37(2):121-9.

[39] Ballingall KT, Ellis SA, MacHugh ND, Archibald SD, McKeever DJ. The DY genes of the cattle MHC: expression and comparative analysis of an unusual class II MHC gene pair. Immunogenetics. 2004;55(11):748-55.

[40] Ballingall KT, McKeever DJ. Conservation of promoter, coding and intronic regions of the non-classical MHC class II DYA gene suggests evolution under functional constraints. Animal Genetics. 2005;36(3):237-9.

[41] Ballingall K, MacHugh N, Taracha E, Mertens B, McKeever D. Transcription of the unique ruminant class II major histocompatibility complex-DYA and DIB genes in dendritic cells. European Journal of Immunology. 2001;31(1):82-6.

[42] FAO. Animal Genetic Resources and Resistance to Disease. Rome, Italy: Food and Agriculture Organization of the Uniated Nations (FAO); 2015.

[43] Weigel KA, Freeman AE, Kehrli ME, Jr., Stear MJ, Kelley DH. Association of class I bovine lymphocyte antigen complex alleles with health and production traits in dairy cattle. Journal of Dairy Science. 1990;73(9):2538-46.

[44] Dietz AB, Cohen ND, Timms L, Kehrli ME, Jr. Bovine lymphocyte antigen class II alleles as risk factors for high somatic cell counts in milk of lactating dairy cows. Journal of Dairy Science. 1997;80(2):406-12.

[45] Sharif S, Mallard BA, Wilkie BN, Sargeant JM, Scott HM, Dekkers JC, et al. Associations of the bovine major histocompatibility complex DRB3 (BoLA-DRB3) with production traits in Canadian dairy cattle. Animal Genetics. 1999;30(2):157-60.

[46] Glass EJ. Genetic variation and responses to vaccines. Animal Health Research Reviews/ Conference of Research Workers in Animal Diseases. 2004;5(2):197-208.

[47] Glass EJ, Baxter R, Leach RJ, Jann OC. Genes controlling vaccine responses and disease resistance to respiratory viral pathogens in cattle. Veterinary Immunology and Immunopathology. 2012;148(1-2):90-9.

[48] Raadsma HW, Gray GD, Woolaston RR. Breeding for disease resistance in Merino sheep in Australia. Revue Scientifique et Technique. 1998;17(1):315-28.

[49] Duangjinda M, Jindatajak Y, Tipvong W, Sriwarothai J, Pattarajinda V, Katawatin S, et al. Association of BoLA-DRB3 alleles with tick-borne disease tolerance in dairy cattle in a tropical environment. Veterinary Parasitology. 2013;196(3-4):314-20.

[50] Shyma KP, Gupta JP, Singh V. Breeding strategies for tick resistance in tropical cattle: a sustainable approach for tick control. Journal of Parasitic Diseases. 2015;39(1):1-6.

[51] Untalan PM, Pruett JH, Steelman CD. Association of the bovine leukocyte antigen major histocompatibility complex class II DRB3*4401 allele with host resistance to the Lone Star tick, Amblyomma americanum. Veterinary Parasitology 2007;145(1-2):190-5.

[52] Maillard JC, Chantal I, Berthier D, Thevenon S, Sidibe I, Razafindraibe H. Molecular immunogenetics in susceptibility to bovine dermatophilosis: a candidate gene approach and a concrete field application. Annals of the New York Academy of Sciences. 2002;969:92-6.

[53] Juliarena MA, Poli M, Sala L, Ceriani C, Gutierrez S, Dolcini G, et al. Association of BLV infection profiles with alleles of the BoLA-DRB3.2 gene. Animal Genetics. 2008;39(4):432-8.

[54] Miyasaka T, Takeshima SN, Jimba M, Matsumoto Y, Kobayashi N, Matsuhashi T, et al. Identification of bovine leukocyte antigen class II haplotypes associated with variations in bovine leukemia virus proviral load in Japanese Black cattle. Tissue Antigens. 2013;81(2):72-82.

[55] Nagaoka Y, Kabeya H, Onuma M, Kasai N, Okada K, Aida Y. Ovine MHC class II DRB1 alleles associated with resistance or susceptibility to development of bovine leukemia virus-induced ovine lymphoma. Cancer Research. 1999;59(4):975-81.

[56] Xu A, van Eijk MJ, Park C, Lewin HA. Polymorphism in BoLA-DRB3 exon 2 correlates with resistance to persistent lymphocytosis caused by bovine leukemia virus. Journal of Immunology1993. p. 6977-85.

[57] Schwab AE, Geary TG, Baillargeon P, Schwab AJ, Fecteau G. Association of BoLA DRB3 and DQA1 alleles with susceptibility to Neospora caninum and reproductive outcome in Quebec Holstein cattle. Veterinary Parasitology. 2009;165(1–2):136-40.

[58] Glass EJ, Crutchley S, Jensen K. Living with the enemy or uninvited guests: functional genomics approaches to investigating host resistance or tolerance traits to a protozoan parasite, Theileria annulata, in cattle. Veterinary Immunology and Immunopathology. 2012;148(1–2):178-89.

[59] Buitkamp J, Filmether P, Stear MJ, Epplen JT. Class I and class II major histocompatibility complex alleles are associated with faecal egg counts following natural, predominantly Ostertagia circumcincta infection. Parasitology Research. 1996;82(8):693-6.

[60] Stear MJ, Bairden K, Bishop SC, Buitkamp J, Epplen JT, Gostomski D, et al. An ovine lymphocyte antigen is associated with reduced faecal egg counts in four-month-old lambs following natural, predominantly Ostertagia circumcincta infection. International Journal for Parasitology. 1996;26(4):423-8.

[61] Liu LX, Zhao SG, Lu HN, Yang QL, Huang XY, Gun SB. Association between polymorphisms of the swine MHC-DQA gene and diarrhoea in three Chinese native piglets. International Journal of Immunogenetics. 2015;42(3):208-16.

[62] Bao WB, Ye L, Zi C, Liu L, Zhu J, Pan ZY, et al. Relationship between the expression level of SLA-DQA and Escherichia coli F18 infection in piglets. Gene. 2012;494(1):140-4.

[63] Goto RM, Wang Y, Taylor RL, Jr., Wakenell PS, Hosomichi K, Shiina T, et al. BG1 has a major role in MHC-linked resistance to malignant lymphoma in the chicken. Proceedings of the National Academy of Sciences of the United States of America. 2009;106(39):16740-5.

[64] Briles WE, Stone HA, Cole RK. Marek's disease: effects of B histocompatibility alloalleles in resistant and susceptible chicken lines. Science. 1977;195(4274):193-5.

[65] Lillehoj HS, Ruff MD, Bacon LD, Lamont SJ, Jeffers TK. Genetic control of immunity to Eimeria tenella. Interaction of MHC genes and non-MHC linked genes influences levels of disease susceptibility in chickens. Veterinary Immunology and Immunopathology. 1989;20(2):135-48.

[66] Banat GR, Tkalcic S, Dzielawa JA, Jackwood MW, Saggese MD, Yates L, et al. Association of the chicken MHC B haplotypes with resistance to avian coronavirus. Developmental and Comparative Immunology. 2013;39(4):430-7.

[67] Maclachlan NJ, Dubovi EJ. Chapter 14: Retroviridae. In: Press A, editor. Fenner's Veterinary Virology. 4th ed.: Elsevier Science; 2011. p. 243-74.

[68] USDA. Bovine Leukosis Virus (BLV) on U.S. Dairy Operations, 2007. 2008.

[69] Samagh BS, Kellar JK, editor. Seroepidemiological survey of bovine leukaemia virus infection in Canadian cattle. Fourth International Symposium on Bovine Leukosis; 1982.

[70] Lorenz RJS, O.C. The epidemiology of enzootic bovine leukosis. In: Burny AaM, M., editor. Developments in Veterinary Virology: Enzootic Bovine Leukosis and Bovine Leukemia Virus. Boston: Martinus Nihoff; 1987. p. 52-68.

[71] Maresca C, Costarelli S, Dettori A, Felici A, Iscaro C, Feliziani F. Enzootic bovine leukosis: report of eradication and surveillance measures in Italy over an 8-year period (2005–2012). Preventive Veterinary Medicine. 2015;119(3–4):222-6.

[72] Nuotio L, Rusanen H, Sihvonen L, Neuvonen E. Eradication of enzootic bovine leukosis from Finland. Preventive Veterinary Medicine. 2003;59(1–2):43-9.

[73] Schwartz I, Levy D. Pathobiology of bovine leukemia virus. Veterinary Research. 1994;25(6):521-36.

[74] Hasselschwert DL, French DD, Hribar LJ, Luther DG, Leprince DJ, Van der Maaten MJ, et al. Relative susceptibility of beef and dairy calves to infection by bovine leukemia virus via tabanid (Diptera: Tabanidae) feeding. Journal of Medical Entomology. 1993;30(2):472-3.

[75] Mirsky ML, Olmstead CA, Da Y, Lewin HA. The prevalence of proviral bovine leukemia virus in peripheral blood mononuclear cells at two subclinical stages of infection. Journal of Virology. 1996;70(4):2178-83.

[76] Panei CJ, Takeshima SN, Omori T, Nunoya T, Davis WC, Ishizaki H, et al. Estimation of bovine leukemia virus (BLV) proviral load harbored by lymphocyte subpopulations in BLV-infected cattle at the subclinical stage of enzootic bovine leucosis using BLV-CoCoMo-qPCR. BMC Veterinary Research. 2013;9:95.

[77] Radostitis O, Gay C, Hinchcliff K, Constable P. Chapter 21: Disease associated with viruses and chlamydia I. In: Elsevier, editor. Veterinary Medicine. 10th ed.: Elsevier; 2007. p. 1209-21.

[78] Hopkins SG, DiGiacomo RF. Natural transmission of bovine leukemia virus in dairy and beef cattle. Veterinary Clinics of North America: Food Animal Practice. 1997;13(1):107-28.

[79] Buxton BA, Schultz RD. Factors affecting the infectivity of lymphocytes from cattle with bovine leukosis virus. Canadian Journal of Comparitive Medicine. 1984;48(4):365-9.

[80] Bartlett PC, Sordillo LM, Byrem TM, Norby B, Grooms DL, Swenson CL, et al. Options for the control of bovine leukemia virus in dairy cattle. Journal of the American Veterinary Medical Association. 2014;244(8):914-22.

[81] Buxton BA, Hinkle NC, Schultz RD. Role of insects in the transmission of bovine leukosis virus: potential for transmission by stable flies, horn flies, and tabanids. American Journal of Veterinary Research. 1985;46(1):123-6.

[82] Erskine RJ, Bartlett PC, Byrem TM, Render CL, Febvay C, Houseman JT. Herd-level determinants of bovine leukaemia virus prevalence in dairy farms. Journal of Dairy Research. 2012;79(4):445-50.

[83] Kobayashi S, Hidano A, Tsutsui T, Yamamoto T, Hayama Y, Nishida T, et al. Analysis of risk factors associated with bovine leukemia virus seropositivity within dairy and beef breeding farms in Japan: a nationwide survey. Research in Veterinary Science. 2014;96(1):47-53.

[84] Ooshiro M, Konnai S, Katagiri Y, Afuso M, Arakaki N, Tsuha O, et al. Horizontal transmission of bovine leukemia virus from lymphocytotic cattle, and beneficial effects of insect vector control. Veterinary Record. 2013;173(21):527.

[85] Romero CH, Cruz GB, Rowe CA. Transmission of bovine leukaemia virus in milk. Tropical Animal Health and Production. 1983;15(4):215-8.

[86] Dimmock CK, Chung YS, MacKenzie AR. Factors affecting the natural transmission of bovine leukaemia virus infection in Queensland dairy herds. Australian Veterinary Journal. 1991;68(7):230-3.

[87] Lassauzet ML, Johnson WO, Thurmond MC, Stevens F. Protection of colostral antibodies against bovine leukemia virus infection in calves on a California dairy. Canadian Journal of Veterinary Research. 1989;53(4):424-30.

[88] Ott SL, Johnson R, Wells SJ. Association between bovine-leukosis virus seroprevalence and herd-level productivity on US dairy farms. Preventive Veterinary Medicine. 2003;61(4):249-62.

[89] Rodriguez SM, Florins A, Gillet N, de Brogniez A, Sanchez-Alcaraz MT, Boxus M, et al. Preventive and therapeutic strategies for bovine leukemia virus: lessons for HTLV. Viruses. 2011;3(7):1210-48.

[90] Gutierrez SE, Dolcini GL, Arroyo GH, Rodriguez Dubra C, Ferrer JF, Esteban EN. Development and evaluation of a highly sensitive and specific blocking enzyme-linked immunosorbent assay and polymerase chain reaction assay for diagnosis of bovine leukemia virus infection in cattle. American Journal of Veterinary Research. 2001;62(10):1571-7.

[91] Juliarena M, Gutierrez S, Ceriani C. Chicken antibodies: a useful tool for antigen capture ELISA to detect bovine leukaemia virus without cross-reaction with other mammalian antibodies. Veterinary Research Communications. 2007;31(1):43-51.

[92] Juliarena MA, Gutierrez SE, Ceriani C. Determination of proviral load in bovine leukemia virus-infected cattle with and without lymphocytosis. American Journal of Veterinary Research. 2007;68(11):1220-5.

[93] Dube S, Abbott L, Dube DK, Dolcini G, Gutierrez S, Ceriani C, et al. The complete genomic sequence of an in vivo low replicating BLV strain. Virology Journal. 2009;6:120.

[94] Burny A, Cleuter Y, Kettmann R, Mammerickx M, Marbaix G, Portetelle D, et al. Bovine leukaemia: facts and hypotheses derived from the study of an infectious cancer. Cancer Surveys. 1987;6(1):139-59.

[95] Juliarena MA, Lendez PA, Gutierrez SE, Forletti A, Rensetti DE, Ceriani MC. Partial molecular characterization of different proviral strains of bovine leukemia virus. Archives of Virology. 2013;158(1):63-70.

[96] Croshaw JE, Jr., Abt DA, Marshak RR, Hare WC, Switzer J, Ipsen J, et al. Pedigree studies in bovine lymphosarcoma. Annals of the New York Academy of Sciences. 1963;108:1193-202.

[97] Ferrer JF. Bovine lymphosarcoma. Advances in Veterinary Science and Comparitive Medicine. 1980;24:1-68.

[98] Lewin HA, Bernoco D. Evidence for BoLA-linked resistance and susceptibility to subclinical progression of bovine leukaemia virus infection. Animal Genetics. 1986;17(3):197-207.

[99] Palmer C, Thurmond M, Picanso J, Brewer AW, Bernoco D, editor. Susceptibility of cattle to bovine leukemia virus infection associated with BoLA type. 91st Annual Meeting of the United States Animal Health Association; 1987; Richmond, VA, EUA: Animal Health Association.

[100] Lewin HA, Wu MC, Stewart JA, Nolan TJ. Association between BoLA and subclinical bovine leukemia virus infection in a herd of Holstein-Friesian cows. Immunogenetics. 1988;27(5):338-44.

[101] Stear MJ, Dimmock CK, Newman MJ, Nicholas FW. BoLA antigens are associated with increased frequency of persistent lymphocytosis in bovine leukaemia virus infected cattle and with increased incidence of antibodies to bovine leukaemia virus. Animal Genetics. 1988;19(2):151-8.

[102] Lewin HA. Disease resistance and immune response genes in cattle: strategies for their detection and evidence of their existence. Journal of Dairy Science. 1989;72(5):1334-48.

[103] Zanotti M, Poli G, Ponti W, Polli M, Rocchi M, Bolzani E, et al. Association of BoLA class II haplotypes with subclinical progression of bovine leukaemia virus infection in Holstein-Friesian cattle. Animal Genetics. 1996;27(5):337-41.

[104] Zavala-Ruiz Z, Sundberg EJ, Stone JD, DeOliveira DB, Chan IC, Svendsen J, et al. Exploration of the P6/P7 region of the peptide-binding site of the human class II major histocompatability complex protein HLA-DR1. The Journal of Biological Chemistry. 2003;278(45):44904-12.

[105] Tiwari JL, Terasaki PI. HLA-DR and disease associations. Progress in Clinical and Biological Research. 1981;58:151-63.

[106] Aida Y. Influence of host genetic differences on leukemogenesis Induced by bovine leukaemia virus. AIDS Research and Human Retroviruses 2001; 17 (supplement 1), S12. doi:10.1089/088922201750252223.

[107] Mirsky ML, Olmstead C, Da Y, Lewin HA. Reduced bovine leukaemia virus proviral load in genetically resistant cattle. Animal Genetics. 1998;29(4):245-52.

[108] Juliarena M. Contribution to the study of the role of virus and host in the infection profile caused by Bovine Leukemia Virus. Doctoral Thesis FCV-UNCPBA. 2008.

[109] Esteban EN, Poli M, Poiesz B, Ceriani C, Dube S, Gutierrez S, et al. Bovine leukemia virus (BLV), proposed control and eradication programs by marker assisted breeding of genetically resistant cattle. In: Rechi LJ, editor. Animal Genetics. Hauppauge, NY, USA: Nova Science Publishers, Inc.; 2009. p. 107-30.

[110] Juliarena MA, Poli M, Ceriani C, Sala L, Rodriguez E, Gutierrez S, et al. Antibody response against three widespread bovine viruses is not impaired in Holstein cattle carrying bovine leukocyte antigen DRB3.2 alleles associated with bovine leukemia virus resistance. Journal of Dairy Science. 2009;92(1):375-81.

[111] Rhodes JK, Pelzer KD, Johnson YJ. Economic implications of bovine leukemia virus infection in mid-Atlantic dairy herds. Journal of the American Veterinary Medical Association. 2003;223(3):346-52.

[112] Esteban EN, Thorn RM, Ferrer JF. Characterization of the blood lymphocyte population in cattle infected with the bovine leukemia virus. Cancer Research. 1985;45(7):3225-30.

[113] Bendixen HJ. Bovine enzootic leukosis. Advances in Veterinary Science 1965;10:129-204.

[114] Revelli GRS, O.A. Prevalencia de leucosis enzoótica bovina en la zona noroeste de Santa Fe y sur de Santiago del Estero, Argentina. Revue de Médecine Vétérinaire (Bogotá). 2004;85(4):135-8.

[115] Barrios CN, Rensetti DE, Revelli GR, Ceriani MC, Trabattoni E, Esteban EN, Juliarena M, editor. En 2012, al norte del paralelo 34°S, el virus de la leucosis bovina infectaría más del 99% de los tambos con endemias en rodeos de carne. Reunión Anual de la Sociedad Argentina de Virología; 2012.

[116] Juliarena MA, Barrios CN, Ceriani MC, Esteban EN. Hot topic: Bovine leukemia virus (BLV)-infected cows with low proviral load are not a source of infection for BLV-free cattle. Journal of Dairy Science. 2016;99(6):4586-9.

[117] Juliarena MA, Rensetti D, Favier P, Morán PE, Pérez SE, Carignano HA, Basigalupe D, Poli M, Esteban EN, Gogorza LM. Study of the association between the presence of BoLA DRB3*0902 and infection by bovine viral diarrhea virus, bovine herpesvirus-4 and neosporacaninum. Revista Argentina de Microbiología. 2011;Supl 1:140.

[118] Lützelschwab CM, Forletti A, Cepeda R, Esteban EN, Confalonieri O, Gutiérrez SE. Co-infection with Mycobacterium bovis does not alter the response to bovine leukemia virus in BoLA DRB3*0902, genetically resistant cattle. Research in Veterinary Science. http://dx.doi.org/10.1016/j.rvsc.2016.09.002

[119] Dietz AB, Detilleux JC, Freeman AE, Kelley DH, Stabel JR, Kehrli ME, Jr. Genetic association of bovine lymphocyte antigen DRB3 alleles with immunological traits of Holstein cattle. Journal of Dairy Science. 1997;80(2):400-5.

[120] Rupp R, Hernandez A, Mallard BA. Association of bovine leukocyte antigen (BoLA) DRB3.2 with immune response, mastitis, and production and type traits in Canadian Holsteins. Journal of Dairy Science. 2007;90(2):1029-38.

[121] Kelm SC, Detilleux JC, Freeman AE, Kehrli ME, Jr., Dietz AB, Fox LK, et al. Genetic association between parameters of inmate immunity and measures of mastitis in periparturient Holstein cattle. Journal of Dairy Science. 1997;80(8):1767-75.

[122] Bojarojc-Nosowicz BK, E. Somatic cell count and chemical composition of milk in naturally BLV-infected cows with different phenotypes of blood leukocyte acid phosphatase. Archiv Tierzucht, Dummerstorf. 2006;49(1):17-28.

[123] Abdalla EA, Weigel KA, Byrem TM, Rosa GJM. Short communication: Genetic correlation of bovine leukosis incidence with somatic cell score and milk yield in a US Holstein population. Journal of Dairy Science. 2016;99(3):2005-9.

[124] Yoshida T, Furuta H, Kondo Y, Mukoyama H. Association of BoLA-DRB3 alleles with mastitis resistance and susceptibility in Japanese Holstein cows. Animal Science Journal. 2012;83(5):359-66.

Section 4

Veterinary Genetics and Future

Chapter 7

New Advances in NGS Technologies

Edo D'Agaro

Additional information is available at the end of the chapter

http://dx.doi.org/10.5772/66924

Abstract

In the next-generation sequencing (NGS) methods, a DNA molecule of an individual is broken down into many small fragments to make up the so-called sequencing library. These small fragments serve as a template for the synthesis of numerous complementary fragments (called reads). Every small piece of the original DNA is copied many times in a variable number of reads. Depending on the desired accuracy level, it is possible to set the system to achieve a certain level of coverage, i.e., a number of reads per fragment. A level of 30X coverage is already sufficient for the routine diagnosis of most of the Mendelian diseases. All the sequences are then transferred into a computer and aligned with a reference sequence available in the international databases. By this way, all sequences of reads can be recomposed as a fine puzzle to obtain the sequence of a single gene or whole genome. The NGS machines, available today, are very flexible devices. In fact, an NGS sequencer can be used for different types of applications: (1) whole-genome sequencing (WGS): analysis of the entire genome of an individual; (2) whole exome sequencing (WES): analysis of the entire coding genes of an individual; (3) targeted sequencing: analysis of a set of genes or a single gene; (4) transcriptome analysis: analysis of all the RNA produced by specific cells.

Keywords: genomics, NGS, genetic screening, animal diseases, bioinfomatics

1. Introduction

The next-generation sequencing (NGS) technologies, with the capability to produce, at a low price, millions of DNA sequences per analysis, have changed the way to make the genetic analysis in the veterinary and animal fields. In the past few years, the observed reduction of cost and time required to obtain the genomic information (whole genome, whole exome or targeted gene sequencing) have had several repercussions in various disciplines such as animal selection, animal research, genetic disease diagnosis and control, cancer research, and metagenomic studies. The focus of this chapter is to give an updated overview of the next-generation techniques, analyzing the general framework, the bioinformatic analysis pipeline, present applications in the genetic disease detection, problems and future possible developments.

2. Patterns of transmission of genetic diseases

2.1. The hereditary transmission

The hereditary traits are transmitted from the DNA (deoxyribonucleic acid) contained in the chromosomes and in the mitochondria. The gene is formed by regions that encode proteins, the exons, and segments that are not translated, the introns. Genetic diseases are due to inherited mutations, which are changes in DNA sequence and transmitted in familiars in different ways. Several diseases are inherited in a simple way and follow the Mendel's law. These are monogenic or Mendelian diseases. Monogenic diseases can be classified according to their mechanisms of inheritance: autosomal dominant and recessive, X-linked and mitochondrial diseases.

2.2. Autosomal dominant

In the case of dominant disease, the most common genotype is the heterozygous genotype. The disease is transmitted to an average of 50% of the offspring regardless of their sex. The most common cross is between a heterozygous affected (Aa) and a homozygous unaffected (aa). A typical pedigree of an autosomal dominant disease has the following distinguish features:

(a) vertical segregation, with affected individuals in all generations, both males and females;

(b) an equal number of affected males and females;

(c) each affected individual have at least one affected parent.

An autosomal dominant disease may also arise from a new mutation. A risk factor of a new mutation is the parental age. The frequency of new mutations increases proportionally with the age of the parents. One feature of the dominant autosomal diseases is to show a variable expression among the affected individuals, even in the same family. Some autosomal dominant diseases exhibit the phenomenon of anticipation, which consists of an earlier onset and an aggravation of symptoms with the passing generations. Another characteristic of the autosomal dominant diseases is the penetrance, which is the percentage of animals expressing the phenotype over the total number of individuals which carry the mutation. Other genes or the environment can interfere with an occurrence of a disease resulting in a lack of penetrance. In this case, the subject that carries the dominance mutation will not be affected but, 50% of the offspring will manifest the disease with varying degrees.

2.3. Autosomal recessive diseases

The presence of two recessive alleles at the same locus causes the disorders. The most frequent cross is between heterozygous individuals for the mutated allele (healthy carriers of an autosomal recessive disease). A typical pedigree of an autosomal recessive disease has the following distinguish features:

(a) unaffected parents could have affected offspring;

(b) equal number of males and females;

(c) all offspring are affected when parents are affected.

The heterozygous parents will show a risk of 25% to get affected offspring. Inbreeding is the most important risk factor for the occurrence of an autosomal recessive disease.

2.4. Disease linked to the chromosome X

The X chromosome contains hundreds of genes. The dominant or recessive effect is determined in the females because they have two chromosomes. Males have only one X chromosome and therefore they express the recessive mutations (called hemizygous). In this case, the recessive trait is always expressed. If the alleles are different, a female is heterozygous, i.e., a carrier. A typical pedigree of an x-linked dominant disease has the following distinguish features:

(a) each generation usually has an affected individual;

(b) all daughters of an affected male are affected;

(c) all males and females of a heterozygous are affected.

The family tree study shows a zig-zag or diagonal pattern, with a variable number of affected males in the following generations.

A typical pedigree of an x-linked recessive disease has the following distinguish features:

(a) all males of an affected female are affected;.

(b) affected males never transmit the trait to their male offspring;

(c) unaffected parents may have affected offspring.

2.5. Multifactorial diseases

Some genetic diseases show a polygenic and/or multifactorial inheritance. The multifactorial traits can be continuous and measurable, such as the weight, height, blood pressure, or discontinuous, such as congenital heart disease, diabetes, osteoporosis, and cardiovascular disease.

2.6. Mitochondrial disease

The defects in the mitochondrial DNA show a maternal inheritance because mitochondria are transmitted to the offspring by the egg cell. Characteristics of mitochondrial diseases are incomplete penetrance, variable expressivity, and pleiotropy. The phenotypic expression of mitochondrial disorders depends on the ratio of normal and mutated mtDNA present in the cells of various tissues. The organ impairment and its severity depend on the percentage of mutated mitochondria, which is variable in different tissues. Mitochondria are distributed in cells throughout the body and are therefore responsible for pathologies with impairment of different organs and apparatuses.

3. Mutations

A mutation is defined as a stable and heritable modification of the genetic material. The mutation can occur at different levels and change the attitude of the entire genome showing a variation in the number of chromosomes (genomic mutation), a variation in a single chromosome (mutation chromosome) or, it may involve a single gene (gene mutation). Mutations can be spontaneous or induced. The most common causes of mutation can be physical, chemical, or biological factors (called mutagens). The gene mutation can be lethal to the cell or, when the gene is expressed, give rise to senseless, inactive, or less active proteins or, although much rarely, resulted in products with a greater or different activity. Most of the mutations are harmful and only a small percentage appears to be advantageous. The carrier of an unfavorable gene may die before to reproduce (lethal disease). Natural selection tends to reduce mutated genes. Sometimes, however, due to the changing environment, insignificant mutations can be expressed or even turn out to be advantageous and to be favored by natural selection. Genomic and chromosomal mutations, when they are compatible with life, give rise to a more complex phenotypic pattern, because they involve a large number of genes. On the contrary, gene mutations affect the sequence of a single gene and therefore they have an effect only on the functionality of a single protein. A *transition mutation* is one substitution of a purine with a purine or pyrimidine with a pyrimidine while a *transversion mutation* is a substitution between a purine and a pyrimidine. At phenotypic level, effects of mutations can vary from the complete neutrality to a range of events whose gravity depends on the interaction with other genes and with the environment. At the molecular level, a gene mutation consists in a variation of the sequence of a nucleotide of the gene. The normal DNA sequence may change as a result of insertion or deletion of one or more bases. A gene mutation, if it concerns a single point of DNA, i.e., one or a few bases, it is called a point mutation or SNP. The first element to be considered, in assessing the effects of a gene mutation, is what part of the gene has changed. The sequence of a gene is made, in addition to a promoter, of a number of exons interspersed with introns. As is known, the entire sequence of the gene is transcribed, but the intronic fragments are removed during the process of splicing. The exon region of a gene is characterized by the presence of a coding region, which contains the information for the synthesis of the coded protein, and two noncoding regions that are located at the beginning and end of the mRNA molecule (5'UTR and 3'UTR that are transcribed but not translated). Mutations that modify the coding region may have important effects on the translation of the proteins, mutations at the junction between intron and exon can interfere with the recognition of splice sites causing the production of modified transcripts while mutations in the untranslated regions (UTRs) and the introns are often neutral or in some cases may alter the regulatory functions of these regions. The mutations that show (most frequently) phenotypic effects are those affecting the coding regions. Therefore, in this chapter, we will focus on them. In the case of a *silent mutation*, the replacement of a base causes a change in the codon without a change of the amino acid (the genetic code is degenerated and the same amino acid can be coded by more than one codon). For example, if a mutation changes the codon CUA in CUG, as both codons code for the same amino acid leucine, the amino acid does not change. For this reason, a silent mutation has no effect at the level of the protein and thus on the phenotype. In the case of a *missense mutation*, the substitution of a base of a codon with a different base causes the change in the codon function. For example, if the codon AGC, which codes for the amino acid serine, becomes AGA, encoding for the amino acid arginine, during the protein synthesis, an arginine will be inserted instead of a serine. The substitution of an amino acid may therefore change the protein function. Based on the amino acid substitution, the missense mutations are divided into: (a) conservative substitutions: the new amino acid has similar characteristics to the replaced one (neutral mutation); (b) nonconservative substitutions: the new amino acid has different characteristics [e.g. GAG (Glu) changing to GTG (Val)]. The consequences of a missense mutation are more or less serious depending on the physical-chemical characteristics of the two amino acids involved. Characteristics of the amino acids present in the primary structure determine the secondary and tertiary structures of the proteins by means of ionic and hydrophobic interactions. In turn, the correct folding of the protein chain determines its biological functionality. The maintenance of the protein functions depends on the amino acid position and its structural role. In the case of sickle cell disease, due to a missense mutation in the gene of the beta-globin, a polar amino acid (water-soluble, glutamic acid) is replaced by an insoluble apolar amino acid valine. This causes the production of a beta-globin chain resulting in an altered hemoglobin solubility, which in turn causes the characteristic shape of the sickle red blood cells. A gene mutation can change a codon sense in a noncodon sense (*nonsense mutation*). For example, if the codon AAG, coding for lysine, becomes UAG, which is a stop codon, then, the protein synthesis will end prematurely. The synthesized protein is therefore incomplete and, in most cases, it will not be functional. An elongation mutation arises when, a nonsense triplet present in the wild gene, following a base substitution, becomes a triplet "sense," encoding for an amino acid. In this case, the stop triplet is eliminated and the mRNA translation will continue with the formation of a longer protein. Deletions and insertions of bases in the coding region of a gene cause a slippage of the reading code system (*frameshift mutations*). The inclusion or loss of one or more bases causes a slip, resulting in loss of sense of the whole protein. All codons downstream of the mutation change and from that point they are then incorporated into the protein, giving rise to an abnormal protein and almost always nonfunctional. A deletion of an entire portion of a gene can severely alter the three-dimensional protein structure, the chemical properties and functionality. Even in this case, the deletion may lead to a slip of reading (frameshift), determining the loss of a part of the protein. A mutation in a gene can also determine a quantitative variation (not qualitative) of the protein. This occurs when the mutation falls in a regulatory region (i.e., the sequence of the promoter) and modifies the transcription of the gene. A point mutation (by substitution or by insertion/deletion of bases), both in coding and noncoding regions, can give rise to an RFLP (polymorphism of length of the restriction fragments) and to an SNP (single nucleotide polymorphism).

4. DNA sequencing

Over the last 60 years, it has observed a significant increase in the knowledge of animal genomes and the genetic code, starting from the discovery of the structure of DNA in 1953 until the publication of the first draft of the human genome in 2001 [1, 2]. The Sanger sequencing [3], also known as sequencing of the first generation, was the method used to sequence the genome within the project "Human Genome' bringing the entire genome sequence in 2003, after 13 years from the beginning of the project with a cost of $3 billion and the contribution of six different nations. In the recent years, several animal and plant genome sequencing projects have been carried out thanks to the implementation of both molecular biology and computer science innovations [4]. The evolution in parallel of these two sectors has enabled the advent of several next-generation sequencing (NGS) platforms. Nowadays, by means of this new technology, which is more efficient and economic compared to the previous methods, it is possible to sequence a new genome at the cost of less than one thousand euros in a very short time (1–2 days). Furthermore, the cost and time can be greatly reduced by analyzing only the coding regions (exomes). Despite the fact that the exomes are only 1% of the entire genome, by mean of this method, it is possible to identify the 85% of the monogenic diseases.

4.1. Last-generation sequencing (NGS) possible

All NGS methods are characterized by two important phases: a molecular biology step, which goes from the preparation of the sample to the sequencing phase, which allows to carry out, at the same time, more than one reaction and with less dexterity than the Sanger method, and a computerized stage for the analysis of the data. The first part of the process is divided into three steps: *sample preparation, amplification*, and *sequencing*. Sample preparation, which is the common passage for all platforms, is the fragmentation of DNA (dimensions vary from 100 to 800 base pairs (bp) in relation to the platform and the adapters used). The amplification is based on two methods: emulsion or solid PCR amplifications. In the emulsion PCR method, described for the first time by Tawfik Griffiths, the individual molecules of DNA are clonally amplified in micro-compartments consisting of mixtures of water and oil [5]. The adapters bound to individual DNA molecules, hybridize to complementary sequences coating the surface. Cycles of upcoming amplification allow to the formation of "clusters" of folded fragments clonally amplified. All the NGS platforms are characterized by the ability to sequence and massively parallel amplifying the DNA molecules in a clonal or single way. Unlike the Sanger method, where the fragments of different sizes from individual sequencing reactions were separated by electrophoresis, in the NGS technologies, sequencing is accomplished through the repetition of nucleotide extension cycles or oligonucleotide ligations. The principles of sequencing and image acquisition are the peculiar steps that characterize the different platforms on the market. To date, different methods of sequencing are known. The cyclic reversible termination (CRT) sequencing method uses reversible labeled nucleotides. Each sequencing cycle comprises: the incorporation of the nucleotide, the acquisition of the fluorescence, and the cutting of the nucleotide. The subsequent washing step allows the elimination of all nonincorporated nucleotides. At this point, the image for identifying the incorporated nucleotide is captured, followed by a cleavage step that removes the terminator group and the fluorophore. After the elimination, the polymerase can continue the reaction of extension and tie the second nucleotide. This process is used by two types of trading platforms: Illumina and Helicos, which differ in the templates of sequencing. While Illumina uses clonally amplified fragments on a solid surface, Helicos is currently the only commercial platform able to use single DNA molecules. In addition, the acquisition platform of Illumina uses a four-color (the four reversible nucleotides are labeled with a different fluorophore and are dispensed at the same time in the sequencer), while in the Helicos platform, all nucleotides they are labeled with the same fluorophore and are dispensed into the sequencer in a determined hierarchical order.

4.2. Commercial systems for NGS

We describe here the main platforms used for the last-generation sequencing:

Roche 454 system was the first genome sequencer to be marketed in 2004. This system uses the sequencing by synthesis technology known as pyrosequencing. Initially, the 454 sequencing method used reads of 100–150 bp, producing about 200,000 reads, with an output of 20 Mb for each run. In 2008, a new sequencer the 454 GS FLX titanium was produced (reads of 700 bp, with an accuracy after filtering of 99.9%, with an output of 0.7 Gb for run in 24 hours). In 2009, the GS Junior and 454 GS FLX platforms were used to set up a new sequencer with an output of 14 Gb for run. Further developments have led to the production of the GS FLX +, which is able to sequence reads up to 1 kb. The high speed of analysis combined with the long reads is the positive characteristics of this platform. However, the cost of reagents remains a problem to be solved.

Ion Torrent. The method used by Ion Torrent Genome Machine (PGM) is very similar to the Roche 454 system. This platform, instead of using images to capture the incorporated nucleotide, detects the change of pH. The output per run is of 270 Mb with reads of 100–200 bp.

AB SOLiD system. The Applied Biosystems method was first marketed in 2006. This system uses the ligation sequencing method (in both directions) to ligate fluorescently labeled octomers to the DNA fragment. Initially, the length of the reads was only 35 bp and the output of 3 Gb for run. In 2010, the 5500x1 SOLiD platform was released (reads with length of 85 bp, precision of 99.99% and output 30 Gb per run). The main problem of this method is the low length of the reads.

Illumina GA/HiSeq system. In 2006, the Solexa company released the Genomic Analyzer (GA) and in 2007, the company was bought by Illumina. The system uses the sequencing by synthesis method (SBS) and the amplification bridge which is an alternative method of the PCR. At the beginning, the analyzer's output was of 1 Gb for run, after upgraded to 50 Gb. In 2010, the HiSeq 2000 was released with an output of 600 Gb for run and reads of 200 bp. The basic method is to generate a great number of polonies (generated DNA colonies) that are simultaneously sequenced in parallel reactions occurring on the surface of a flow cell. The cost of sequencing is lower compared to the competitors. **Table 1** presents the main NGS platforms.

4.2.1. Third-generation sequencing technologies.

Helicos single-molecule sequencing device: Heliscope method was presented for the first time in 2007. This platform uses a technique that individually analyzes the molecules achieving a greater accuracy. Using this system, you can obtain an output in the order of 28 Gb. However, the main disadvantage of this method remains the low capacity to correctly identify indels,

Platform	Type
Illumina	Sequencing by synthesis
454 Roche	Pyrosequencing
Ion Torrent	Ion semiconductor
ABI Solid	Ligation based sequencing (color spaced)
Oxford nanopore	Nanopore sequencing
Pacific biosciences	Single molecule real time (SMRT)

Table 1. List of sequencing platforms.

with a consequent increase in errors. Another problem is the length of the reads, which has never exceeded 50 bp.

Oxford Nanopore Miniontechnology. Most of the nanopore sequencing technologies are based on the transit of DNA molecules, after the application of an electric potential, through an array of protein nanopores located in a high-salt buffer. Single bases are identified according to the electric change. Several methods have been proposed based on the nanopore technique. Among these, one is produced by Oxford Nanopore (exploits the combination of three molecules), one based on MSpa (a protein). This method can be very useful for identifying infectious diseases and to analyze environmental samples (metagenomic analysis of bacteria, viruses and fungi) without a previous knowledge of the sample composition.

An additional advantage of the third-generation sequencing methods is the production of long reads (>than 10,000 pb and up to 100,000 bp) enabling to analyze insertions, deletions, and translocations [6–9]. Using these technologies and mapping methods, it is possible to study entire chromosome arms.

4.3. NGS data analysis

Although the various sequencing technologies use different methods, they all provide as output the FASTQ sequences. The FASTQ string is the type of information used in molecular biology to store genetic sequences and the related quality scores, namely the score that the algorithm assigns to the string and which is then used to choose the best match against the reference genome. At this point, the bioinformatics analysis is divided into three steps: *alignment*, which search of correspondences between the reads and the reference genome and the *variant calling* that attempts to separate the differences due to genetic mutations and instrumental errors made during the analysis and *filtration and annotation*, which attempt to align the reads to the reference genome.

4.3.1. Alignment

The alignment is the process by which you map short reads to a reference genome. It is a complex task, since the software must compare each reads in all of the reference DNA positions

[8, 10, 11]. It is a computationally challenging passage and wasteful in terms of time. The SAM (sequence alignment map) and BAM (binary alignment map) are the standard file formats for storing the data obtained using the next-generation technologies (NGS). There are many commercially available software, free or on sale, to perform this task. Most software use a method based on indices, which are very fast in the search for all alignment positions (without gaps) in the reference genome. Other algorithms, instead, allow the search for alignments with gaps. The various methods to solve the problem include the use of hash tables (e.g., MAQ, ELAND), algorithms based on Burrows-Wheeler transformation (e.g., BWA, Bowtie, SOAP2), an algorithm that uses a reversible compression method commuting the order of the characters without changing the values; genome-based hash (e.g., Novoalign, SOAP). Some software can take into account of gaps (e.g., BWA, Bowtie2) while others do not (e.g., MAQ, Bowtie).

4.3.2. Variant calling

After the alignment, the DNA sequence can be compared to the reference genome, identifying the possible changes. These variations can be due to genetic diseases or they can be only noise. The complexity of this subject lies in the difficulty to distinguish between the true variations and the sequencing errors [12]. The continuous development and improvement of NGS technologies has brought continuous advantages in this area, improving the quality of analysis [13, 14]. The main difficulty in this kind of analysis is the presence of indels, i.e., phenomena of inserts (insertion) or cancelation (deletion) of DNA segments. In fact, indels are the major cause of false-positives. The number of false-positives increases when using algorithms that do not take it into account of gaps. Another source of errors arises during the preparation of sequences and the PCR analysis. In order to reduce the errors, it is advisable to increase the sensitivity of the PCR analysis, use updated alignment software and a big reference database for getting wider comparisons.

4.3.3. Filtering and annotation

After the alignment and variant calling steps, a list of thousands of potential differences is generated between the genome under study and the reference genome. The next step is then to determine which of these variations are due to sequencing errors. The use of specific filters allows to remove variants that do not follow the models under study and to make annotations. The comparison of reads against a genetic reference tree will find all elements of known function. In addition to the filtration step, the annotation process provides another tool to select and restrict the test sample, applying specific functional models [15]. The low cost of these new instruments is leading to the discovery of a great number of genetic variants and identifying various diseases [16]. For example, it has been observed that about 1300 positions of a gene or a sequence within a chromosome are associated with 200 diseases [17].

4.3.4. Definitions of DNA sequence variants

In general, there are three principal categories of variants:

(a) Causative variants

Variants showing a clear pathogenetic role and associated with a phenotype disease.

(b) Unrelated variants

The most commonly used definition to define this class of variants is "incidental findings."

(c) Variants with undefined functional and clinical effects (variants of uncertain significance, VUS).

Table 2 reports some useful Internet sites for the genetic variant discovery analysis.

SAMTools	http:// mamtools.sourceforce.net
	http//htslib.org
GATK	https://www.broadinstitute.org/gatk
Platypus	http://www.well.eox.ac/platypus
Freebayes	http://github.com/ekg/freebayes
BreakDancer	http://breakdancer.souceforge.net
Dindel	https://sanger.ac.uk/resources/software/dindel

Table 2. List of variant discovery resources (Internet sites).

4.3.5. Example of a variant calling analysis using the galaxy platform (www.galaxy.org)

The protocol in a nutshell:

- Inspect the reads;
- Raw data cleanup/quality trimming;
- Align reads to a reference genome;
- Mark duplicates;
- Combine samples into a single file;
- Realign reads around insertions and deletions (indels);
- Correct inaccurate base qualities (optional);
- Make variant calls, SNVs, indels;
- Annotate the results.

(a) Read quality control

Steps involved and suggested tools:

NGS: QC and manipulation → FastQC

Command line: fastqc

http://dx.doi.org/10.5772/66924

Some of the important outputs of FastQC for our purposes are:

- Quality encoding type: important for quality trimming software;
- Total number of reads: gives you an idea of coverage;
- Presence of highly recurring k-mers;

(b) Quality trimming/cleanup of read files

NGS: QC and manipulation → trimmomatic

Suggested trimmomatic functions:

- Adapter trimming;
- Sliding window trimming;
- Trailing bases quality trimming;
- Leading bases quality trimming;
- Minimum read length.

(c) Genome alignment

Suggested tools:

NGS: Mapping → BWA

NGS: Picard → MarkDuplicates

NGS: SAM Tools → Merge BAM Files

NGS: GATK Tools → Indel Realigner

NGS: GATK Tools → Count Covariates

NGS: GATK Tools → Table Recalibration

(d) Variant calling

NGS: GATK Tools → Unified Genotyper

Possible alternative software:

Varscan http://varscan.sourceforge.net/

(e) Annotation

NGS: GATK Tools → Variant Annotation

Figure 1 shows an example of a variant analysis workflow.

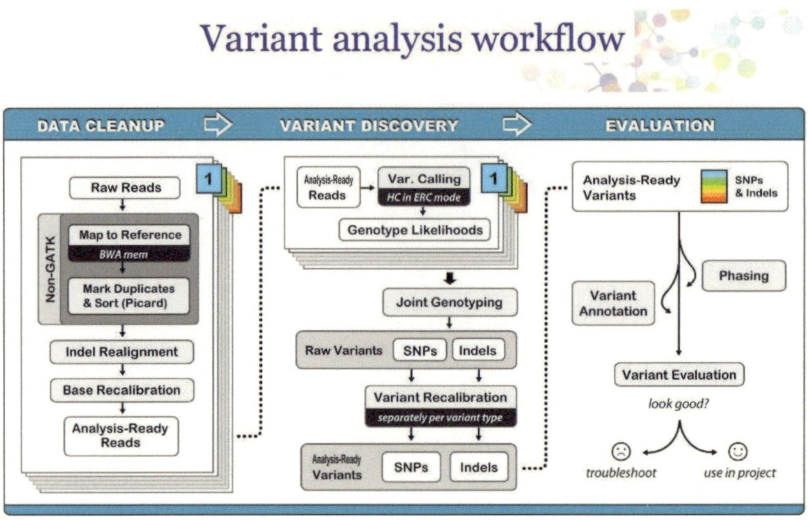

Figure 1. Example of a variant analysis workflow.

4.3.6. Bioinformatic analysis of the NGS data

Genetic testing based on NGS analysis can be divided depending on the width of the portion of the analyzed genome:

(a) sequencing the entire genome (whole genome sequencing; WGS);

(b) sequencing the entire exome (whole exome sequencing; WES) [18];

(c) targeted gene sequencing.

The choice of the different method will take into account several factors:

- *Costs*: since the introduction of the NGS practice, the use of specific panels has been privileged for economic reasons. Nowadays, the cost of the different methods has gradually narrowed and today this aspect is not, in most of the cases, the primary choice element. WES may be, in fact, less expensive of sequencing a panel of genes and, similarly, the cost of WGS is getting closer to that of WES;

- *Purpose*: in general, the NGS techniques find the best applications in the case of high heterogeneity genetic diseases or for the Mendelian diseases in which the gene is not yet been identified;

- *Diagnosis:* direct clinical applications are more and more frequent, especially for the congenital diseases;

- *Sensitivity*: the higher the number of reads of a specific region, the greater will be the sensibility for that particular stretch of DNA. In principle, in the analysis of specific panels, the smaller is the portion of the genome analyzed, the greater is the coverage and then the sensitivity. This is the reason why, for a mosaic alteration, the analysis of known genes shows a greater sensitivity than the WES analysis;

- *Data storage*: in relation to the increasing number of sequenced genomes and data to be analyzed, new bioinformatic platforms for storage and data analysis are needed.

The amount of data generated by NGS platforms is on the order of terabytes (Tb). Software used for data analysis differ according to the NGS technology but, all follow a "pipeline" system of data analysis converting the luminescence images or fluorescence data to "reads" sequences. In this process, defined, "base calling," a quality score value is set for each nucleotide, indicating the probability of an error associated with it. The "quality score" is an important value for selecting the reads during the analysis process. If they fall below a specific level, they are eliminated improving the accuracy of the alignment process. In order to get an adequate efficiency of the alignment, this value should not be below 30. Another limitation for the alignment process is represented by the repeated sequences. The error rates associated with the NGS technologies seem to be higher than the traditional Sanger method. However, the accuracy of the NGS sequencing is increased by means of a repeated and massive reading of each gene fragment, which determines the "coverage" of the genome. The latter parameter represents an essential value in the NGS analysis (value ranging between 20 and 50 times, in relation to the platform used) determining the presence of false negatives (for heterozygous individuals) in the detection of nucleotide variants. At the end of the variant annotation process, the number of identified variants varies in relation to the application of various filters, used to reduce the number of candidates. The filters most commonly used are based on:

- inheritance pattern (autosomal/X-linked, dominant/recessive);
- sharing equal variations in well-characterized families;
- removal of variants already known through the use of public databases (dbSNP);
- based on the potential effect of the change (no sense, missense, changes in splicing sites or insertions and deletions that modify the reading frame);
- prediction of the functional effects of changes through the use of *in silico* bioinformatic tools (SIFT, POLYPHEN, and ANNOVAR software).

4.3.6.1. Advantages of using the NGS technology

Although, in previous decades, the development of the Sanger method has brought many findings in chemistry, automation and miniaturization of the process, only the advent of NGS technologies has led to a significant improvement of quality and speed of the genome analysis [19]. The release of new sequencing platforms and the reduction of costs associated with the NGS technology is the consequence of three factors:

(1) Thousands/millions of sequencing reactions can be conducted in parallel exceeding the limit of 1–96 possible reactions obtainable with a traditional sequencer;

(2) Cloning or amplification of the DNA fragment is, in the new technologies, not necessary or completely automated within the platforms;

(3) Ability to detect the minor allele with high accuracy. This in term allows a better identification of a variant in mosaic sample or heterozygous deletions. The number of times that a DNA fragment is amplified and sequenced is proportional to the abundance of such segment in the original sample.

4.3.6.2. Limits of NGS technology

The NGS technology has, however, some limitations related mostly to the magnitude of data products. In fact, in the NGS results we can observe false positives and false negatives.

False positives can result from:

- an incorrect alignment with the reference sequence. You can overcome this problem using different alignment software;
- systematic sequencing errors. This type of error can be identified in all the samples and removed from the final list [20];
- technical errors of the sequencer. For example, with the pyrosequencing method, a common error was observed using homopolymers longer using the pyrosequencing method, was observed when reading homopolymers longer than 5–6 bases;

False negatives instead come from:

- low coverage;
- low coverage in regions of interest;
- alignment of repeated regions.

The reduction of errors can be obtained increasing the coverage and the quality of DNA fragmentation (fragments of greater size). The implementation of the "paired-end" sequencing, that is able to sequence fragments of a greater length by both ends, allows the analysis of fragments of 5–10 kb. The use of the Sanger method is, however, required at the end of the analysis because the results, obtained using the NGS methods, require to be validated.

4.3.7. Applications of NGS technology

The genome can be assessed globally, only in the coding regions or in target regions. The main interest of the veterinary genetic sector is to study the coding regions as the greater number of diseases is caused by mutations or exonic splicing which alter the correct amino acid sequence of the protein. Indeed, exomes, while constituting only 1% of the genome, are the location of 85% of pathogenetic mutations. The number of mutations known to be associated with a genetic disease exceeds 110,000 variants, in most of 3700 different genes. It was estimated that only half of the Mendelian diseases have a known genetic basis. For these reasons, the scientific research focused mostly on exomes for the identification of new genes [21]. The approach, commonly used in the past, was to identify the transmitted loci associated with the phenotype by means of the segregation or linkage analysis, identifying shared genes of affected individuals in large size families. The advent of WES technology has triggered a rapid growth of the sector (identification of new disease), having the advantage of requiring a limited number of samples. The first successful application of this method has led to the identification of the gene DHODH as causative of Miller syndrome. Since 2010, a large amount of studies have identified new disease-causing mutations, through the exome sequencing method using a reduced number of affected individuals, in various types of diseases including cases of neuropathy, poikiloderma associated with neutropenia, familial exudative vitreoretinopathy, immune disorders, and tumor predisposition. The use of WES allowed to identify some causative mutations also in diseases with high phenotypic heterogeneity where the traditional linkage analysis approach is more difficult. A new area of the development of NGS technology is linked to the identification of new biomarkers or pharmagenomics with the development of personalized therapies. The impact of next-generation sequencing technology on genomics has in turn led to a new revolution in the genetic field changing the nature of genetic trials. The production of a large number of low cost NGS platforms is useful for many applications. These include: new variants discovered by targeted resequencing regions of interest or whole genomes; *de novo* assemblies of bacterial genomes and lower eukaryotes; cataloging of cell, tissues and organism transcriptomes (RNA-Seq); profiling of genome-wide epigenetic marks and chromatin structure using seq-based methods (Chip-seq and Methyl-seq); classification of species and/or discovery of the gene using metagenomic studies. NGS technologies can also accelerate exploration of the natural world [22, 23]. Despite a dramatic increase in the number of complete genome sequences available in public databases, most of the biological diversity, in our world, remains to be explored. Nowadays, *de novo* assembly of NGS data requires the development of new software tools that can overcome the technical limitations of these technologies. In fact, the main limitation is a rapid deterioration in the quality of assembly as the length of reading decreases.

4.3.8. *De novo assembly*

De novo genome assembly is often compared to solving a great puzzle without knowing the picture that we are trying to rebuild [7, 21, 24]. Mathematically, the issue *de novo* assembly is difficult regardless of the method of sequencing. During the *de novo* assembly process, a high number of repeated segments in the genome may cause several errors. The assembler tool should guess the right genome, starting from a great number of alternative options (the number of attempts increases exponentially with a high pattern of repetitions in the genome) [25]. As the technology has evolved, new methods for assembling genomes have continuously changed [26]. Genome sequencers have never been able to read more than a relatively short stretch of DNA at once, with read lengths gradually increasing over time.

Assembly quality: High coverage is necessary to sequence polymorphic alleles within diploid or polyploidy genomes. However, using shorter reads, the coverage should be increased in order to balance the low connectivity of the system and to obtain an optimal assembly. However, some times, a poor assembly process cannot be improved by a higher coverage. In fact, in the case of a high number of long repeated sequences in the genome, a high coverage will never fully compensate for the increasing errors and gaps which are produced during the editing phase. Using paired end technology gaps can be crossed and eliminated [5].

Assembly methods aim to create the most comprehensive reconstruction as possible without introducing errors. The central challenge of assembling the genome is to solve the problem of repetitive sequences. If the DNA reads are random, than the expected number of cases of each sequence will decrease exponentially and the number of repeats in the genome is reduced. However, several genomes may share highly repeated structures which do not allow an easy assembly process [27].

Scaffolding: The phase of scaffolding focuses on repeats to fix linking contig initials in data-driven scaffolds. A scaffold is a collection of contig linked by pair partners, where gaps between contigs between contig might be repeats, in which the gap can in theory be filled or outright gaps that original sequencing project does not capture [6]. If the distances are long enough, the assembler is able to connect contig in nearly all repetitions. Assembler tools may vary in the method how they call the contigs. The great majority of them are based on a combination of two factors: contig length and a number of reads. A contig containing too many reads is called as a repetition. High-copy-number patterns are easy to be identified. On the contrary, the identification of two copies is more difficult) [25]. If the contigs are overlapping in a scaffold, the assembler can merge at this point. Otherwise, the assembler will record a gap inside the scaffold.

Example of de novo assembly using the galaxy platform (www.galaxy.org)

(a) Read quality control

Steps involved and suggested tools:

NGS: QC and manipulation → FastQC: comprehensive QC

Command line: fastqc

Some of the important outputs of FastQC for our purposes are:

- Read length: Will be important in setting maximum k-mer size value for assembly;
- Quality encoding type: Important for quality trimming software;
- % GC: High GC organisms don't tend to assemble well and may have an uneven read coverage distribution;
- Total number of reads: Gives you an idea of coverage;
- Dips in quality near the beginning, middle, or end of the reads: Determines possible trimming/cleanup methods and parameters and may indicate technical problems with the sequencing process/machine run;
- Presence of highly recurring k-mers: May point to contamination of reads with barcodes, adapter sequences, etc.;
- Presence of large numbers of Ns in reads: May point to poor quality sequencing run. You need to trim these reads to remove Ns.

(b) Quality trimming/cleanup of read files

Steps involved and suggested tools:

NGS: QC and manipulation > trimmomatic

Command lines:

- Adapter trimming
- Sliding window trimming
- Trailing bases quality trimming
- Minimum read length

(c) Assembly

Steps involved and suggested tools:

NGS-Assembly → Velvet Optimizer

Possible alternative software:

Spades

SOAP-denovo

MIRA

ALLPATHS

Possible tools for improving your assemblies:

QUAST – http://bioinf.spbau.ru/quast

Mauve

InGAP-SV – https://sites.google.com/site/nextgengenomics/ingap

Semi-automated gap fillers:

Gap filler – http://www.baseclear.com/landingpages/basetools-a-wide-range-of-bioinformatics-solutions/gapfiller/

IMAGE – http://sourceforge.net/apps/mediawiki/image2/

Genome visualizers and editors:

Artemis – http://www.sanger.ac.uk/resources/software/artemis/

IGV – http://www.broadinstitute.org/igv/

Geneious – http://www.geneious.com/

CLC BioWorkbench – http://www.clcbio.com/products/clc-genomics-workbench/

Automated and semi-automated annotation tools:

Prokka – https://github.com/tseemann/prokka

RAST – http://www.nmpdr.org/FIG/wiki/view.cgi/FIG/RapidAnnotationServer

JCVI – http://www.jcvi.org/cms/research/projects/annotation-service/.

Figure 2 shows an example of a genome assembly workflow.

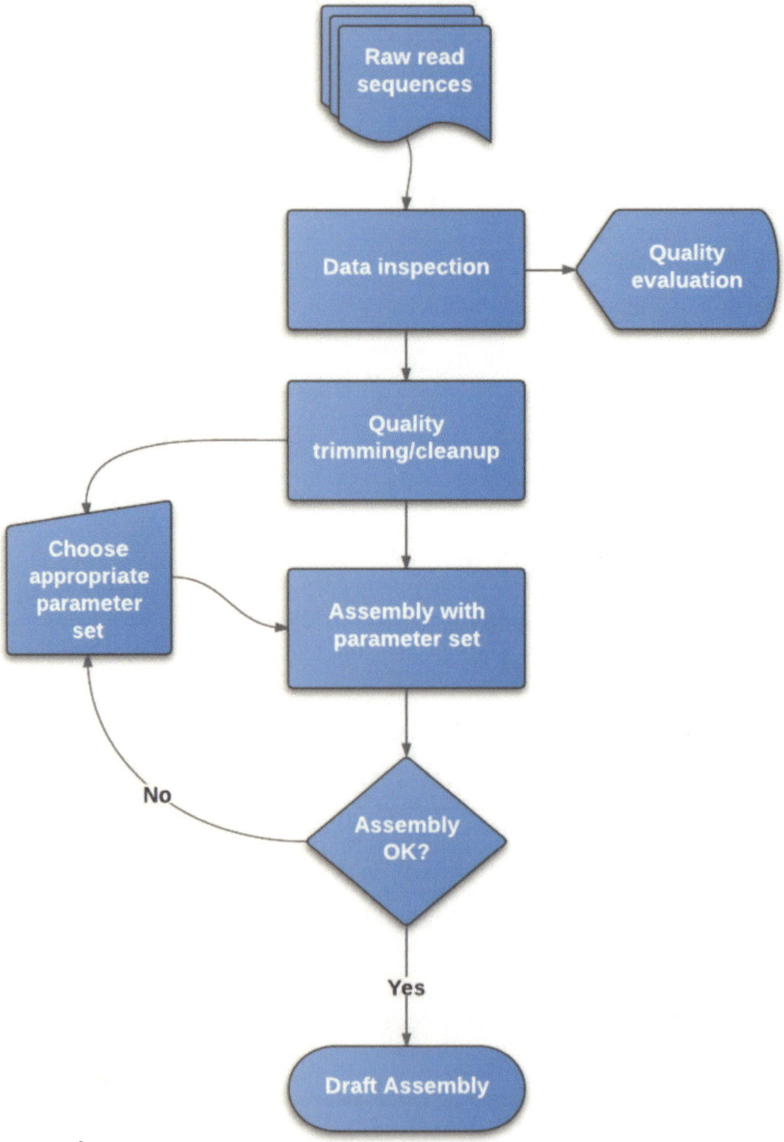

Figure 2. Example of a genome assembly workflow.

4.3.9. RNA-seq method

The transcriptome is the totality of the transcripts present in a cell, each with their abundance and varies depending on the age stage and physiological conditions of the animals. The study of the transcriptome allow to interpret the functional genome elements identifying the different types of transcripts (mRNA, coding RNA, and small RNAs), to determine their level of expression and their structure (terminations to the 5' and 3', exon-intron structure, alternative splicing). The introduction of NGS methods has revolutionized the characterization and quantification of transcriptomes overcoming limitations of previous methods (for example, microarrays or RT-PCR), as the need for a previous knowledge of the genomic sequence, the background noise (due to cross-hybridization), and the limited dynamic range. Starting from the mRNA, a cDNA library is constructed and specific adapters to both ends of each sequence are used. Each molecule is then sequenced after the PCR amplification. The sequencing produces a series of short reads, which can be aligned to the genome or the reference transcriptome. These are used to construct an expression profile for each gene, with a resolution that can reach up to a single base. If the reads are short and very numerous (up to several million per run) you can identify transcripts with a low level of expression. The RNA-seq is highly reproducible and requires less RNA for the synthesis library, since it lacks the step of cloning. Nc RNAs (noncoding RNA) are small molecules which are not translated into proteins. This class of RNAs includes several RNAs as the transfer RNA (tRNA), ribosomal RNA (rRNA), small nuclear and small nucleolar RNA, micro RNA and small interfering RNA (miRNA and siRNA). Micro RNAs (21-nucleotide-long RNAs) are very important posttranscriptional regulators of genes in animals. **Table 3** reports the most important Internet reference databases.

NCBI–RefSeq	htttp://www.ncbi.nlm.nih.gov/refseq
UCSC	http://genome.ucsc.edu
Ensembl	http://www.ensembl.org/index.html
dbSNP	htpp://www.ncbi,nlm.nih.gov/SNP/index.html
dbVar	http://www.ncbi.nlm.nih.gov/dbvar
	http://ncbi.nlm.gov/dbvar/content/overview
dbGaP	www.ncbi.nlm.nih.gov/gap
DNA Data of Japan	http://www.dbbj.nig.ac.jp
ExPASy	http://ca.expasy.org
GenAtlas	http://citi2.fr/GENATLAS/
GenBamk	http://wwww.ncbi.nlm.nih.gov/
SNP consortium	http://snp.shl.org
Stanford microarray	http://genome.stanford.edu/microarray
Swiss-Protein	http://www.expasy/sprot

Table 3. List of reference databases (Internet sites).

5. Other methods for screening the genetic diseases

5.1. Mendelian disorders

Karyotyping and *in situ* fluorescent hybridization technique (FISH) were traditionally used to detect the large genetic disorders. In the last decade, microarrays have been used to improve the resolution. Nowadays, NGS technologies can be used to sequence all the exomes or targeted exome regions.

5.2. Microarrays or SNP chip

SNP array is a specific type of chip array which is used to identify the single point mutations. After the DNA extraction, DNA is fragmented and processed by means of biochemical methods and labeled with a fluorescent dye. The DNA spots (20–100 bp) are attached to a solid surface (glass, plastic, or silicone) and the hybridization is performed using the samples of DNA to be tested. For each SNP to be genotyped, several DNA probes are designed with similar sequences but variable at one position corresponding to a polymorphism. The measure of the fluorescence, at each spot, allows us to detect the presence/absence of a specific allele. Two individual are identical at 99.9% of the genome and the wide linkage disequilibrium (LD) observed throughout the genome reduces the number of needed SNPs. If many SNPs are linked together in one region, only one maker is needed to be accurately measured. The ability to detect SNPs using array-based approaches is often limited by the density of the array.

5.3. Epigenetics

Methylation effects and histone modifications explain most of the epigenetic and posttranscriptional modifications. Chip-seq (chromatin-immuno-precipitation and direct sequencing) is used at the whole-genome level [28].

5.4. Analysis of a nucleotide sequence

The operations to be carried out in the molecular laboratory are as follows:

- extracting DNA from a tissue, usually the blood;
- DNA amplification. It consists in amplifying selectively the DNA;
- DNA sequencing. Once you obtained the various DNA fragments amplified by PCR, you run the "sequencing reaction";
- Analysis of the nucleotide sequences and search for gene mutations.

Specific software is used to perform an alignment between the nucleotide sequences of an individual showing a monogenic disease (from which you want to search for the mutation) and those of a control healthy individual (i.e., which does not have one specific disease). From this comparison, if the animal has a monogenic disease, may emerge one or more differences in the nucleotide sequence. These mutations (silent mutations, missense, not sense, frameshift, and splicing) shall be individually analyzed and evaluate the effects. The prediction of the effects of a missense mutation in the protein structure level is a complex process, in which we must take into account all the characteristics of the amino acids protein chain and their mutual interactions. Currently, some programs are available (such as SwissPdbViewer, for free on the websitehttp://www.expasy.org/spdbv/text/download.htm), able to process all of these data and provide a prediction of how the mutation will affect the three-dimensional structure of the protein. The automated sequencer provides the data files that can be displayed in the form of electropherograms with specific programs such as MT-Navigator (Applied Biosystems). The succession of peaks that make up the electropherogram is the result of the detection the fluorescence emitted by the fluorophores linked to the four ddNTPs used in the reactions of sequence. For each fluorochrome, and then to each nucleotide, it is conventionally associated a different color (A = green, T = red, C = blue, and G = black), thus facilitating the reading of the sequence. The reference sequences for the comparison may be obtained from the National Database Center for Biotechnology Information (NCBI, website: http://www.ncbi.nlm.nih.gov). The individual mutations are recognizable on the basis of several peak patterns. The substitutions of a single nucleotide or more nucleotides can be recognized because of its presence in a specific point of different color peaks corresponding to the replaced bases. One individual homozygous shows only one peak while a heterozygous shows two peaks corresponding to two alleles. A mutation can be localized in correspondence of the first base of the junction of splicing (GT becomes TT). In fact in most eukaryotic genes, introns begin with the "GT" bases and end with "AG."

6. Clinical applications in domestic animals

Animal geneticist, whose role consisted only once in calculating the probability of transmission hereditary of a given genetic disease in a given individual, is now an active figure throughout the clinical process, from diagnosis to treatment. The collection of family history is a central point in clinical genetics. It, in fact, can help to arrive at a correct diagnosis. In addition, through early diagnosis, it is possible to prevent or delay the onset of the disease through a suitable therapy. This possibility is often about relatives of an individual and can take to extend the analysis beyond the individual subject. Even for a correct formulation of the prognosis, it is important to be able to refer to the specific form assumed by a given disease in a certain family. For example, in some cases, analysis of family history has allowed to recognize some individuals with less aggressive forms of a disease, a less severe clinical picture, and then improved life expectancy.

7. Genetic counseling

Genetic counseling is a communication process that aims to provide to individual pet owners or farmers the risk of genetic diseases in order to help these people to analyze the consequences and to make responsible decisions. The first task of the genetic counselor is to identify the individual's needs and provide information with an appropriate manner to the degree of its culture and its beliefs. In addition to information about the disease, it must present the possible available genetic tests, highlighting their reliability. Finally, it should discuss the implications of the various choices.

Author details

Edo D'Agaro

Address all correspondence to: edo.dagaro@uniud

Department of Agricultural, Food, Environment and Animal Sciences, University of Udine, Udine, Italy

References

[1] Mardis, E R. The impact of next-generation sequencing technology on genetics. Trends Genet. 2008; **24**: 133–141.

[2] Schatz M C, Delcher A L, Salzberg, S L. Assembly of large genomes using second – generation sequencing. Genome Res. 2010; **20**: 1165–1173.

[3] Dong Y. Sequencing and automated whole-genome optical mapping of the genome of a domestic goat (*Capra hircus*). Nat. Biotechnol. 2013; **31**: 135–141.

[4] Narzisi G, Mishra B, Schatz MC. Algorithms for computational biology. Lecture Notes in Computer Science. 2014; **21**: 183–195.

[5] Gnerre S. High-quality draft assemblies of mammalian genomes from massively parallel sequence data. Proc. Natl. Acad. Sci. USA. 2011; **108**: 1513–1518.

[6] Berlin K. Assembling large genomes with single-molecule sequencing and locality – sensitive hashing. Nat. Biotechnol. 2015; **33**: 623–633.

[7] Chaisson, M J, et al. Resolving the complexity of the human genome using single-molecule sequencing. Nature. 2015; **517**: 608–611.

[8] Pendleton M. Assembly and diploid architecture of an individual human genome via single-molecule technologies. Nat. Methods. 2015; **12**: 780–786.

[9] Sharon, D., Tilgner, H., Grubert, F., Snyder, M. A single-molecule long-read survey of the human transcriptome. Nat Biotechnol. 2013; **31**: 1009–1014.

[10] Gordon D. Long-read sequence assembly of the gorilla genome. Science. 2016; **352**: aae0344.

[11] Koren S. Reducing assembly complexity of microbial genomes with single-molecule sequencing. Genome Biol. 2013; **14**: R101.

[12] Sebat J. Large-scale copy number polymorphism in the human genome.Science. 2004; **305**: 525–528.

[13] Browning S R, Browning B L. Haplotype phasing: existing methods and new developments. Nat. Rev. Genet. 2011; **12**: 703–714.

[14] Zheng G X. Haplotyping germline and cancer genomes with high-throughput linked-read sequencing. Nat. Biotechnol. 2016; **34**: 303–311 (2016).

[15] Phillippy A M, Schatz M C, Pop M. Genome assembly forensics: finding the elusive mis-assembly. Genome Biol. 2008; **9**: R55.

[16] Baker M. Structural variation: the genome's hidden architecture. Nat. Methods. 2012; **9**: 133–137.

[17] Hosomichi K, Shiina T, Tajima A, Inoue I. The impact of next-generation sequencing technologies on HLA research. J. Hum. Genet. 2015; **60**: 665–673.

[18] Kuleshov V. Whole-genome haplotyping using long reads and statistical methods. Nat. Biotechnol. 2014; **32**: 261–266.

[19] Chen X. The architecture of a scrambled genome reveals massive levels of genomic rearrangement during development. Cell. 2014; **158**: 1187–1198.

[20] Ross M G. Characterizing and measuring bias in sequence data. Genome Biol. 2014; **14**: R51.

[21] Cao H. Rapid detection of structural variation in a human genome using nanochannel-based genome mapping technology. GigaScience. 2014; **3**: 34.

[22] Oulas A. Metagenomics: tools and insights for analyzing next–generation sequencing data derived from biodiversity studies. Bioinform. Biol. Insights. 2015; **9**: 75–88.

[23] Voskoboynik A. The genome sequence of the colonial chordate, *Botryllus* schlosseri. eLife. 2013; **2**: e00569.

[24] Li R. The sequence and de novo assembly of the giant panda genome. Nature. 2010; **63**: 311–317.

[25] Church D M. Extending reference assembly models. Genome Biol. 2016; **16**: 13.

[26] Putnam NH. Chromosome-scale shotgun assembly using an in vitro method for long-range linkage. Genome Res. 2016; **26**: 342–350.

[27] Paszkiewicz K, Studholme DJ. *De novo* assembly of short sequence reads. Brief Bioinform. 2010; **11**(5):457–72.

[28] Fang G. Genome-wide mapping of methylated adenine residues in pathogenic *Escherichia coli* using single-molecule real-time sequencing. Nat. Biotechnol. 2012; **30**: 1232–1239.